NATURAL PRODUCTS AND THERAPEUTICS

WHAT TO KNOW ABOUT ESSENTIAL OILS

NATURAL PRODUCTS AND THERAPEUTICS

Additional books and e-books in this series can be found on Nova's website under the Series tab.

Library of Congress Cataloging-in-Publication Data

Names: Kjeldsen, Malene M., editor.
Title: What to know about essential oils / Malene M. Kjeldsen, editor.
Identifiers: LCCN 2020019485 (print) | LCCN 2020019486 (ebook) | ISBN 9781536179866 (hardcover) | ISBN 9781536179873 (adobe pdf)
Subjects: LCSH: Essences and essential oils--Therapeutic use. | Essences and essential oils--Physiological effect.
Classification: LCC RM666.A68 W47 2020 (print) | LCC RM666.A68 (ebook) | DDC 615.3/219--dc23
LC record available at https://lccn.loc.gov/2020019485
LC ebook record available at https://lccn.loc.gov/2020019486

Published by Nova Science Publishers, Inc. † New York

NATURAL PRODUCTS AND THERAPEUTICS

WHAT TO KNOW ABOUT ESSENTIAL OILS

MALENE M. KJELDSEN
EDITOR

nova
Medicine & Health
New York

CONTENTS

PREFACE

Cardiovascular diseases remain a leading cause of morbidity and mortality worldwide, with hypertension standing out as one of the most relevant risk factors. As such, in this compilation, an update on the hypotensive and vasorelaxant effects of essential oils and isolated compounds is presented.

The authors determine the chemical constituents and evaluate the anti-pain properties of essential oils from Thuja plicata var.

The chemical composition, antimicrobial activity and mosquito larvicidal action of essential oils from the leaves, pseudo-stem, rhizome and fruits of Alpinia malaccensis grown in Vietnam is also discussed.

Essential oils are explored in the context of their ethnobotanical survey in the treatment of one or more gastrointestinal troubles.

The medicinal benefits of lemon, lavender and peppermint essential oils are described. Further research should be performed to discover more uses for these oils so that we can gain the most benefit from use.

Later, the medicinal uses of essential oils from ancient times to the present are highlighted, particularly their mosquito repellent activities, toxicity and side effects.

The in vitro and in vivo pharmacological activities of Jasminum grandiflorum are assessed, and current insights are provided with regards to clinical efficacy and safety.

A critical overview is provided focusing on the diverse roles of the most abundant compounds in essential oil samples as determinants of the influence of impact notes and biological activities, calling for genuine and reproducible characterisation of such dominant compounds.

In the penultimate chapter, an integrated summary of the authors' experimental findings from an analysis of the community of fluorescent Pseudomonas strains in the rhizosphere of commercially grown Mentha piperita is presented.

Chapter 1 - Cardiovascular diseases (CVD) remain a leading cause of morbidity and mortality worldwide, with hypertension standing out as one of the most relevant risk factors. Indeed, hypertension affects 1.13 billion people worldwide and this number is expected to rise due to ageing population, increasing urbanization, and increases in age-specific related conditions. Furthermore, hypertension is a major economic burden for national health-care systems accounting for a huge percentage of the annual drug expenditure worldwide.

Despite the significant scientific and medical investment in new antihypertensive drugs, more than half of the patients do not follow the medication as prescribed, mainly due to undesired side effects. In this scenario, secondary metabolites from aromatic and medicinal plants emerge as potential new alternative and/or complementary antihypertensive drugs. Indeed, several scientific-based reports highlight beneficial effects such as the hypotensive and vasorelaxant properties of essential oils and their isolated compounds (terpenes, phenylpropanoids, sulphur and nitrogen containing compounds). In this review, an update on the hypotensive and vasorelaxant effects of essential oils and isolated compounds is presented together with putative mechanisms of action and composition/structure-activity relations. Overall, this compilation aims to provide a comprehensive revised state of the art on the antihypertensive potential of these compounds, thus paving the way for the development of new preventive/therapeutic plant-based approaches.

Chapter 2 - This study was designed to determine the chemical constituents and evaluate the anti-pain properties of the essential oils from *Thuja plicata* var. Excelsa Van den Berk (Cupressaceae), *Alstonia boonei*

De Wild (Apocynaceae), *Curcuma longa* L. (Zingiberaceae) and *Allium sativum* L (Alliaceae). The essential oils were isolated using hydrodistillation method in an all glass Clevenger-type apparatus and characterized by gas chromatography (GC-FID) and gas chromatography-mass spectrometry (GC-MS). The hot plate method was used to determine the anti-nociceptive property while the anti-inflammatory activity was established by means of carrageenan induced and formalin models. The yields of the essential oils were 1.31%, 1.49%, 0.80% and 0.75% (v/w) respectively, calculated on a dry weight basis. The major constituents of T. plicata var. Excelsa were δ-3-carene (31.6%), α-pinene (20.3%), cedrol (7.3%) and β-caryophyllene (6.7%). Its carrageenan-induced inflammation study showed a high activity consistent with dose and time. Inflammatory mediators were significantly suppressed within the 1st to the 3rd h at a level of $p < 0.001$ by the 200 and 400 mg/kg. In addition, the activity of the 100 mg/kg rises steadily from $p > 0.05$ (non-significant) to $p < 0.001$ for the 1st to the 3rd h respectively. The oil only displayed a slight inhibition of heat latency activity at 90th and 120th min ($p < 0.05$) by the 400 mg/kg. The main constituents of *A. boonei* were cedrol (32.2%), α-humulene (18.9%), β-caryophyllene (17.2%) and α-pinene (13.4%). The hot plate model (maximal pain threshold) displayed significant activity ($p < 0.001$) for the 200 and 400 mg/kg within the 60th and the 90th min. Inflammation was significantly inhibited by all doses at the 3rd and 4th h. The 100 mg/kg of *A. boonei* essential oil displayed a steady activity at the 1st and 2nd h ($p < 0.01$) and increased at 3rd and 4th h ($p < 0.001$). 200 mg/kg of the essential oil also showed steady activity at the 3rd and 4th h ($p < 0.01$). The result showed that 400 mg/kg of the essential oil was significant at the 1st h ($p < 0.05$) but there was a total loss of activity at the 2nd h ($p > 0.05$) then it was highly significant at the 3rd and 4th h ($p < 0.001$).

Formalin model showed high inhibition (100% maximal) at the inflammatory phase than the neurogenic phase. The main constituents of the oil of C. *longa* were ar-tumerone (28.6%), β-atlantone (21.9%) and curlone (18.8%) while diallyl trisulfide (53.9%), diallyl disulfide (15.7%), diallyl tetrasulfide (11.7%), methylallyl trisulphide (9.2%) were the compounds identified in *A. sativum* oil. The essential oils of *A. sativum* and *C. longa* inhibited the proliferation of anti-nociceptors induced by hot plate method. There was prolonged activity ($p < 0.001$) independent of the time and the dose except for a reduced activity of the 400 mg/kg at the 90th min ($p < 0.001$ to $p < 0.05$) for *A. sativum.* The anti-inflammatory activity of the essential oils of *A. sativum* were only significant for the 100 mg/kg at the 2nd h (p < 0.001) and 3rd h (p < 0.05) of the analysis. Activity observed could be attributed to effect of absorption rate and inflammation mediators' modulation.

In conclusion, results in this study indicated that the essential oils could be considered as potential alternative source for amelioration of inflammation and pain disorders.

Chapter 3 - The chemical compositions, antimicrobial activity and mosquito larvicidal action of essential oils from the leaves, pseudo-stem, rhizome and fruits of *Alpinia malaccensis* grown in Vietnam are being reported. The essential oils were obtained by hydrodistillation of the different parts of the plant using Clevenger-type apparatus. The oils were separately analysed using gas chromatography-flame ionization detector (GC-FID) and gas chromatography coupled with mass spectrometry (GC-MS). The Minimum inhibitory concentration (MIC) values of the antimicrobial activity of the essential oils were determined by the micro-dilution broth susceptibility assay using eight standardized American Type Culture Collection (ATCC) strains. The mortality rate and larvicidal activity of the essential oils against fourth-instar larvae of *Aedes albopictus* and *Culex quinquefasciatus* were evaluated according to World Health Organization protocol. The yields of the essential oils were 0.23%, 0.19%, 0.25% and 0.40% (v/w), for the leaf, pseudo-stem, rhizome and fruit of the plant respectively, calculated on dry weight basis. The main constituents of the leaf oil were β-eudesmol (33.3%), β-pinene (22.5%) and δ-cadinene (8.9%). The quantitatively significant compounds of the pseudo-stem oil were β-pinene (40.8%), τ-muurolol (10.7%), α-phellandrene (9.1%) and β-phellandrene (9.1%). However, β-pinene (24.3%), β-phellandrene (16.7%), benzyl salicylate (8.9%) and farnesol (8.1%) were the most abundant compounds in the rhziome oil. Moreover, the principal constituents in the fruit oil were methyl cinnamate (16.5%), germacrene D (16.4%) and δ-cadinene (11.8%).

The results of antimicrobial study indicated that the studied essential oil samples exhbited potent and varying activity towards the tested microorganisms with MIC vaues ≤ 50.0 μg/mL. The pseudo-stem and fruits of *A. malaccensis* inhibited the growth of *Escherichia coli* (ATCC 25922; MIC 50 μg/mL) and *Saccharomyces cerevisiae* (ATCC 16404; MIC < 50 μg/mL). Only the fruit essential oil displayed microbial action against *Pseudomonas aeruginosa* (ATCC 25923; MIC < 50 μg/mL). Essential oils from fruits and rhizome exhibited antimicrobial activity on *Staphylococcus aureus* subsp. *aureus* (ATCC 11632; MIC < 50 μg/mL). The leaf, pseudo-stem and fruit oils also showed activity against *Aspergillus niger* (ATCC 9763; MIC 50 μg/mL). Only the rhizome oil displayed potential antimicrobial action against *Fusarium oxysporum* (ATCC 48112; MIC 50 μg/mL). However, all the oil samples did not inhibited the growth of *Bacillus subtilis* (ATCC 11774) and *Candida albicans* (ATCC 10231). All the tested essential oils displayed mortality (100%) against the mosquito vectors. In addition, the essential showed potential larvicidal action with reasonable minimum lethal concentrations (LC_{50} and LC_{90}) values at 24 h and 48 h comparable with established standards.

In conclusion, the antimicrobial and larvicidal activities of essential oils from different parts of *A. malaccensis* revealed that the oils could be considered as a potentially alternative source for developing novel formulation for controlling diseases.

Chapter 4 - The rate at which ignorance of hygiene and sanitary practices is being neglected in the suburban and rural areas of developing regions of the world never seem to reduce. Lack of adequate sanitation and health facilities together with deficiency in educating these rural dwellers on how to maintain proper hygiene has made the prevalence and impact of helminthiasis on public health and animal production a great socio-economic problem. Often associated with these problems are conditions such as anaemia, malnutrition, vitamin deficiencies, poor cognitive ability, less intellectual and mental development which are prominent in underage children and pregnant women. Animal health care and husbandry has also been hit as a result of this inadequate hygiene and sanitary practices which thus pose great challenge in food production. Most of the domestic animals serve as primary host to infectious helminths (worms) from which they are transmitted into humans. However, many naturally occurring secondary metabolites (phytochemicals) of plants such as terpenoids from essential oils, alkaloids, flavonoids, glycosides and tannins have been explored as leads to develop medicines for a disease-free and healthy society. Plant essential oils are ingredients present in formulations used ethno-medicinally, pharmaceutically, in food and cosmetic industries due to their potential bioactive and therapeutic activities against a wide spectrum of pathogenic organisms. Results from many reported researches as well as from the authors' research findings, using the essential oils of plants from the Fabaceae species, showed the efficacy of some of these plant constituents as anthelmintics against various test organisms. The essential oils explored from plants of choice premised on their ethnobotanical survey in the treatment of one or more gastrointestinal troubles (GIT). The different essential oils studied demonstrated varying inhibitory activities (*in vitro* and *in vivo*) against different classes of helminth parasites (nematodes, cestodes, trematodes) and annelids which could be a lead to developing potent anthelmintics. As a result of these findings, the discovery of natural plant constituents should be kept on-going.

Chapter 5 - The purpose of this chapter is to describe the medicinal benefits of lemon, lavender and peppermint essential oils. Essential oils are liquid extracts from aromatic plants that possess a variety of uses. In order to extract the liquid oil from plants, the most common extraction processes are steam distillation, cold press and enfleurage. Quality assurance testing should be performed on the oils before they are used by consumers to minimize risk and maximize benefit. To obtain the benefits for the body, essential oils can be used by topical application, inhalation and ingestion as well as other techniques. Many studies have been performed to find the statistical significance behind therapeutic claims about these oils. Lemon oil has been proven to help with morning sickness, bacterial infections, skin inflammation, pain and cognitive function. Lavender oil has proven use for alopecia, postpartum depression, hypertension, insomnia, and skin conditions. Peppermint oil has shown use for irritable bowel syndrome, motion sickness, nausea, pruritus, migraines, chest pain, dysphagia, and to treat bacterial and fungal infections. Lemon, lavender and peppermint oils can treat some of the same conditions, such as anxiety and depression. These oils have an abundance of uses that have been studied and proven to have statistically significant outcomes. Essential oil use has been proven to be an influential holistic approach to treatment of various disease states and symptoms. Further research should be performed to discover even more uses for these oils so that we can gain the most benefit from use.

Chapter 6 - Essential oils are secreted in the glands of plants as volatile oils and are responsible for the scents emitted from different plant parts. When plant parts are used as spices, the essential oil present in them enhances the palatability of the cooked food. Irrespective of the high price of most essential oils, it remains an important item needed for human daily living as it is used in the production of soaps, creams, lotions, perfumes, roll-ons and deodorizers. It improves mood, enhances self-esteem, ignites romance and helps to relieve stress. In addition, essential oils have a variety of applications such as preservation of food and drinks, control of insects and pests, air freshener, and the treatment of diseases and infections. The therapeutic value of essential oils cannot be over emphasized. They have been used to cure diseases for several centuries. In this article, the medicinal use of essential oils from ancient times to the present are highlighted. Irrespective of their history, caution must be taken when using essential oils as they are easily absorbed by the skin and then find their way into the blood stream. Thus, indiscriminate use of essential oils may lead to serious health hazards. This article therefore highlights various usage, its mosquito repellent activities, and reaction of bees to essential oil (EO) volatiles, toxicity, side effects and applications of EO.

Chapter 7 - *Jasminum grandiflorum* essential oil has received a great interest worldwide for its multiple biological activities due to its chemical constituents. Indeed, the application of *jasminum grandiflorum* essential oil in cosmetic and personal hygiene products is gradually increasing. Also, it has been widely used in the traditional medicine for centuries, in the treatment of respiratory diseases, common cold, influenza, and sinus congestion. This review addressed chemical composition and ethno-pharmacological aspects of *jasminum grandiflorum* plants, as also its *in vitro* and *in vivo* pharmacological activities, and current insights with regards to clinical efficacy and safety.

Chapter 8 – The authors are giving a critical overview of the diverse roles of the most abundant compounds in essential oil (EO) samples as determinants of important features such as the influence of impact notes and biological activities displayed. It calls for genuine and reproducible characterisation of such dominant compounds. Essential oils (EOs) are complex odoriferous compounds, which are distillable exudates in natural products. Their ubiquitous content includes mono-terpenes, sesqui-terpenes and their oxygenated derivatives with varied functional groups such as esters, alcohols, ketones, carboxylic acids, and aromatic derivatives. Essential oils obtained from different parts (leaves, stem and stem bark, root and root bark, fruits parts, etc.) of the same plant do vary uniquely and significantly. They are important in medicine, perfumery, and flavouring which are commercially utilized in pharmaceutical, cosmetics, paints, petroleum and food industries as inhalants, germicides, stimulants, antiseptics, perfumes, toiletries, additives, preservatives and artificial flavours in foods and drinks. Characterised components have been reported to exhibit a broad spectrum of bioactivities such as larvicidal, anti-inflammatory and antimicrobial relevant for several therapeutic interventions. The values and importance of essential oils depend mainly on the type and quantity of impact compounds it contains. The dominance of some compounds in the essential oils has a great influence on the characteristics including bioactivity exhibited by the plant. They determine the nature of the EO and are usually responsible for impacting the characteristic notes of each EO sample. On the suitability of EOs, their most abundant compounds have characteristic impact notes, which are utilized on finished products industrially and for commercial purposes. There are earlier reports on dominant compounds in essential oils such as Limonene for the cashew fruity odour and β-caryophyllene for Hog plum fruity odour. Fragrances perceived and aroma exhibited by such abundant compounds play major roles in acceptability, accessibility (judging) and bioactivities expressed by the EOs. Most abundant compounds in EOs are important and reliable in chemotaxonomic studies of plants. Some of these the authors will be examining.

Chapter 9 - Peppermint (*Mentha piperita*) is one of the most important EO (essential oil crops) and is cultivated worldwide. It is composed primarily of monoterpenes, whose medicinal properties are mainly due to their EO composition, accumulated in glandular trichomes. Nowadays, agriculture relies heavily on the use of synthetic chemicals, such as fertilizers and pesticides, to achieve high yields but without taking into account their deleterious effects on the environment. However, there is an interesting biotechnological alternative using microorganisms to increase the availability and intake of nutrients by crops and to control phytopathogenic organisms and herbivorous insects. The group of bacteria termed plant growth-promoting rhizobacteria (PGPR) colonizes the rhizosphere and stimulates plant growth and development by direct or indirect mechanisms. Thus, in the search for new strategies of plant production to optimize essential oil (EO) yield, inoculation with PGPR is an interesting candidate. The authors present here an integrated summary of their experimental findings from an analysis of the community of fluorescent Pseudomonas strains in the rhizosphere of commercially grown *Mentha piperita*, including the effects of inoculation and co-inoculation with different PGPR strains (native and wild type) on total EO yield and glandular trichome density. The qualitative and quantitative compositions of the main monoterpenes (menthol, menthone, pulegone, limonene and linalool) were also determined to analyze the effects of the volatiles emitted by PGPR rhizobacteria on EO production. The various PGPR strains (*Bacillus amyloliquefaciens* GB03, *Pseudomonas fluorescens* WCS417r, *Azospirillum brasilense* SP7, *Pseudomonas putida* SJ04-SJ25-SJ48) and co-inoculations evaluated produced significant increases in the production of EO in peppermint plants, but at different magnitudes. Bacterial inoculants are thus an effective biotechnological tool for stimulating the secondary metabolism in plants. Application of these techniques may contribute to environmental conservation, increased crop productivity and sustainable agricultural practices.

Chapter 10 - Certain plants produce some essential oils containing phenylpropanoids/terpenoids (e.g., (*E*)-anethole, estragole, eugenol, (E)-isoeugenol, safrole, (*E*)-/(*Z*)-citral, (*R*)-/(*S*)-citronellal, (*E*)-/(*Z*)-geraniol and carvacrol) as main constituents (relative amounts >50%), which are isolated of different parts from star anise/aniseed, winter tarragon/ Mexican tarragon, clove tree, sassafras, lemongrass, lemon balm, citronella grass, palm rose, and Cuban oregano. These EO/molecules have many and different bioactivities (e.g., antimicrobial, antiparasitic, antioxidant, anti-inflammatory, anticancer/chemopreventive, cytotoxic/toxic, anesthetic/ analgesic, antinociceptive, antispasmodic, pro-cholinergic, anticonvulsant, hypotensor/vasorelaxant, antidiabetic, insecticidal, larvicidal, fumigant and repellent, among other) and are used as flavoring/preserving/active ingredients in foods and beverages, personal care and cosmetics, perfumery, etc., as well as raw materials. Since the 1950s, the EO have been sources of substances as starting materials for different chemical synthesis; however, with the emergence of green chemistry, the EO and their main constituents (as biomass) have become attractive to the scientific community, as starting/raw material for fine chemical synthesis. Some examples are the preparation/obtaining of tetrahydroquinoline, isoindoloquinolinone, dihydrobenzofuranol, iridoid, octahydroacridine, trioxane, oxirane and benzochrome derivatives, from EO isolated of star anise fruit, clove bud, citronella and palm rose grasses, and Cuban oregano leaves. These hemisynthetic derivatives showed interesting biological properties, e.g., antiparasitic, antimicrobial, antiviral, antioxidant, and anticancer.

In: What to Know about Essential Oils
Editor: Malene M. Kjeldsen
ISBN: 978-1-53617-986-6

Chapter 1

ARE ESSENTIAL OILS POTENTIAL ANTIHYPERTENSIVE AGENTS?

Jorge M. Alves-Silva[1,2,3,4,*], Carla Marques[2,3,4], Lígia Salgueiro[1,5], Henrique Girão[2,3,4] and Mónica Zuzarte[2,3,4]

[1]Faculty of Pharmacy of the University of Coimbra, University of Coimbra, Coimbra, Portugal

[2] University of Coimbra, Coimbra Institute for Clinical and Biomedical Research (iCBR), Faculty of Medicine, Azinhaga de Sta Comba, Coimbra, Portugal

[3] University of Coimbra, Center for Innovative Biomedicine and Biotechnology (CIBB), Portugal

[4]Clinical Academic Centre of Coimbra (CACC), Coimbra, Portugal

[5] University of Coimbra, CIEPQPF, Department of Chemical Engineering, Faculty of Sciences and Technology, Coimbra, Portugal

[*] Corresponding Author's Email: jmasilva@student.ff.uc.pt.

ABSTRACT

Cardiovascular diseases (CVD) remain a leading cause of morbidity and mortality worldwide, with hypertension standing out as one of the most relevant risk factors. Indeed, hypertension affects 1.13 billion people worldwide and this number is expected to rise due to ageing population, increasing urbanization, and increases in age-specific related conditions. Furthermore, hypertension is a major economic burden for national health-care systems accounting for a huge percentage of the annual drug expenditure worldwide.

Despite the significant scientific and medical investment in new antihypertensive drugs, more than half of the patients do not follow the medication as prescribed, mainly due to undesired side effects. In this scenario, secondary metabolites from aromatic and medicinal plants emerge as potential new alternative and/or complementary antihypertensive drugs. Indeed, several scientific-based reports highlight beneficial effects such as the hypotensive and vasorelaxant properties of essential oils and their isolated compounds (terpenes, phenylpropanoids, sulphur and nitrogen containing compounds). In this review, an update on the hypotensive and vasorelaxant effects of essential oils and isolated compounds is presented together with putative mechanisms of action and composition/structure-activity relations. Overall, this compilation aims to provide a comprehensive revised state of the art on the antihypertensive potential of these compounds, thus paving the way for the development of new preventive/therapeutic plant-based approaches.

Keywords: cardiovascular diseases, hypertension, aromatic plants, volatile extract, terpenes, phenylpropanoids

1. INTRODUCTION

Cardiovascular disease (CVD) is a general term used to describe a plethora of pathological conditions in which the heart and/or the blood vessels are affected. According to the World Health Organization (WHO), CVDs account for 31% of total deaths worldwide [1] and this number is expected to rise mainly due to population ageing as well as an increase in associated risk factors. Very often, the management of CVDs includes therapeutic approaches that target the associated risk factors. These approaches tend to avoid disease progression and prevent additional complications but do not tackle the CVD itself. Moreover, the therapy is easily compromised by the existence of several side effects mainly due to polymedication and drug-drug interactions [2]. Some risk factors such as genetic background, age and ethnicity are non-modifiable while other risk factors, like high blood pressure (BP) or hypertension, high cholesterol and diabetes are generally treatable. Additional modifiable risk factors include inactivity, diet, alcohol misuse and tobacco that lead to high BP, overweight and several other complications that promote the onset of early CVDs [3,4]. Bearing in mind the huge impact of these risk factors, the WHO has launched several initiatives such as the MPOWER package to reduce tobacco use and the SHAKE package to decrease the consumption of salt [5].

Despite these efforts, hypertension still remains the leading risk factor for CVD-associated mortality. Indeed, in 2016, half of the deaths due to chronic diseases were attributed to CVDs with hypertension being the leading risk factor [6]. Moreover, elevated BP is associated with increased risk of heart, brain and kidney diseases [7] and the majority of hypertensive patients, concomitantly show other risk factors [8]. Indeed, in the Framingham Heart Study, 80% of the enrolled hypertensive patients had at least one coexisting risk factor, whereas 55% of them had two or more risk factors [9]. It has been shown that in patients that have hypertension associated with other risk factors, the risk for CV events increases exponentially rather than the sum of individual risks, being this association also true for low values of BP [8]. Indeed, in prehypertensive individuals the risk for 10-year absolute risk for CVD is increased by 10% however when diabetes is also present, this risk is increased by 40% [10].

Hypertension has a significant economic impact on healthcare systems, with antihypertensive drugs accounting for 10% of the annual drug expenditure in the US alone [11]. In addition, more than half of the patients do not follow the medication as prescribed mainly due to undesired side effects that include vision problems, shortness of breath and insomnia [12]. Also polymedication compromises the adherence to therapies. For these reasons, the development of innovative and more effective therapeutic/preventive strategies is an urgent need [13]. In this scenario, several approaches have emerged, namely plant-based ones [14]. In fact, plant-based therapies still remain a primary health care solution for around 80% of the world's population [15]. Furthermore, the Mediterranean plant-based diet is widely advised due to its documented beneficial effects directly on CVDs or, indirectly, by reducing associated risk factors such as atherosclerosis, high cholesterol and hypertension [16]. Also, several aromatic plants and their essential oils have been described as effective in the management of borderline hypertension, thus highlighting the potential of these compounds in the management of CVDs [17]. In addition, these compounds are relevant in drug development, being used directly as therapeutic agents, or as starting materials and models for the synthesis of other drugs [18].

Considering the huge socioeconomic burden and health impact of hypertension worldwide, the present review aims to gather the scientific information on the antihypertensive effects of essential oils and their isolated compounds including monoterpenes, sesquiterpenes, phenylpropanoids and, in less extent, sulphur and nitrogen-containing compounds. In addition, when known, the putative mechanisms of action underlying these effects are pointed out as well as an attempt to establish a chemical composition/ structure-activity relation. The research was conducted using popular search engines, namely *Pubmed*, *Scopus*, *Web of Science* and *Google Scholar* using keyword combinations such as "essential oil" and "hypertension." Papers that assessed the antihypertensive effects of essential oils or volatile isolated compounds published between 2000 and 2019 were considered.

2. HYPERTENSION

2.1. General Considerations

BP refers to the pressure of circulating blood on the walls of blood vessels [19]. This pressure is expressed in terms of systolic pressure (maximum when the heart contracts and sends the blood to the arteries) over diastolic pressure (minimum when the heart relaxes and refills with blood)

[20]. The WHO defines BP as 120 mmHg for systolic pressure and 80 mmHg for diastolic pressure, however lower BP values, up to 105 mmHg and 60 mmHg for systolic and diastolic values, respectively, are not harmful [19]. On the other hand, hypertension is defined as a systolic and diastolic BP higher than 140 and 90 mmHg, respectively, with different grades recognized as shown in Table 1 [19,21].

Table 1. Values of BP. Adapted from ESC/ESH guidelines [21]

Category	**Systolic BP (mmHg)**		**Diastolic BP (mmHg)**
Optimal	<120	and/or	<80
Normal	120 – 129	and/or	80 – 84
High normal	130 – 139	and/or	85 – 89
Grade 1 hypertension	140 – 159	and/or	90 – 99
Grade 2 hypertension	160 – 179	and/or	100 – 109
Grade 3 hypertension	≥ 180	and/or	≥ 110
Isolated systolic hypertension	≥ 140	and/or	< 80

Hypertension can be divided into systemic hypertension or pulmonary hypertension. The first refers to a condition in which the BP in the body arteries is persistently elevated while the later indicates a BP increase specifically in pulmonary arteries [22,23]. Another division considers primary hypertension that has no single known cause but is related to several risk factors detailed below and secondary hypertension that refers to high BP caused by another medical condition that affects for example the kidneys, arteries, heart or the endocrine system [24].

2.2. Prevalence and Burden of Hypertension

In 2005 an estimate predicted that by 2025 the burden of hypertension would reach 1.6 billion people, rising from the 0.9 billion diagnosed in 2000 [6,11]. However, the burden of this condition was already 1.13 billion in 2015 [25], thus advising that by 2025 the estimated number will be largely exceeded. According to the WHO, around two-thirds of hypertensive people (ca. 1.04 billion) live in low- and middle-income countries [26,27]. In 2005 a study pointed out Asia and the Pacific Islands as the regions with lower prevalence of hypertension whereas Latin America and the Caribbean islands were the places with the highest numbers. Also, in Africa the prevalence of hypertension is alarming, reaching around 46% of the population [28], with higher numbers registered in Nigeria, Cameroon and Tanzania [29–31]. In Europe, in 2010, hypertension prevalence was highest in Central and Eastern European countries whereas in the Northern and Southern ones it was the lowest. Among the European Union (EU) countries, Estonia accounted for the highest prevalence (32%) while in the United Kingdom hypertension was less common (15%). Regarding non-EU countries, Israel, Norway and Switzerland had all a prevalence of 18% while in Moldova it was around 31% [32]. Interestingly, in 2014, a decrease in the prevalence of hypertension was observed in most European countries, however Luxembourg, the Netherlands and Portugal had an opposite trend, with hypertension increasing between 2010 and 2014. Regarding the United States of America (USA), the American Heart Association estimated that between 2011 and 2014 approximately 86 million adults aged over 20 years had hypertension [33].

Hypertension remains a major economic burden for national health-care systems accounting for a huge percentage of the annual drug expenditure worldwide. Costs include direct health-care expenses, such as medication, laboratory tests and hospitalizations as well as indirect costs due to the loss of productivity resulting from premature mortality and disability [34]. Health-care system costs with hypertension vary greatly according to the region. For example, high BP accounts for 22.6% of all healthcare expenses in Eastern Europe and Central Asia, but only 7.2% of health costs in East Asia and Pacific [34]. Strikingly, in 2010 the financial burden of high BP was 370 billion US dollars and it was predicted to increase to nearly 1 trillion US dollars in a 10-year period [34]. In 2006, the financial burden of cardiovascular diseases in the EU was rated at €110 billion, which accounted for 10% of the total health-care expenditure [35]. Of those €51.3 billion were attributed to hypertension, being the main reason for these numbers the low adherence of patients to therapeutics. Indeed, it has been foreseen, that increasing therapeutic adherence to 70% would reduce direct costs of hypertension by €332 million [35].

2.3. Hypertension Risk Factors

Several risk factors for high BP are related to lifestyle and behavioural aspects such as diet, abusive consumption of alcohol, physical inactivity and poor stress management [36]. Indeed, social causes including globalization, urbanization, ageing, income, education and housing can lead to elevated BP since they influence people´s lifestyle, thus affecting the development of hypertension. For example, unemployment or fear of unemployment, that increase stress levels, may lead to high BP. In addition, living and working conditions can delay diagnosis and effective treatments leading to the development of hypertension-related complications. Furthermore, a rapid and unplanned urbanization with associated sedentarism also tend to promote the development of hypertension due to the abusive consumption of fast food, tobacco and alcohol.

Although hypertension is predominantly associated to adults, childhood hypertension is an emerging health problem, with prehypertension and hypertension affecting 3.4% and 3.6%, respectively, of the population aged between 3 and 18 years [37]. In these cases, treatments rely mainly on lifestyle modifications, such as healthy food intake, with low sodium and high potassium levels, physical activity, as well as tobacco and alcohol avoidance. Women during pregnancy may also develop gestational hypertension or preeclampsia when other health complications arise such as proteinuria or fetus growth delay [38]. The risk of hypertension tends to increase with age due to the stiffening of blood vessels. It has been demonstrated that young men have higher BP than women, but BP variation is higher in women than in men [27,39]. Other relevant risk factors include metabolic factors like diabetes, high cholesterol and overweight or obesity [40]. The genetic background also plays a relevant role in the development of hypertension. Indeed, race and ethnicity are major risk factors for hypertension, due to sociodemographic, environmental and behavioural factors [41]. For example, in the USA a study that analysed data from 2015 to 2016 reported a significantly higher age-standardized prevalence of hypertension in non-Hispanic Black individuals (57.3%) when compared to non-Hispanic White individuals (43.8%) and Hispanic-Americans (44.7%) [42]. On the other hand, high BP is particularly common among people of African heritage, often developing this condition at an early age [43].

2.4. Hypertension Management

Hypertension is a serious medical condition that significantly increases the risks of heart, brain and kidney diseases. Indeed, uncontrolled high BP can lead to several complications like heart failure, stroke, aneurism, compromised kidney function, vision loss, memory deficits, vascular dementia and metabolic syndrome [7], thus pointing out the need to effectively prevent or control increased BP.

Hypertension and higher BP in general, can be controlled by two well-established approaches, lifestyle modifications and/or treatment with antihypertensive drugs [21]. Adopting a healthy and active lifestyle is a trend that is growing especially in modern societies with the reduction in salt consumption and the practice of physical exercise being the most relevant for hypertension. It is well-known that excessive salt consumption creates a pressor effect and is associated with an increased prevalence of high SBP and hypertension [21]. Indeed, a recent meta-analysis demonstrated that decreasing the salt consumption by 4.4 g per day leads to a decrease of 4.2 mmHg SBP and 2.1 mmHg in DBP, in normotensive individuals, being this effect more noticeable in hypertensive individuals (SBP and DBP decrease by 5.4 and 2.8 mmHg, respectively) [44].

In addition to lifestyle modifications, pharmacotherapy is still a major cornerstone in the treatment of hypertension [45]. It has been shown that lowering SBP by 10 mmHg or DBP by 5 mmHg leads to a decrease in all CV events by 20%, all-cause mortality by 10%, stroke by 35%, coronary events by 20% and heart failure by 40% [21]. There are four classes of antihypertensive drugs (diuretics, blockers of the renin-angiotensin system, calcium antagonists and beta-blockers) that have-antihypertensive effects by lowering BP [45].

Diuretics have been widely used to prevent stroke, coronary artery disease and decrease the risk of heart failure. They include several subgroups such as hydrochlorothiazide, chlorthalidone, indapamide, aldosterone antagonists and loop diuretics. Despite being the first line of therapeutics for hypertension, several side effects are recognized. For example, the thiazide class of diuretics are responsible for biochemical (e.g., hypokalaemia, hyperuricemia, and increased risk for diabetes) and clinical (e.g., weakness, impotence, gout attacks) signs, and the antialdosterone class can lead to hyperkalaemia, dizziness, sexual disturbances and vomiting [45].

Inhibitors of the renin-angiotensin system (RAS) are the most widely used antihypertensive drugs in developed countries. Several classes including angiotensin converting enzyme (ACE) inhibitors, angiotensin receptor blockers (ARBs) or renin inhibitors are known. Care must be taken when administering ACE inhibitors and ARBs since both can cause hyperkalaemia and increase serum creatinine. In addition, ACE inhibitors can also cause persistent dry cough, angio-edema, dry mouth and rash whereas ARBs lead to dry mouth, nausea and abdominal pain [45].

Calcium antagonists are classified according to structural differences in phenylalkylamine (verapamin), benzothiazepine (diltiazem) and dihydropyridine (nifedipine). These drugs differ in their cardiac and vascular selectivity, being dihydropyridines the most used to lower BP due to their higher selectivity towards smooth muscle cells. Patients under calcium antagonist's therapy report an array of side effects that include peripheral edema, headache and constipation for non-dihydropyridines, and bradycardia, headache and arrythmia for dihydropyridines [45].

Finally, the use of beta blockers has fallen in the last years since it has been shown that these drugs are less effective than the other classes of antihypertensives. Besides weak effects on central systolic BP and pulse pressure, beta blockers can lead to increased levels of triglycerides and lower levels of high-density lipoprotein. Furthermore, patients under this therapy report an aggravation of asthma, bradycardia, fatigue, and insomnia [45].

All classes of antihypertensive drugs, as previously pointed out, have a wide array of undesired side effects that tend to increase in older patients and with longer treatments [2]. Furthermore, most of these drugs are only effective in combined therapies, thus decreasing patient adherence and treatment efficacy [45]. This leads to increased hospitalizations that reflect the socio-economic burden associated with hypertension [35].

2.5. Disease Models of Hypertension

Hypertension prevalence and ineffective treatment is quite concerning and has attracted researchers' attention in the last years. Indeed, several animal models, either genetic or induced models, of disease have been developed in order to understand the pathogenesis of this condition and to develop new approaches to prevent and lower high BP [46]. These models are useful to address prevention and treatment strategies as well as hypertension-associated comorbidities [47].

The genetic models include the Spontaneously Hypertensive Rat (SHR), the Dahl Salt-Sensitive (DSS) rat, the Fawn-Hooded Hypertensive (FHH) rat, the Milan hypertensive strain, the Lyon hypertensive rat, the Sabra hypertensive rat, the genetically hypertensive rat, and the inherited stress-induced arterial hypertension rat [46]. Amongst these, the SHR model is the most used, being widely applied in primary hypertension [46]. In this type of hypertension, the patients develop some hypertensive end-organ damage like cardiac hypertrophy, cardiac failure and renal dysfunction, which are mimicked by the SHR animal model. However, another important end-organ damage is stroke that is not displayed by this model [48]. To overcome this, a sub-strain was developed named SHR stroke prone (SHR-SP) that shows a higher BP than SHR and has a natural tendency to die due to stroke [46,48].

In what concerns the induced models of hypertension, this condition can be triggered using two main strategies, a surgical approach or a chemical one. The first type includes the renovascular model in which the blood flow to the kidney is affected and the renoprival model in which the kidney or part of the kidney is removed, thus leading to organ failure. The most common surgical model is the Goldblatt-hypertension model (renovascular) that was the first to be used and contributed to a better understanding of hypertension´s pathophysiology by linking the kidney to BP control [46, 48].

Chemical induction using angiotensin II (Ang II), mineralocorticoid-salts or nitric oxide synthase inhibitors can also induce hypertension in animals. The administration of Ang II leads to an increase in BP similar to that observed in patients with uncontrolled grade II hypertension. The Ang II models rely on the fact that the renin-angiotensin-aldosterone system (RAAS) plays an important role in sodium homeostasis with this system being largely activated in humans with primary hypertension. This model also leads to the development of end-organ damage, namely cardiac hypertrophy, vascular remodeling and chronic kidney disease [49–52]. The use of mineralocorticoid-salts, particularly DOCA-salt is used generally in combination with high salt diets to develop hypertension. This model mimics patient´s severe hypertension with some characteristics of low-renin hypertension. It discloses the role of mineralocorticoids in the setting of resistant hypertension. Inhibition of nitric oxide (NO) production catalyzed by endothelial nitric oxide synthase using N^{G}-monomethyl-L-arginine (L-NMMA) or N^{ω}-nitro-L-arginine methyl ester (L-NAME) causes an increase in BP with concomitant renal vasoconstriction and hypoperfusion [53–55]. With disease progression, the L-NAME treated rats develop renal dysfunction, renal hypertensive microangiopathy, cardiac, vascular and renal fibrosis as well as malignant hypertension.

Despite the *in vivo* effectiveness of antihypertensive drugs, some controversy has raised due to very low success in human trials [47]. To avoid this, all current candidate drugs for hypertension have to decrease BP in at least one of the most common models of hypertension, namely the SHR, the DSS or the mineralocorticoid-salt model [48,56].

3. Effect of Essential Oils and Isolated Compounds on Hypertension

3.1. Essential Oils

The International Standard Organization on Essential Oils [57] and the European Pharmacopoeia [58] define an essential oil as the product obtained from plant raw material by hydrodistillation, steam distillation or dry distillation or by a suitable mechanical process (for *Citrus* fruits). These volatile mixtures are synthesised and stored in specialized secretory structures such as secretory cells, secretory cavities, secretory ducts, glandular trichomes, osmophores or epidermal cells that can be found in all plant organs [59]. Essential oils play relevant roles in plant ecophysiology, being involved for example in the attraction of pollinators and seed dispersers, in plant protection against microorganisms and insects and in allelopathic interactions [60]. Their chemical profile is variable and depends upon several extrinsic (ecological and environmental aspects) and intrinsic (sexual, seasonal, ontogenetic, and genetic variations) factors [61]. Genetic variations in plants are quite relevant since they can lead to significant chemical variations in essential oil composition, allowing the identification of intraspecific categories named chemotypes. The hyphenation of gas chromatography (GC) with mass spectrometry is the analytical technique mostly used for accurate compound identification [62,63]. Moreover, analytical guidelines such as the European Pharmacopoeia and International Standard Organization establish standardized chemical profiles for several essential oils to guarantee quality control of both commercialized oils and plants from which they are obtained [64].

In general, monoterpenes ($C_{10}H_{16}$) and sesquiterpenes ($C_{15}H_{16}$) are the main group of compounds found in essential oils. In some cases, other compounds such as phenylpropanoids are also relevant. Moreover, fatty acids and their esters as well as nitrogen and sulphur derivatives can also occur [62] Terpenoids are synthetized via the mevalonate and non-mevalonate (deoxyxylulose phosphate) biosynthetic pathways while phenylpropanoids are formed through the shikimate pathway [64].

Aromatic plants and their essential oils have been used for centuries is different cultures, being also valued as raw materials in the food, pharmaceutical, perfumery and cosmetic industries [65]. Although more than 3,000 essential oils are known only ca.150 have commercial relevance in global markets [66]. It is important to point out that several aromatic species are included in the Generally Recognized as Safe (GRAS) list fully approved by the US Food and Drug Administration (FDA) and Environmental Protection Agency (EPA, USA) for addition to food and beverages, thus highlighting their industrial relevance. This interest is mainly due to essential oil´s organoleptic properties and/or bioactive potential. Indeed, several biological properties have been described for these compounds including fungicidal, bactericidal, anti-inflammatory, antioxidant, anticarcinogenic and cardioprotective effects [60,67,68].

3.2. Antihypertensive Effects of Essential Oils

The development of new antihypertensive drugs is in need with plant metabolites emerging as potential candidates. Some of these compounds can be used directly as antihypertensive drugs or, indirectly, as lead compounds for the development of new effective drugs [18]. Several systematic reviews have highlighted the beneficial effect of these metabolites on the cardiovascular system [67–70] and more specifically, essential oils have been described as effective in the management of borderline hypertension [17]. For this reason, the present review focuses on the beneficial effects on these volatile extracts and their isolated compounds in hypertension management. The main direct effect assessed in these compounds is their hypotensive potential using both normotensive animals or hypertensive models, namely the DOCA-salt hypertensive rat model or, in less extent, the Goldblatt-hypertension or the renoprival models. Since it has been described that impaired vasodilation causes increased BP leading to hypertension [71], the vasorelaxant activity of these extracts and their isolated compounds will also be considered in this review. For this purpose, *ex vivo* models are preferred namely the aortic rings (pre)contracted with different vasoconstrictor agents, such as phenylephrine (Phe) or high potassium concentrations. In this review the hypotensive and vasorelaxant effect of several essential oils are pointed out as well as the underlying mechanism of action. In order to disclose essential oil's mechanism of action, several inhibitors can be employed. For instance, to unveil the importance of the parasympathetic nervous system, atropine and its derivative, methylatropine, can be used [72] as well as bilateral vagotomy or bivagotomy [73]. Whereas, hexamethonium is used to inhibit the sympathetic nervous system [74]. L-NAME acts as an eNOS inhibitor, thus excluding the role of the nitric oxide system on the reported effect [75]. The effect of prostaglandins is removed by the addition of indomethacin [76]. Capsaicin, in turn, inhibits the activity of vanilloid receptor subtype 1 (TRPV1), which acts as an ion channel [77]. Other ion channel blockers can also be used, namely glibenclamide (ATP-sensitive potassium channels, [78]), tetraethylammonium chloride (voltage-dependent potassium channels, [79]) and nifedipine (L-type calcium channels, [80]). Then, relevant clinical trials validating the potential of these extracts are mentioned followed by a section addressing possible chemical/structural-activity relations.

3.2.1. Hypotensive Effects

The hypotensive effects of essential oils have been addressed in several species from distinct families. Next, examples of studies carried out in species from the Anacardeaceae, Euphorbiaceae, Lamiaceae, Lauraceae, Poaceae and Zingiberaceae families are pointed out.

The essential oil obtained from the aerial parts of *Schinus areira* L. [(Anacardiaceae); syn. *Schinus mole* L. var. *areira* (L.) DC.] induced a decrease in SBP while showing a tachycardic effect in conscious normotensive rabbits [81].

The essential oil obtained from the aerial parts of *Croton zehntneri* Pax et Hoffm. (Euphorbiaceae), rich in estragole (46%), E-anethole (42.1%) and germacrene B (4.8%) when applied to conscious and normotensive rats decreased mean arterial pressure (MAP) and heart rate (HR) in phase I, however the presence of the essential oil led to a pressor effect while maintaining its bradycardic effect [82]. These effects were also observed using DOCA-salt hypertensive rats [83]. Furthermore, in anesthetized rats the essential oil induced hypotension associated with bradycardia [84] which was abolished by the presence of capsaicin. Another study reported the effect of the essential oil obtained from the aerial parts of a different *Croton* species, *C. argyrophylloides* Muell. Arg. (Euphorbiaceae), rich in spathulenol (26.65%), caryophyllene oxide (13.13%), β -elemene (12.15%), β -caryophyllene (10.94%). The oil administered to both conscious and anesthetized normotensive rats evoked a hypotensive effect that was dose-dependent while eliciting tachycardia [85]. Both effects of the essential oil were reduced with a pretreatment of methylatropine in conscious rats, whereas hexamethonium pretreatment transformed the tachycardic effect into bradycardia without having any effect on the hypotensive properties of the essential oil. On anesthetized rats, cervical bivagotomy had no effect on the hypotensive effect of the essential oil.

Regarding the Lamiaceae family, the essential oil from the leaves of *Ocimum gratissimum* L. (Lamiaceae), rich in eugenol (43.7%), 1,8-cineole (32.7%) and *trans*-caryophyllene (4.1%) induced hypotension on conscious DOCA-salt-hypertensive rats which was unaffected by the pre-treatment with propranolol [86]. Treatment of uni-nephrectomized or DOCA-salt hypertensive rats with the essential oil of *O. gratissimum* elicited a dose-dependent hypotension associated with bradycardia [87], with a more preeminent effect on the latter. On anesthetized and conscious rats, *O. gratissimum* essential oil caused an immediate decrease in MAP and HR [88]. The bradycardic effect was dependent on the parasympathetic system since the effect was reduced by bilateral vagotomy or with methylatropine and hexamethonium. Also, the essential oil from leaves of *Hyptis fruticosa* Salzm., ex Benth (Lamiaceae), composed by α-pinene, caryophyllene and 1,8-cineole, when administered to conscious normotensive rats, induced hypotension associated with tachycardia [89]. Two essential oils from the leaves of *Mentha* x *villosa* Huds. (Labiatae), with distinct amounts of piperitone oxide, 95.87% (sample 2) and 62.32% (sample 1), were able to decrease both MAP and HR in a dose-dependent manner in anesthetized rats [90]. Sample 2 had a more preeminent effect when compared to sample 1. The hypotensive effect was not affected by bilateral vagotomy, methylatropine and hexamethonium whereas the bradycardic effect was decreased by the presence of hexamethonium. In another study, an essential oil with a composition similar to sample 2 induced hypotension with associated bradycardia in conscious, normotensive rats [91]. However, both effects were abolished by the presence of atropine. The same essential oil induced hypotension and bradycardia in conscious DOCA-salt hypertensive rats as well as in uni-nephrectomized rats [92]. Similarly, to the previous study, the presence of hexamethonium was able to reduce the bradycardic effect without affecting hypotension. The essential oil from *Pogostemon elsholtzioides* Benth. (Lamiaceae) leaves, rich in curzerene (46.1%), benzophenone (8.6%), germacrone (6.3%) and α-cadinol (5.7%), decreased SBP (84.18 vs 100.12 mmHg), DBP (21.69 vs 64.77 mmHg), MAP (45.78 vs 88.39%) and HR [150.52 vs 176.73 beats per minute (bpm)] in anesthetized rats [93].

The essential oil from the trunk wood of *Aniba rosaeodora* var *amazonica* Ducke (Lauraceae), rich in (-)-linalool (50.6%) and (+)-linalool (49.4%) when given to anesthetized rats induced biphasic hypotension and bradycardia which was not observed in rats submitted to bilateral vagotomy or pretreated with capsaicin [94]. On the other hand, the oil administered to conscious rats, induced a monophasic hypotensive and bradycardic effect which was lost in the presence of methylatropine. In addition, the essential oil obtained from the bark of *Aniba canelilla* (H.B.K.) Mez [(Lauraceae); syn. *Aniba elliptica* A. C. Sm., *Cryptocarya canelilla* Kunth] rich in 1-nitro-2-phenylethane (52.4%) and methyleugenol (38.6%), induced hypotension associated with bradycardia, in both anesthetized and conscious normotensive rats [95]. The bradycardic effect was reduced after bilateral vagotomy, in the latter, and by hexamethonium, in the former and both treatments had no effect on the hypotensive properties. In conscious rats, the hypotensive effect was lost after L-NAME treatment without affecting bradycardia. Furthermore, methylatropine reduced both the hypotensive and bradycardic effects of *A. canellila* essential oil.

The administration of essential oil obtained from the leaves of *Cymbopogon winterianus* Jowitt (Poaceae), characterized by geraniol (40.06%), citronellal (27.44%) and citronellol (10.45%) to conscious rats elicited an intense yet transitory hypotensive effect associated with tachycardia in a dose dependent manner [96]. In the higher dose tested (20 mg/Kg), the authors reported a bradycardic effect prior to tachycardia.

The essential oil from the leaves of *Alpinia zerumbet* K. Schum (Zingiberaceae), characterized by the presence of terpinen-4-ol (28.1%), 1,8-cineole (15.1%) and γ-terpinene (13.7%) induced a dose-dependent hypotensive effect in both conscious and anesthetized rats [97]. In addition, at high doses (10 and 20 mg/Kg), the oil decreased heart rate in anesthetized rats, while in conscious rats the effect was not uniform, with some animals showing bradycardia, others tachycardia or tachycardia followed by bradycardia. The effect of this oil has also been assessed in other models. For example, in uni-nephrectomized, normotensive rats, the oil showed a hypotensive effect in a dose-dependent manner [98]. In DOCA-salt hypertensive rats, the essential oil led to a stepper effect in MAP when compared to normotensive rats, and this effect was not affected by methylatropine nor hexamethonium. Furthermore, a methanolic fraction obtained from the essential oil of *A. zerumbet*, characterized by terpinen-4-ol (57.35%) and 1,8-cineole (27.81%), also decreased MAP, systolic arterial pressure (SAP) and diastolic arterial pressure (DAP) 26 days after L-NAME-induced hypertension [99].

3.2.2. Vasorelaxant Effects

Regarding the vasorelaxant effects of essential oils, several *Croton* species have been assessed namely, *C. zehntneri*, C. *argyrophylloides*, *C. nepetaefolius* and *C. zambesicus*. Both *C. zehntneri* and *C. argyrophylloides* oils induced vasorelaxation in a dose-dependent manner in aortic rings containing endothelium (IC_{50} = 202.0 μg/mL and 25.31 μg/mL, respectively) [83,85]. For *C. argyrophylloides* the observed effect was independent from the presence of endothelium (IC_{50} = 189.0 vs 202.0 μg/mL) and atropine (IC_{50} = 158.6 vs 202.0 μg/mL) [83], while *C. zehntneri* lost its relaxant effect after endothelium removal (IC_{50} = 76.22 vs 25.31

μg/mL) or by the pretreatment with atropine (IC_{50}= 197.20 vs 25.31 μg/mL), indomethacin (IC_{50}= 90.60 vs 25.31 μg/mL) and glibenclamide (IC_{50}= 64.46 vs 25.31 μg/mL). Nevertheless, it was unaffected by the presence of L-NAME (IC_{50} = 41.75 vs 25.31 μg/mL) and tetraethylammonium chloride (TEA, IC_{50}= 25.64 vs 25.31 μg/mL) [85]. In a different study, the essential oil from *C. argyrophylloides* induced relaxation in intact aortic rings (IC_{50} = 126.7 μg/mL) and mesenteric bed preparations (IC_{50} = 46.0 μg/mL) precontracted with Phe [100]. Also, *C. nepetaefolius* Baill. (Euphorbiaceae), composed by 1,8-cineole (25.4%), methyleugenol (14.9%), xanthoxilin (10.1%), β-caryophyllene (9.66%), sabinene (5.2%) showed a relaxant effect on intact aortic rings precontracted with K^+ in a dose-dependent manner (IC_{50} = 26.7 μg/mL) and dependent on the presence of endothelium (IC_{50} = 105.6 μg/mL) and NOS (IC_{50} = 52.7 μg/mL after L-NAME pretreatment) [101]. In intact aortic rings precontracted with Phe, the essential oil induced relaxation in a soluble guanylate cyclase (sGC)-dependent manner. Moreover, in mesenteric bed preparations, the presence of the essential oil reverted the flow decrease evoked by K^+ in a NOS-dependent manner. *C. nepetaefolius* characterized by 1,8-cineole (25.37%), methyleugenol (14.90%), bicyclogermacrene (11.06%) and xanthoxilin (10.10%) induced relaxation in aortic rings isolated from DOCA-salt hypertensive rats precontracted with Phe, in a dose-dependent manner, with a reduction more significant than that observed in uni-nephrectomized controls (IC_{50}= 16.4 vs 112.9 μg/mL) [102]. The essential oil from the leaves of *C. zambesicus* collected at different time periods, characterized by *ent*-trachyloban-3-one (1.4 28.0%), caryophyllene oxide (2.9% – 25.9%) and longifolene (0.4 – 26.4%) induced relaxation in a dose-dependent manner in intact aortic rings (IC_{50} = 5.6 – 11.8 μg/mL) [103].

The essential oil from the flower calices of *Ocotea quixos* (Lam.) Kosterm. (Lauraceae), composed by *trans*-cinnamaldehyde (27.8%), methyl cinnamate (21.6%) and limonene (8.1%) caused relaxation on Phe-induced contractions in aortic rings with (IC_{50} = 86 μg/mL) and without (IC_{50} = 110 μg/mL) endothelium [104].

The vasorelaxant effect of the essential oil from *O. gratissimum* is partially dependent on the endothelium (IC_{50} = 226.9 μg/mL vs IC_{50} = 417.2 μg/mL, respectively, in the presence or absence of endothelium). Furthermore, in Ca^{2+}-free medium, increasing concentrations of $CaCl_2$ evoked contractions which were reduced by the essential oil [86].

The essential oil from the leaves of *O. gratissimum*, composed mainly by eugenol (52.1%), 1,8-cineole (29.2%), β-selinene (5.6%) caused vasorelaxation on Phe-contracted aortic rings independent of the presence of endothelium, but dependent of NOS [105]. In mesenteric vascular beds the essential oil elicited a decrease in the perfusion pressure evoked by noradrenaline in a NOS-dependent pathway.

Santo et al. [106] showed that the essential oil obtained from the aerial parts of *Alpinia speciosa* K. Schum (Zingiberaceae), rich in terpinen-4-ol (38%), 1,8-cineole (18%) and γ-terpinene (12%), when applied to rat left atria decreased the force of contraction in a dose-dependent manner (IC_{50} = 292.2 μg/mL) as well as the sinus rhythm (IC_{50} = 595.4 μg/mL). In a different study, two essential oils from *A. zerumbet*, with a distinct chemical composition, one rich in 1,8-cineole (33.3%), terpinen-4-ol (19.4%) and *p*-cymene (11.4%) and other characterized by β-phellandrene (16.4%), β-pinene (15.1%) and 1,8-cineole (11%), showed a distinct vasorelaxant effect. The former induced an incomplete relaxation in aortic rings with endothelium that were pre-contracted with Phe [107] whereas the latter induced full relaxation in aortic rings contracted either with KCl and norepinephrine [108]. Similarly, the essential oil from the aerial parts of *Artemisia campestris* L. (Asteraceae), with spathulenol (10.19%) as the main component, followed by β-eudesmol (4.05%), *p*-cymene (3.83%) and δ-cadinene (3.67%), induced almost full relaxation in intact aortic rings precontracted with Phe [109]. This effect seemed to be independent of the NOS/GC pathway and potassium channels; however, the authors suggest that the vasorelaxant effect of *A. campestris* might be dependent of L-type Ca^{2+}-channels and the activation of SERCA pumps.

The contraction evoked by high potassium in isolated rabbit aortic rings was revoked by the presence of the essential oil of *Citrus aurantifolia* (Christm) Swingle (Rutaceae), composed mainly by limonene (58.4%) and β-pinene (15.4%) by activating Ca^{2+} channels [110]. In intact aortic rings precontracted with $PGF_{2\alpha}$, the presence of the oil from *Citrus aurantium* L. var. *amara* (Rutaceae) [linalool (23.2%), β-pinene (9.6%), limonene (8.54%)] and *Citrus bergamia* Risso (Rutaceae) [D-limonene (43.5%), linalyl acetate (25.5%)] induced relaxation [111,112]. Using mesenteric artery rings, de Menezes et al. [96], showed that the essential oil of *C. winterianus* induced relaxation in an endothelium-independent manner (E_{max} = 125% vs 117%, with and without endothelium, respectively). In addition, the same oil also induced relaxation in endothelium-denuded rings precontracted with high K^+ (E_{max} = 121%). The essential oil from *Hyptis fruticosa* decreased the contractions evoked by Phe (E_{max}= 64% vs 122%, respectively, with or without endothelium) as well as by $CaCl_2$ (E_{max} = 12% vs 81%) [89]. The leaves of *Lippia thymoides* Mart. & Schauer (Verbenaceae) collected in the four seasons and characterized by β-caryophyllene (17.22 – 26.27%), borneol (4.45 – 7.36%), camphor (3.22 – 8.61%), camphene (2.64 – 5.66%), and germacrene D (4.72 – 6.18%) were tested for their vasorelaxant activity, being able to induce relaxation in endothelium-intact (IC_{50} = 305 – 544 μg/mL) and endothelium-denuded (IC_{50} = 150 – 283 μg/mL) rings [113]. The presence of the essential oil of *Menta* x *villosa* in atrial preparations had a negative chronotropic (IC_{50} = 229 μg/mL) and ionotropic (IC_{50} = 120 μg/mL) effect that were dose-dependent [91]. In aortic rings, the essential oil caused relaxation in rings contracted with Phe (IC_{50} = 255 μg/mL), $PGF_{2\alpha}$ (IC_{50} = 174 μg/mL) and KCl (IC_{50} = 165 μg/mL). The vasorelaxant capacity of *M.* x *villosa* was also shown in aortic rings with (IC_{50} = 61 μg/mL) and without (IC_{50} = 109 μg/mL) endothelium contracted with KCl [92]. Pereira et al. [114] showed that the essential oil from the aerial parts of *Pectis brevipedunculata* (Gardner) Sch. Bip. (Asteraceae), characterized mainly by citral (81.7%: neral 32.5% and geranial 49.2%) induced vasorelaxation on endothelium-intact (IC_{50} = 0.044%) and endothelium-denuded (IC_{50} = 0.093%) rings, dependent on the NO/sGMP pathway since the pretreatment with L-NAME reduced the vasorelaxant activity of the essential oil. Opposing, the essential oil of *P. elsholtzioides* induced vasorelaxation in aortic rings precontracted with Phe, in a NO/cGMP independent pathway [93]. In an *ex vivo* model of mice hearts, the essential oil from *S. areira* decreased the contractility induced by Phe [81]. The essential oil from the seeds of *Trachyspermum ammi* [L.] Sprague (Apiaceae), rich in thymol (38.1%), limonene (33.3%) and *p*-cymene (23.1%), decreased the contraction of aortic rings induced by Phe (IC_{50} = 54.4 µg/mL), KCl (IC_{50} = 49 µg/mL), as well as, in the presence (IC_{50} = 46.6 µg/mL) and absence (IC_{50} = 45.2 µg/mL) of endothelium [115]. This effect was independent of NO/cGMP pathway but dependent on the extracellular Ca^{2+} flux, since pretreatment with nifedipine, a calcium channel blocker, reduced the relaxant activity of the essential oil. The essential oil obtained from the leaves of *Xylopia langsdorfiana* A. St.-Hil. &Tul. (Annonaceae) and characterized by germacrene D (22.9%), *trans*-β-guaiene (22.6%), β-caryophyllene (15.7%), weakly inhibited the contractions induced by Phe [116]. The essential oil isolated from the oleo-gum resin from *Ferula assa-foetida* L.(Apiaceae), characterized by di-(2-methyl-1,3-oxathiolanyl)methane (22.43%), *trans*-propenyl sec butyl disulfide (14.59%), thiophene, 2-ethyltetrahydro- (10.61%), *trans*, *trans*-dibenzylideneacetone (10.07%), *cis*-propenyl sec butyl disulfide (8.78%), 2-methyl-2 methylthiopropionic acid (8.07%) and disulfide, methyl 1-(methylthio)propyl (5.54%) was able to induce vasorelaxation precontracted with high K^+ both in the presence (IC_{50} = 1.6 µL/L) and absence (IC_{50} = 19.2 µL/L) of endothelium [117]. This effect appears to be partially mediated by NOS and COX activity since the presence of L-NAME and indomethacin decreased the relaxation induced by the essential oil. In addition, the presence of the essential oil, in Ca^{2+}-free medium reduced the contraction induced by Ca_2Cl, thus suggesting that the oil blocks the calcium influx. The fruit of *Psidium guajava* L. (Myrtaceae) was submitted to steam distillation and yielded an essential oil characterized by butanoic acid methyl ester, 3-methyl glutaric anhydride, 1-butanol, 3-hexenal, cinnamyl alcohol, 1-hexanol and hexane, that caused relaxation in rabbit aortic rings precontracted with Phe (EC_{50} = 6.23 mg/mL) and high K^+ (EC_{50} = 5.52 mg/mL) [118]. The essential oil obtained from the bark of

Aniba canelilla relaxed mesenteric arteries isolated from SHRs contracted by K^+ (IC_{50} = 294.19 μg/mL) or Phe (IC_{50} = 11.07 μg/mL) [119]. Under Ca^{2+}-free conditions, the essential oil reduced the contractions evoked by phorbol dibutyrate and Phe but failed to do so in caffeine-induced contractions. Furthermore, in Ca^{2+}-free and high K^+ conditions, the contractions elicited by $CaCl_2$ or $BaCl_2$ were reduced and even abolished by the essential oil. In a different study, the same essential oil reduced the contraction evoked by high K^+ in intact aortic rings (IC_{50} = 64.5 μg/mL). This effect was abolished by the addition of atropine (IC_{50} = 109.5 μg/mL) and by endothelium removal (IC_{50} = 139.1 μg/mL) [95]. In addition, Ca_2Cl-induced contractions in Ca^{2+}-free medium were reduced by 100 μg/mL and abolished by 600 μg/mL of the essential oil. The oil from *Nigella sativa* L. (Ranunculaceae) seeds elicited a dose-dependent relaxation in intact aortic rings precontracted with noradrenaline and high K^+ in a NO-independent way [120]. In addition, the oil abolished the tension created by increasing levels of Ca^{2+}, thus suggesting that the essential oil might induced relaxation by blocking both voltage-sensitive and receptor operated calcium channels. The essential oil obtained from the petals of *Rosa indica* L. (Rosaceae), characterized by methylsantonilate, butanoic acid, 2-methyl-5-oxo-1-cyclopentene-1-yl ester, santolina epoxide and artemiseole, induced relaxation in isolated rabbit aortic rings precontracted with high K^+ (EC_{50} = 5.80 mg/mL) and Phe (EC_{50} = 7.39 mg/mL) [121]. The essential oil distilled from the bulbs of *Allium macrostemon* Bunge (Amaryllidaceae), rich in dimethyl trisulfide (34.93%), dimethyl disulfide (11.61%), 2,3,5,6-tetramethylpyrazine (7.32%) and 1,3-dithiane (7.18%), induced relaxation in a endothelium-dependent manner (relaxation of 59.56% vs 9.31%, after endothelium removal) in pulmonary arteries [122]. In addition, the effect was dependent on eNOS (59.56% vs 12.75%, after L-NAME treatment) but not on COX (59.56% vs 50.98%, after indomethacin treatment). In pulmonary artery endothelial cells, the authors showed that the presence of the essential oil induced the phosphorylation of eNOS at serine 1177 without affecting the total levels of the protein. This effect was reverted by the presence of Protein Kinase A Inhibitor (PKI). In addition, the essential oil failed to increase the intracellular Ca^{2+} levels in the absence of extracellular calcium. These results suggest that the essential oil from *A. macrostemon* leads to eNOS phosphorylation via intracellular Ca^{2+}/PKA/eNOS pathway.

3.2.3. Clinical Trials

Despite several *in vivo* studies highlighting the beneficial therapeutic effects of essential oils in CVDs, and more specifically in hypertension [123], very few clinical trials validate these effects. Moreover, the majority of the clinical trials are non-randomized trials and they include a reduced number of patients. Further clinical trials should be preferably randomized, multi-centered and gather a larger pool of patients in order to produce significant results regarding the potential of essential oils as new therapeutic agents for hypertension. Next, examples of clinical trials are mentioned. Of notice, the majority include mixtures of essential oils, with lavender oil standing out as one of the most studied.

A randomized, cross-over clinical trial included 30 prehypertensive middle aged women, who received a mixture of lavender and jojoba oils via inhalation (2 minutes, 3 times a day for 5 days) and through a topical administration by spreading the mixture on the parotid areas (once daily for 5 days) followed by one week washout period. In general, the treatment decreased both SBP and DBP when compared to the placebo [124], thus highlighting the hypotensive effect of the extracts.

In another non-randomized clinical trial with 60 patients with essential hypertension those who received a mixture of lavender:ylang-ylang:bergamot (ratio of 5:3:2) by inhalation for 5 minutes per day for 4 weeks showed an improvement in their SBP and DBP when compared to both placebo and control groups [125].

A different trial on 47 patients with hypertension showed that those who received only lavender essential oil, or a mixture of lavender:roman chamomile (1:1), or lavender:roman chamomile:sandalwood (3:1:1) by inhalation during 5 minutes didn´t show any significative improvements on SBP and DBP values [126].

Furthermore, another non-randomized clinical trial in 43 hypertensive patients showed that those who inhaled for 5 min the essential oil of lavender, or a mixture of lavender:marjoram (1:1) or of lavender:marjoram:ylang-ylang (4:3:3) had an improvement of SBP 5, 30 and 60 min after inhalation, whereas DBP only decreased 60 min after administration [127].

In a clinical trial, with 20 patients with hypertension, those who received ylang-ylang:clary sage:marjoram (1:1:1) by inhalation followed by a 45 minute massage, failed to show–any improvement when comparing to the placebo group [128].

Moreover, a non-randomized clinical trial compared the effect of a mixture of lavender:ylang-ylang:marjoram:neroli (20:15:10:2) essential oils with placebo (artificial fragrance). The results showed that 10 minutes after inhalation, the aromatherapy group had a decrease in home-measured SBP (132.3 to 127.6 vs 133.3 vs 134.2 mmHg, for aromatherapy and placebo, respectively) and in home-measured DBP (85.7 to 84.5 vs 85.0 to 84.7, for treated group and placebo, respectively). The decrease of SBP was similar amongst prehypertensive and hypertensive patients whereas the decrease of DBP was more significant on hypertensive individuals. For ambulatory BP, the aromatherapy had a decrease in daytime SBP (140.6 to 129.9 vs 132.6 to 136.0 mmHg, compared to placebo) and daytime DBP (90.5 to 83.3 vs 84 to 85.6 mmHg, compared to placebo). However, no effects were detected at nighttime SBP and DBP values [129].

Finally, a clinical trial (NCT02656004) sponsored by Universidade Federal do Vale do São Francisco (Brazil) aimed to assess the effect of eucalyptus essential oil on cardiovascular responses, although the trial ended in 2016, no results have yet been revealed [130].

3.2.4. Chemical Composition-Activity Relation

Bearing in mind the chemical complexity of essential oils, the activity of the volatile extract may not be due to the presence of a single major compound, since synergistic effects between different compounds of the mixture may occur or minor compounds may have a relevant role in the bioactivity of the oil. Indeed, for example, the essential oil of *Allium macrostemon* is mainly characterized by the presence of dimethyl trisulfide (34.93%) and dimethyl disulfide (11.61%), however dimethyl trisulfide has a vasoconstrictor activity, in opposition to the essential oil and dimethyl disulfide has a preeminent vasodilator activity. Therefore, the activity described for *Allium macrostemon* is attributed mainly to dimethyl disulfide rather than to its major compound [122]. Nevertheless, in some case the major compounds are those responsible for the activity of the mixture, as occurs with *Ocimum gratissimum* in which the major compounds eugenol and 1,8-cineole are the most active. Indeed, both compounds have been widely reported for their hypotensive and vasorelaxant effects [86–88,114,131–138]. Similarly, the essential oil of *Pectis brevipedunculata* has a vasorelaxant activity that may be attributed to the presence of citral, a mixture of neral and geranial, since these compounds alone are able to induce vasorelaxant effects, however in a less extent than that of the volatile extract [114]. In this case, the activity of the extract may have the contribution of geraniol, the other major compound of *P. brevipedunculata* with both vasorelaxant and hypotensive activities reported [139]. Another example is the activity of cinnamaldehyde and *methyl*-cinnamate that might explain the vasorelaxant effects of *Ocotea quixos* essential oil since both compounds have been reported to be vasorelaxant [140–142]. However, it is likely that the activity is mainly attributed to cinnamaldehyde rather that *methyl*-cinnamate since the latter has a weaker vasorelaxant effect. The reported activity of *Croton zehtneri* and *Foeniculum vulgare* is related to the presence of anethole and estragole, since both compounds have been widely reported as having hypotensive and vasorelaxant activities [82,84,132].

The hypotensive and vasorelaxant effects of several isolated compounds are summarized in Table 2. For this purpose, the main chemical classes of compounds found in essential oils, primarily terpenoids and phenylpropanoids, as well as sulphur and nitrogen-containing compounds were considered. Also, the chemical structure of the compound and the study model used to assess their bioactive effect as well as the main findings are included. The compounds reported herein are commercially available, nevertheless, the plant source where the compound is naturally present in high amounts is mentioned.

Table 2. Hypotensive and vasorelaxant effects of isolated compounds found in essential oils

Chemical class	Compound	Structure	Main Source	Study model	Main findings	Ref
TERPENOIDS						
Monoterpene	Carvacrol	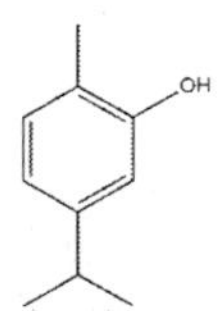	*Origanum vulgare* (oregano)	Isolated rat aortic rings	Induced relaxation in PHE- and KCl-pre-contracted rings; Inhibited the response to PHE and KCl; ↓ $CaCl_2$-induced contractions	[136]
					↓ contraction in PHE-contracted rings and in Pb(II)-induced contraction	[138]
				Isolated rat mesenteric artery rings	↓ PHE-induced contractions with or without endothelium; ↓ $CaCl_2$-induced contractions; Induced relaxation in S(-)-Bay K8644-pre-contracted rings	[143]
				Isolated rat left atria	Demonstrated a negative inotropic and chronotropic effect	
				Isolated canine and human ventricular cardiomyocytes	Suppressed cardiac Ca^{2+} channels	[144]
				Isolated rat cerebral and cerebellar arteries	Induced vasorelaxation	[145]
				Anesthetized, normotensive rats	↓ HR, MAP, SBP and DBP; inhibited L-NAME-induced hypertension	[146]
				Non-anesthetized, normotensive rats	Induced hypotension associated with bradycardia	[143]
	Carvone	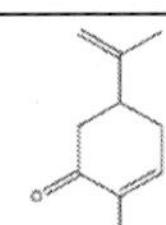	*Mentha spicata* (spearmint)	PHE-pre-contracted isolated aortic segments	Induced relaxation in aortic rings unexposed (66% control) and exposed to As(III) (61% control) and Hs(II) (60% control)	[133]

Chemical class	Compound	Structure	Main Source	Study model	Main findings	Ref
	1,8-Cineole	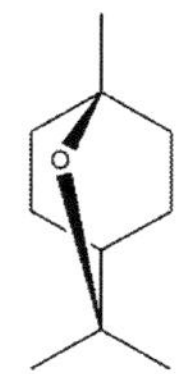	*Alpinia zerumbet* (shell ginger)	Isolated rat left ventricle papillary muscles	↓ isometric contractions, time to peak and relaxation time; ↑ relative potentiation; ↓ tetanic force	[131]
				Isolated aortic rings	Induced endothelium-dependent relaxation	
				Pentobarbital-anesthetized and normotensive rats	↓ MAP and HR	[135]
				Conscious and normotensive rats		
				Rat isolated thoracic aorta preparations	↓ KCl-induced contractions	[114]
	Citral (geranial + neral)	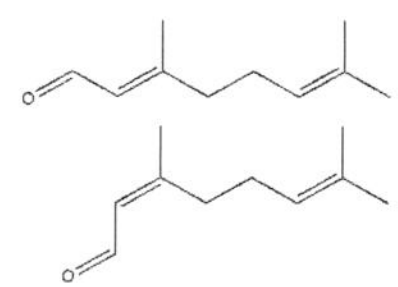	*Pectis brevipedunculata* (cinchweed)	Pre-contracted isolated aortic rings	↓ PHE-induced contraction in endothelium-intact (IC_{50} = 1.42 mM) and endothelium-denuded (IC_{50} = 1.33 mM) aortic rings; ↓ KCl-induced contractions in endothelium-denuded aortic rings; ↓ Ca^{2+}-induced contractions in endothelium-denuded aortic rings	[114]
	(±)-Citronellol	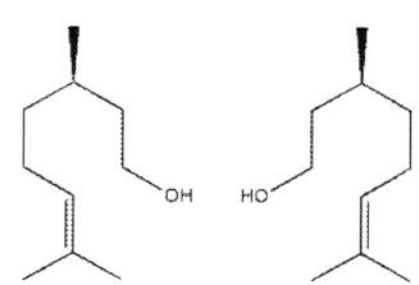	*Cymbopogon citratus* (West Indian lemon grass) *Rosa* spp. (rose)	Non-anesthetized normotensive rats	Induced transitory hypotension associated with tachycardia	[147, 148]
				Endothelium-intact rat mesenteric artery rings	Induced vasorelaxation in PHE- and KCl-pre-contracted rings	[148]
				Endothelium-denuded rat mesenteric artery rings	Induced vasorelaxation in PHE- and KCl-pre-contracted rings; Inhibited $CaCl_2$-induced contractions; Reduced PHE- and Caf-induced contractions in Ca^{2+}-free medium	

Table 2. (Continued)

Chemical class	Compound	Structure	Main Source	Study model	Main findings	Ref
	Geraniol	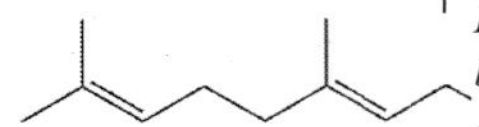	*Pectis brevipedunculata* (cinchweed)	Isolated guinea pig left atria	Induced a negative inotropic effect; ↓ Ca^{2+} influx; Impaired BAY K8644-induced increase in atrial force	[139]
				Isolated mice ventricular cardiomyocytes	↑ APD; ↓ maximal dp/dt	
				Isolated guinea pig heart	↓ LVP; ↑ PRi	
				Ouabain-induced arrhythmias	↓ tonotropic effect; delays arrhythmia onset	
	(±)-Linalool	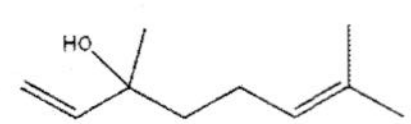	*Croton zambesicus* (lavender croton)	Non-anesthetized normotensive rats	Induced transitory hypotension associated with tachycardia	[147]
				Normotensive conscious rats	Induced hypotension and tachycardia	
				Goldblatt hypertensive conscious rats	↓ MAP without affecting HR	[149]
				Isolated mesenteric artery rings	Induced relaxation in PHE-pre-contracted endothelium-intact and endothelium-denuded rings; Induced relaxation in KCl-pre-contracted endothelium-denuded rings; ↓ contractions induced by $CaCl_2$ in endothelium-denuded rings; Inhibited transient contractions induced by PHE and Caf in endothelium-intact rings in Ca^{2+}-free medium	

Chemical class	Compound	Structure	Main Source	Study model	Main findings	Ref
	(-)-Linalool	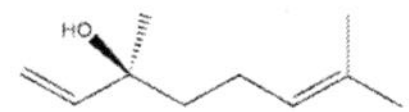	*Coriandrum sativum* (coriander)	Human (inhalation)	↓ SBP, DBP and HR	[150]
	(+)-Linalool	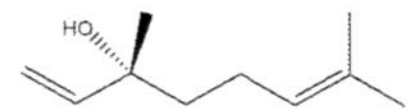	*Lavandula officinalis* (lavender)	Human (inhalation)	↑ SBP, DBP and HR	[150]
				PHE-pre-contracted isolated aortic segments	Induced relaxation in aortic rings unexposed (71% control) and exposed to As(III) (64% control) and Hs(II) (63% control)	[133]
	Menthol	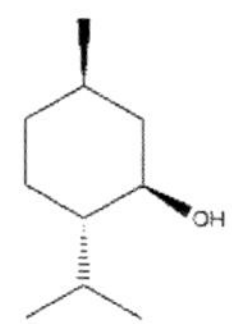	*Mentha* x *piperita* (peppermint)	Rat proximal tail artery, thoracic aorta and mesenteric artery	↓ PHE- and KCl-induced contraction	[151]
				Isolated rat aortic, mesenteric and coronary arteries rings	↓ KCl-induced contractions (E_{max} = 93.72%, 96.52% and 98.48%, respectively) and PHE-induced contractions (E_{max} = 86.39% and 97.59% in aortic and mesenteric rings); ↓ Ca^{2+}-induced contraction in Ca^{2+}-free medium with high K^+ and Ca^{2+} influx	[152]
	(+)-α-Pinene (-)-β-Pinene	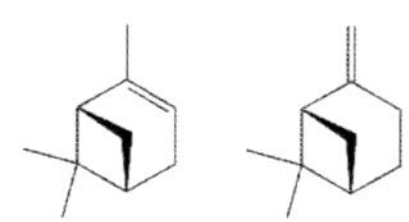	*Pinus* spp. (pine)	Non-anesthetized normotensive rats	Induced transitory hypotension associated with tachycardia	[147]
	Piperitenone oxide	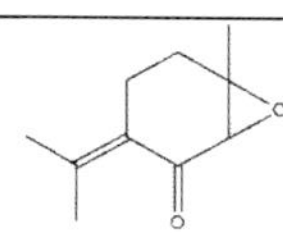	*Mentha x villosa* (Mojito mint)	Anesthetized normotensive rats	↓ MAP and HR	[90]

Table 2. (Continued)

Chemical class	Compound	Structure	Main Source	Study model	Main findings	Ref
	Rotundifolone	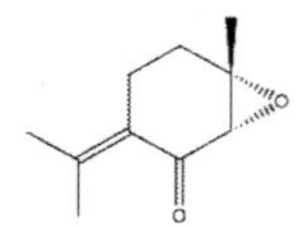	*Mentha x villosa* (Mojito mint)	Non-anesthetized normotensive rats	Induced hypotension and bradycardia	[153]
				Isolated rat atria preparations	Negative inotropic and chronotropic effect on left and right atria, respectively	[153]
				Isolated aortic rings	↓ PHE-induced contractions in a endothelium-dependent manner	[153]
				Isolated aortic rings	Inhibited PHE and KCl contractile effects; ↓ $CaCl_2$-induced contractions	[154]
	Terpinen-4-ol	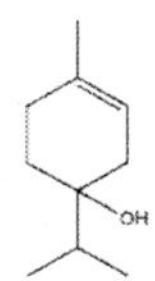	*Alpinia zerumbet* (shell ginger)	DOCA-salt hypertensive rats	↓ MAP	[98]
				Isolated rat aortic rings	Induced relaxation in high K^+ and PHE-pre-contracted endothelium-intact rings; ↓ Ba^{2+}-, PHE- and phorbol 12,13-dibutyrate-induced contractions in Ca^{2+}-free medium; ↓ BAYK-8644-induced contractions	[155]
	α-Terpineol	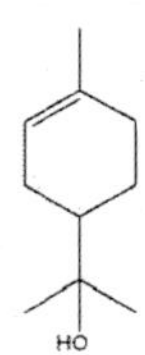	*Croton nepetaefolius* (red quince)	Conscious, normotensive rats	Induced hypotension followed by tachycardia	[156]
				PHE-contracted mesenteric artery rings	Induced an endothelium-dependent relaxation	[156]
				Rabbit aortic endothelial cell line	↑ NO levels	[156]
				Rat mesenteric vascular bed preparations	Induced relaxation of KCl-induced contractions	[101]

Chemical class	Compound	Structure	Main Source	Study model	Main findings	Ref
	Thymol	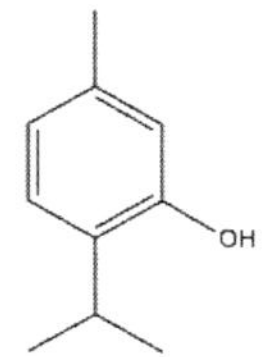	*Trachyspermum ammi* (Ajwain)	Isolated rat aortic rings	Induced relaxation in PHE- and KCl-pre-contracted rings; Inhibited the response to PHE and KCl; ↓ $CaCl_2$-induced contractions	[136]
				Isolated canine and human ventricular cardiomyocytes	Suppressed cardiac Ca^{2+} and K^+ channels	[157]
				Guinea pig and canine heart preparations	Negative inotropic effect; Induced SR Ca^{2+} release and inhibited Ca^{2+} pump activity	[158]
				Isolated canine and human ventricular cardiomyocytes	Suppressed cardiac Ca^{2+} channels	[144]
Sesquiterpene	(-)-α-Bisabolol	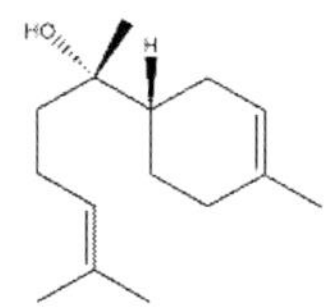	*Matricaria recutita* (German chamomile)	Non-anesthetized normotensive rats	Transitory hypotension associated with bradycardia	[147]
				Isolated rat aortic and mesenteric rings	↓ High K^+- and PHE-induced contractions on endothelium-intact and endothelium-denuded aortic rings and endothelium-intact mesenteric rings	[159]
				Isolated rat aortic rings	↓ KCl- and PHE-induced contractions; ↓ $CaCl_2$-induced contractions in KCl-stimulated rings under Ca^{2+}-free medium	[160]
				Fluo-4 AM-loaded isolated rat mesenteric rings	↓ Tension and Ca^{2+} cytosolic levels in response to K^+	

Table 2. (Continued)

Chemical class	Compound	Structure	Main Source	Study model	Main findings	Ref
	β-Caryophyllene oxide	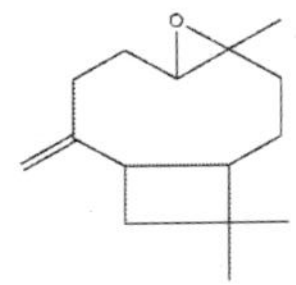	*Syzigium aromaticum* (clove)	Isolated papillary muscle	Induced contraction at 1 Hz contraction frequency (IC_{50} = 36 µmol/L)	[137]
					Induced a negative ionotropic effect at the rested-state contractions (IC_{50} = 28 µmol/L)	
					Block calcium inward current (IC_{50} = 29 µmol/L)	
				Isolated ventricular myocytes	Inhibited outward potassium currents	
	β - Caryophyllene	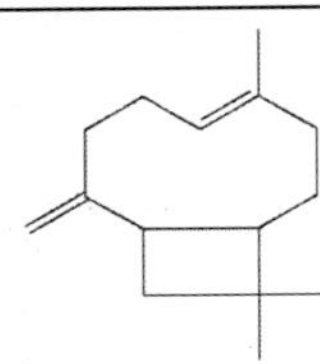		Isolated papillary muscle	Induced a negative ionotropic effect at the rested-state contractions (IC_{50} = 268 µmol/L)	
PHENYLPROPANOIDS						
Phenyl ether	Anethole	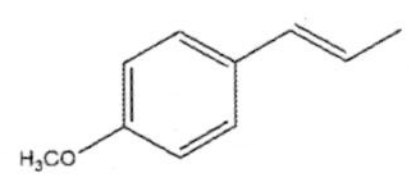	*Croton zehtneri*	Conscious normotensive rats	Induced hypotension and bradycardia (phase I); induced pressor effect associated with delayed bradycardia (phase II)	[82]
				Anesthetized conscious rats	Transient hypotension and bradycardia	[84]
				Isolated aortic rings precontracted with PHE	↓ contraction in rings with (IC_{50} = 9.01 mM) and without (IC_{50} = 4.28 mM) endothelium	[132]

Chemical class	Compound	Structure	Main Source	Study model	Main findings	Ref
Phenyl aldehyde	Cinnamaldehyde	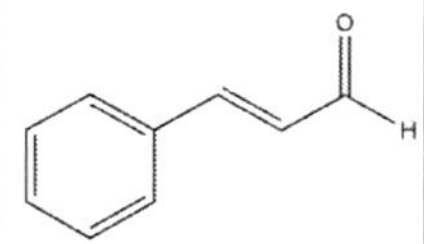	*Cinnamomum* spp.	Porcine coronary artery rings	↓ Thromboxane A_2 agonist-evoked contractions	[141]
					↓ contractions elicited by KCl	
					↓ $CaCl_2$-induced contractions in high K^+ and Ca^{2+}-free medium	
				Aortic rings	↓ contractions induced by prostaglandin $F_{2\alpha}$, norepinephrine and KCl	[140]
Phenyl ester	*methyl*-Cinnamate	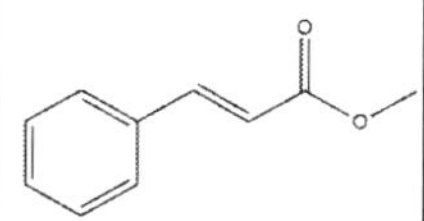	*Ocotea quixos* (Ecuadorian cinnamon)	PHE-contracted aortic rings	Induced relaxation in endothelium-intact (IC_{50} = 877.6 μM) and -denuded (IC_{50} = 725.5 μM)	[142]
					↓ contractions evoked by KCl (IC_{50} = 1147.7 μM)	
					↓ contractions induced by Phe and Ca^{2+} in Ba^{2+}-containing medium	
					Induced relaxation evoked by Ba^{2+} in Ca^{2+}-free medium	
				Mesenteric rings	Abolished KCl-induced contractions (IC_{50} = 314.5 μM)	
Monophenol	Estragole	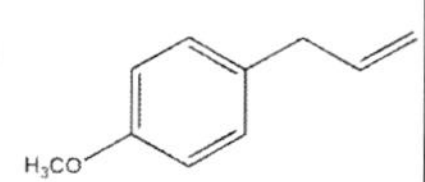	*Croton zehtneri*	Isolated aortic rings precontracted with PHE	↓ contraction in rings with (IC_{50} = 4.34 mM) and without (IC_{50} = 6.70 mM) endothelium	[132]
				Conscious normotensive rats	Induced hypotension and bradycardia (phase I) Induces pressor effect associated with delayed bradycardia (phase II)	[82]
				Anesthetized conscious rats	Transient hypotension and bradycardia	[84]

Table 2. (Continued)

Chemical class	Compound	Structure	Main Source	Study model	Main findings	Ref
Diphenol	Eugenol	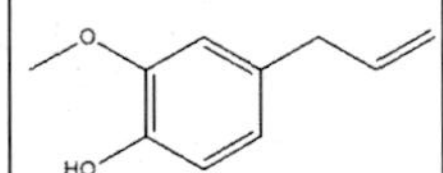	*Ocimum gratissimum* (clove basil)	Isolated aortic rings precontracted with PHE	↓ contraction in rings with (IC_{50} = 1.36 mM) and without (IC_{50} = 2.13 mM) endothelium	[132]
				DOCA-salt hypertensive rats	Induced hypotension and bradycardia	[87]
				Anesthetized and conscious normotensive rats	Induced hypotension and bradycardia	[134]
				Conscious normotensive rats	↓ MAP and HR	[88]
				Aortic rings isolated from DOCA-salt hypertensive rats contracted by PHE	↓ contractions in a dose-dependent manner (IC_{50} = 1.2 mM)	[86]
				Isolated rat aortic rings	↓ contractions in rings unexposed and exposed to Pb(II)	[138]
				Isolated rat aortic rings	↓ hypercontractility associated with As(III) and Hg(II)	[133]
					Induced relaxation in unexposed rings	
				Mesenteric vascular bed	Induced relaxation in K^+-induced contractions	[161]
				Isolated papillary muscle	Induced contraction at 1 Hz contraction frequency (IC_{50} = 127 µmol/L)	[137]

Chemical class	Compound	Structure	Main Source	Study model	Main findings	Ref
					Induced a negative ionotropic effect at the rested-state contractions (IC_{50} = 194 μmol/L)	
					Block calcium inward current (IC_{50} = 226 μmol/L)	
				Isolated ventricular myocytes	Inhibited outward potassium currents	
Diphenol ester	Eugenol acetate	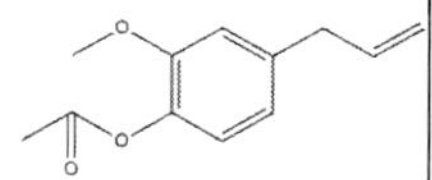	*Syzigium aromaticum* (clove)	Isolated papillary muscle	Induced contraction at 1 Hz contraction frequency (IC_{50} = 298 μmol/L)	
Diphenol	*iso*-Eugenol	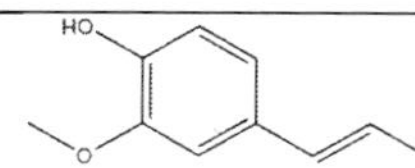	*Cananga odorata* (ylang-ylang)	Isolated aortic rings precontracted with PHE	↓ contraction in rings with (IC_{50} = 3.28 mM) and without (IC_{50} = 3.45 mM) endothelium	[132]
Diphenol derivative	*methyl*-Eugenol	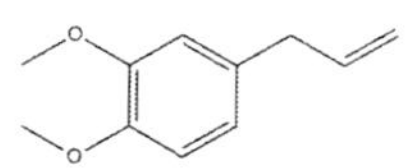	*Croton malambo*	K^+-reduced flow in rat isolated mesenteric bed preparations	Recovery of flow in a dose-dependent manner	[101]
				Anesthetized normotensive rats	↓ MAP and HR at 10 mg/Kg	[162]
				Conscious normotensive rats	↓ MAP	
				Aortic rings precontracted with high K^+	↓ contractions evoked by K^+	

Table 2. (Continued)

Chemical class	Compound	Structure	Main Source	Study model	Main findings	Ref
OTHERS						
Sulphur-containing compounds	Dimethyl disulfide	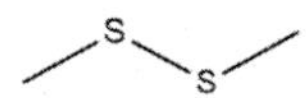	*Allium macrostemon* (long-stamen chive)	Pulmonary artery	Caused dilation in PHE-contracted pulmonary arteries (39.24% dilation)	[122]
					Dilation in DTT-treated pulmonary arteries	
	Dimethyl trisulfide	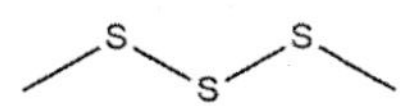			Induced vasoconstriction in PHE-contracted pulmonary arteries (30.84% constriction)	
Nitrogen-containing compounds	1-Nitro-2-phenylethane	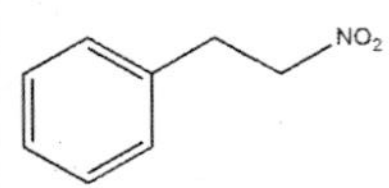	*Aniba canelilla* (precious bark)	Anesthetized normotensive rats	Rapid hypotension and bradycardia (Phase I) Delayed hypotension and bradycardia (Phase II)	[163]
				PHE-contracted aortic rings with intact endothelium	Induced relaxation (IC_{50} = 60.1 μg/mL)	
				Mesenteric artery rings from SHR	↓ contractions evoked by high K^+ (IC_{50} = 501.27 μg/mL), PHE (IC_{50} = 7.91 μg/mL) and phorbol dibutyrate (IC_{50} = 39.13 μg/mL)	[119]
					In Ca^{2+}-free medium, decreased the contractions elicited by Phe	
					In Ca^{2+}-free and high K^+ conditions, induced relaxation in rings contracted by $CaCl_2$ and $BaCl_2$	

APD – Action potential duration; As(III) – Arsenic (III); Ba^{2+} – Barium ion; $BaCl_2$ – Barium chloride; BAY K-8644 – Calcium channel agonist; Ca^{2+} – Calcium ion; $CaCl_2$ – Calcium chloride; Caf – Caffeine; DBP – Diastolic blood pressure; dp/dt - maximal rate of rise of left ventricular pressure; DTT – Dithiothreitol; Hg(II) – Mercury (II); HR- Heart rate; Hz – Hertz; IC_{50} – half maximal inhibitory concentration; K^+ - Potassium ion; KCl – Potassium chloride; L-NAME – N^{ω}-nitro-L-arginine; LVP – Left ventricular pressure; MAP – Mean arterial blood pressure; NO – Nitric oxide; Pb(II) – Plumb (II); PHE – Phenylephrine; PRi – PR interval; SBP – Systolic blood pressure; SR – Sarcoplasmic reticulum.

Chemical structure-activity relations are relevant to design more effective drugs. Following, this relation is endeavored by considering some examples of effective antihypertensive isolated compounds. For example, comparing the activity of two compounds, 1-nitro-2-phenylethane (NP) and 1-nitro-2-phenylethene (NPe), a synthetic derivative, it was shown that the later had an activity 3.3-fold higher than the former (IC_{50} = 10.47 vs 37.65 µg/mL, in Phe-contracted aortic rings, for NPe and NP, respectively) [164]. The reason behind this difference is, according to the authors, a conformational restriction imposed by the alkene moiety in 1-nitro-2-phenylethene [164]. The authors described that 1-nitro-2-phenylethane can have varying dihedral angles between the phenyl and the nitro moieties linked at the ethylene atoms, namely 180º, 120º, 60º and 0º. The most common angles are 180º (*trans* conformation) and 0º (*cis* conformation) for 1-nitro-2-phenylethane, whereas 1-nitro-1-phenylethene only can be in the 180-degree conformation.

Another study compared two isomers of linalool, R-(-)-linalool and S-(+)-linalool [150]. The authors showed that the isomers have opposite effects, with the R-(-) isomer having hypotensive and bradycardic effects and the S-(+) isomer showing hypertensive and tachycardic properties. The authors attributed this difference to the chirality of the compounds, which determines the compounds effect on the sympathetic nervous system as well as their interaction with receptors. Also, when comparing the hypotensive activity of (-)-β-pinene and (+)-α-pinene, the (-)-β isomer was more efficacious than the (+)-α one [147]. The authors hypothesized that the exocyclic double bond in (-)-β-pinene is more active than the endocyclic double bond, present in the other isomer. Furthermore, the authors suggested that the difference in the stereochemistry at the two chiral centers (carbon 1 and 5) might also have impact of the effect. The activity of two acyclic monoterpenes, (±)-citronellol and (±)-linalool, was also assessed, being citronellol, a primary alcohol, the most effective in comparison with linalool, which is a tertiary alcohol [147]. The effect of anethole, estragole, eugenol and *iso*-eugenol on voltage dependent Ca^{2+} channels was unveiled, and the authors found out that anethole and estragole had a more strong effect when compared to eugenol and its isomer *iso*-eugenol, thus suggesting that this activity has some specific structural requirements. Indeed, the authors pointed out this difference might be attributed to position of the methoxy group, which is in *para* position in anethole and estragole but in *meta* position on eugenol and *iso*-eugenol [132].

CONCLUSION

This review highlights the great potential of essential oils and isolated volatile compounds on the management of hypertension, particularly due to their widely reported hypotensive and vasorelaxant effects. Despite several *in vivo* studies addressing these effects, relevant clinical trials are still lacking. Indeed, only a few have been carried out, using mixtures of essential oils, on non-randomized small cohorts. In most of these trials, the essential oil of lavender is used, and the observed beneficial effects seem to be due to the presence of linalool, a monoterpene with both hypotensive and vasorelaxant effects.

Regarding other isolated compounds, several studies show that mono and sesquiterpenes as well as phenylpropanoids have beneficial effects on hypertension, however no clinical trials are known. Interestingly, the mentioned chemical composition-activity relations show that, in some cases, the major compounds found in essential oils play a relevant role in the antihypertensive effect of these extracts. For this reason, new studies assessing the effect of essential oils rich in these compounds should be considered, as for example *Origanum vulgare* and *Thymbra capitata* essential oils that are rich in carvacrol. In addition, studies addressing the structural requirements for antihypertensive effects highlight that new chemical entities based on natural compounds can be designed, originating more effective compounds, such as 1-nitro-2-phenylethene synthetized from 1-nitro-2-phenylethane.

Overall this review paves the way the development of new effective therapies for the management of hypertension that negatively impacts on patient's quality of life and ultimately leads to higher levels of morbidity and mortality.

References

[1] WHO, WHO | Cardiovascular diseases (CVDs). 2017,. http://www.who.int/mediacentre/factsheets/fs317/en/ (accessed February 15, 2018).

[2] Faulx, M. D.; Francis, G. S., Adverse drug reactions in patients with cardiovascular disease. *Curr. Probl. Cardiol.*, 2008, *33* (*12*), 703–768.

[3] Harvey, R. E.; Coffman, K. E.; Miller, V. M., Women-specific factors to consider in risk, diagnosis and treatment of cardiovascular disease. *Women's Heal.*, 2015, *11* (*2*), 239–257.

[4] WHO, Cardiovascular diseases (CVDs). 2017,. http://www.who.int/cardiovascular_diseases/en/.

[5] WHO, WHO | World Heart Day 2017. *WHO.*, 2017,. http://www.who.int/cardiovascular_diseases/world-heart-day-2017/en/ (accessed February 22, 2018).

[6] Egan, B. M.; Kjeldsen, S. E.; Grassi, G.; Esler, M.; Mancia, G., The global burden of hypertension exceeds 1.4 billion people. *J. Hypertens.*, 2019, *37* (*6*), 1148–1153.

[7] Kokubo, Y.; Iwashima, Y., Higher blood pressure as a risk factor for diseases other than stroke and ischemic heart disease. *Hypertension.*, 2015, *66* (*2*), 254–259.

[8] Taddei, S.; Bruno, R. M.; Masi, S.; Solini, A., Epidemiology and pathophysiology of hypertension, in: B. Williams (Ed.), *ESC CardioMed*, Oxford University Press, 2018: pp. 2377–2388.

[9] Kannel, W., Risk stratification in hypertension: new insights from the Framingham study. *Am. J. Hypertens.*, 2000, *13* (*1*), S3–S10.

[10] Egan, B. M.; Stevens-Fabry, S., Prehypertension—prevalence, health risks, and management strategies. *Nat. Rev. Cardiol.*, 2015, *12* (*5*), 289–300.

[11] Nguyen, Q.; Dominguez, J.; Nguyen, L.; Gullapalli, N., Hypertension management: an update. *Am. Heal. Drug Benefits.*, 2010, *3* (*1*), 47–56. http://www.ncbi.nlm.nih.gov/pubmed/25126308.

[12] Tedla, Y. G.; Bautista, L. E., Drug side effect symptoms and adherence to antihypertensive medication. *Am. J. Hypertens.*, 2016, *29* (*6*), 772–779.

[13] Mendis, S.; Puska, P.; Norrving, B., *Global atlas on cardiovascular disease prevention and control*, World Health Organization, Geneva, 2011.

[14] Walden, R.; Tomlinson, B., *Cardiovascular Disease*, 2nd Edition, Taylor & Francis, FL, 2011. http://www.ncbi.nlm.nih.gov/pubmed/22593934 (accessed February 24, 2018).

[15] Cordell, G., Changing strategies in natural products chemistry. *Phytochemistry.*, 1995, *40* (*6*), 1585–1612.

[16] Tuso, P.; Stoll, S. R.; Li, W. W., A plant-based diet, atherogenesis, and coronary artery disease prevention. *Perm. J.*, 2015, *19* (*1*), 62–7.

[17] Buckle, J., Aromatherapy and Cardiovascular Disease, in: R. A. Stein, M. C. Oz (Eds.), Complement. Altern. Cardiovasc. Med., Humana Press, Totowa, NJ, 2004: pp. 239–254.

[18] Wachtel-Galor, S.; Benzie, I. F. F., Herbal medicine: an introduction to its history, usage, regulation, current trends, and research needs, in: S. Wachtel-Galor, I. F. F. Benzie (Eds.), *Herb. Med. Biomol. Clin. Asp.,* 2nd Editio, CRC Press/Taylor & Francis, 2011. http://www.ncbi.nlm.nih.gov/pubmed/22593939 (accessed February 24, 2018).

[19] WHO, Section II: hypertension : the basic facts, in: *A Glob. Br. Hypertens. Silent Kill. Glob. Public Heal. Cris.*, WHO Press, Genève, Switzerland, 2013: pp. 16–22.

[20] Heart Foundation, Is my blood pressure normal? 2017,. https://www.heartfoundation.org.au/your-heart/know-your-risks/blood-pressure/is-my-blood-pressure-normal (accessed December 22, 2019).

[21] Williams, B.; Mancia, G.; Spiering, W.; Agabiti Rosei, E.; Azizi, M.; Burnier, M.; Clement, D. L.; Coca, A.; Brady, A.; et al., 2018 ESC/ESH Guidelines for the management of arterial hypertension. *Eur. Heart J.*, 2018, *39* (*33*), 3021–3104.

[22] Lloyd-Jones, D. M., General population and global cardiovascular risk prediction, in: Hypertens. A Companion to Braunwald's Hear. Dis., Elsevier, 2018: pp. 1–14.

[23] Barst, R. J.; Ertel, S. I.; Beghetti, M.; Ivy, D. D., Pulmonary arterial hypertension: a comparison between children and adults. *Eur. Respir. J.*, 2011, *37* (*3*), 665–677.

[24] Gupta-Malhotra, M.; Banker, A.; Shete, S.; Hashmi, S.S.; Tyson, J. E.; Barratt, M. S.; Hecht, J. T.; Milewicz, D. M.; Boerwinkle, E., Essential hypertension vs. secondary hypertension among children. *Am. J. Hypertens.*, 2015, *28* (*1*), 73–80.

[25] Zhou, B.; Bentham, J.; Di Cesare, M.; Bixby, H.; Danaei, G.; Cowan, M. J.; Paciorek, C. J.; Singh, G.; Zuñiga Cisneros, J.; et al., Worldwide trends in blood pressure from 1975 to 2015: a pooled analysis of 1479 population-based measurement studies with 19.1 million participants. *Lancet.*, 2017, *389* (*10064*), 37–55.

[26] WHO, *Hypertension*. 2019,. https://www.who.int/news-room/fact-sheets/detail/hypertension (accessed February 13, 2020).

[27] Mills, K. T.; Stefanescu, A.; He, J., The global epidemiology of hypertension. *Nat. Rev. Nephrol.*, 2020.

[28] WHO, *A global brief on hypertension*, 2013.

[29] Ogah, O. S., Blood pressure, prevalence of hypertension and hypertension related complications in Nigerian Africans: A review. *World J. Cardiol.*, 2012, *4* (*12*), 327.

[30] Dzudie, A.; Kengne, A. P.; Muna, W. F. T.; Ba, H.; Menanga, A.; Kouam Kouam, C.; Abah, J.; Monkam, Y.; Biholong, C.; Mintom, P.; Kamdem, F.; Djomou, A.; Ndjebet, J.; Wambo, C.; Luma, H.; Ngu, K. B.; Kingue, S., Prevalence, awareness, treatment and control of hypertension in a self-selected sub-Saharan African urban population: a cross-sectional study. *BMJ Open.*, 2012, *2* (*4*), e001217.

[31] Edwards, R.; Unwin, N.; Mugusi, F.; Whiting, D.; Rashid, S.; Kissima, J.; Aspray, T. J.; Alberti, K. G. M. M., Hypertension prevalence and care in an urban and rural area of Tanzania. *J. Hypertens.*, 2000, *18* (2), 145–152.

[32] Wilkins, E.; Wilson, L.; Wickramasinghe, K.; Bhatnagar, P.; Rayner, M.; Townsend, N.; Leal, J.; Luengo-Fernandez, R.; Burns, R., European cardiovascular disease statistics - 2017 Edition, Brussels, Belgium, 2017.

[33] Benjamin, E. J.; Blaha, M. J.; Chiuve, S. E.; Cushman, M.; Das, S. R.; Deo, R.; de Ferranti, S. D.; Floyd, J.; Fornage, M.; Gillespie, C.; Isasi, C. R.; Jiménez, M. C.; Jordan, L. C.; Judd, S. E.; Lackland, D.; Lichtman, J. H.; Lisabeth, L.; Liu, S.; Longenecker, C. T.; Mackey, R. H.; Matsushita, K.; Mozaffarian, D.; Mussolino, M. E.; Nasir, K.; Neumar, R. W.; Palaniappan, L.; Pandey, D. K.; Thiagarajan, R. R.; Reeves, M. J.; Ritchey, M.; Rodriguez, C. J.; Roth, G. A.; Rosamond, W. D.; Sasson, C.; Towfighi, A.; Tsao, C. W.; Turner, M. B.; Virani, S. S.; Voeks, J. H.; Willey, J. Z.; Wilkins, J. T.; Wu, J. H.; Alger, H. M.; Wong, S. S.; Muntner, P., Heart disease and stroke statistics—2017 update: a report from the American Heart Association. *Circulation*., 2017, *135* (*10*),.

[34] Gaziano, T. A.; Bitton, A.; Anand, S.; Weinstein, M. C., The global cost of nonoptimal blood pressure. *J. Hypertens.*, 2009, *27* (*7*), 1472–1477.

[35] Mennini, F. S.; Marcellusi, A.; von der Schulenburg, J. M. G.; Gray, A.; Levy, P.; Sciattella, P.; Soro, M.; Staffiero, G.; Zeidler, J.; Maggioni, A.; Schmieder, R. E., Cost of poor adherence to anti-hypertensive therapy in five European countries. *Eur. J. Heal. Econ.*, 2015, *16* (*1*), 65–72.

[36] Whelton, P. K., Primary prevention of hypertension: clinical and public health advisory from the national high blood pressure education program. *JAMA*., 2002, *288* (*15*), 1882.

[37] Riley, M.; Hernandez, A. K.; Kuznia, A. L., High blood pressure in children and adolescents. *Am. Fam. Physician*., 2018, *98* (*8*), 486–494. http://www.ncbi.nlm.nih.gov/pubmed/30277729.

[38] Braunthal, S.; Brateanu, A., Hypertension in pregnancy: pathophysiology and treatment. *SAGE Open Med.*, 2019, *7* 2050 31211984370.

[39] Gurven, M.; Blackwell, A. D.; Rodríguez, D. E.; Stieglitz, J.; Kaplan, H., Does blood pressure inevitably rise with age? *Hypertension.*, 2012, *60* (*1*), 25–33.

[40] Johnson, H. M.; Thorpe, C. T.; Bartels, C. M.; Schumacher, J. R.; Palta, M.; Pandhi, N.; Sheehy, A. M.; Smith, M. A., Antihypertensive medication initiation among young adults with regular primary care use. *J. Gen. Intern. Med.*, 2014, *29* (*5*), 723–731.

[41] Whelton, P. K.; Einhorn, P. T.; Muntner, P.; Appel, L. J.; Cushman, W. C.; Diez Roux, A. V.; Ferdinand, K. C.; Rahman, M.; Taylor, H. A.; Ard, J.; Arnett, D. K.; Carter, B. L.; Davis, B. R.; Freedman, B. I.; Cooper, L. A.; Cooper, R.; Desvigne-Nickens, P.; Gavini, N.; Go, A. S.; Hyman, D. J.; Kimmel, P. L.; Margolis, K. L.; Miller, E. R.; Mills, K. T.; Mensah, G. A.; Navar, A. M.; Ogedegbe, G.; Rakotz, M. K.; Thomas, G.; Tobin, J. N.; Wright, J. T.; Yoon, S. S.; Cutler, J. A., Research needs to improve hypertension treatment and control in African Americans. *Hypertension.*, 2016, *68* (*5*), 1066–1072.

[42] Dorans, K. S.; Mills, K. T.; Liu, Y.; He, J., Trends in prevalence and control of hypertension according to the 2017 American College of Cardiology/American Heart Association (ACC/AHA) guideline. *J. Am. Heart Assoc.*, 2018, *7* (*11*),.

[43] Lackland, D. T., Racial differences in hypertension: implications for high blood pressure management. *Am. J. Med. Sci.*, 2014, *348* (*2*), 135–138.

[44] He, F. J.; Li, J.; MacGregor, G. A., Effect of longer term modest salt reduction on blood pressure: Cochrane systematic review and meta-analysis of randomised trials. *BMJ.*, 2013, *346* (*apr03 3*), f1325–f1325.

[45] Burnier, M.; Kjeldsen, S.; Heagerty, A.; Williams, B., Drug treatment of hypertension, in: B. Williams (Ed.), ESC CardioMed, Oxford University Press, 2018: pp. 2445–2458.

[46] Lerman, L. O.; Kurtz, T. W.; Touyz, R. M.; Ellison, D. H.; Chade, A. R.; Crowley, S. D.; Mattson, D. L.; Mullins, J. J.; Osborn, J.; Eirin, A.; Reckelhoff, J. F.; Iadecola, C.; Coffman, T. M., Animal models

of hypertension: a scientific statement from the American Heart Association. *Hypertension.*, 2019, *73* (*6*),.

[47] McGonigle, P.; Ruggeri, B., Animal models of human disease: challenges in enabling translation. *Biochem. Pharmacol.*, 2014, *87* (*1*), 162–171.

[48] Pinto, Y., Lessons from rat models of hypertension from Goldblatt to genetic engineering. *Cardiovasc. Res.*, 1998, *39* (*1*), 77–88.

[49] Crowley, S. D.; Gurley, S. B.; Herrera, M. J.; Ruiz, P.; Griffiths, R.; Kumar, A. P.; Kim, H.-S.; Smithies, O.; Le, T. H.; Coffman, T. M., Angiotensin II causes hypertension and cardiac hypertrophy through its receptors in the kidney. *Proc. Natl. Acad. Sci.*, 2006, *103* (*47*), 17985–17990.

[50] Crowley, S. D.; Frey, C. W.; Gould, S. K.; Griffiths, R.; Ruiz, P.; Burchette, J. L.; Howell, D. N.; Makhanova, N.; Yan, M.; Kim, H.-S.; Tharaux, P. L.; Coffman, T. M., Stimulation of lymphocyte responses by angiotensin II promotes kidney injury in hypertension. *Am. J. Physiol. Physiol.*, 2008, *295* (*2*), F515–F524.

[51] Crowley, S. D.; Zhang, J.; Herrera, M.; Griffiths, R.; Ruiz, P.; Coffman, T. M., Role of AT 1 receptor-mediated salt retention in angiotensin II-dependent hypertension. *Am. J. Physiol. Physiol.*, 2011, *301* (*5*), F1124–F1130.

[52] Guzik, T. J.; Hoch, N. E.; Brown, K. A.; McCann, L. A.; Rahman, A.; Dikalov, S.; Goronzy, J.; Weyand, C.; Harrison, D. G., Role of the T cell in the genesis of angiotensin II–induced hypertension and vascular dysfunction. *J. Exp. Med.*, 2007, *204* (*10*), 2449–2460.

[53] Qiu, C.; Engels, K.; Baylis, C., Angiotensin II and alpha 1-adrenergic tone in chronic nitric oxide blockade-induced hypertension. *Am. J. Physiol. Integr. Comp. Physiol.*, 1994, *266* (*5*), R1470–R1476.

[54] Gardiner, S. M.; Kemp, P. A.; Bennett, T.; Palmer, R. M. J.; Moncada, S., Nitric oxide synthase inhibitors cause sustained, but reversible, hypertension and hindquarters vasoconstriction in Brattleboro rats. *Eur. J. Pharmacol.*, 1992, *213* (*3*), 449–451.

[55] Ribeiro, M. O.; Antunes, E.; de Nucci, G.; Lovisolo, S. M.; Zatz, R., Chronic inhibition of nitric oxide synthesis. A new model of arterial hypertension. *Hypertension.*, 1992, *20* (*3*), 298–303.

[56] Zandberg, P., Animal models in experimental hypertension: relevance to drug testing and discovery, in: P. Van Zwieten (Ed.), Pharmacol. Antihypertens. Drugs, Elsevier, Amsterdam, 1984: pp. 6–45.

[57] ISO 9235, Aromatic natural raw materials - vocabulary. 2013,.

[58] Council of Europe, European Pharmacopoeia 7th Edition, Directorate for the Quality of Medicines & HealthCare of the Council of Europe, Strasbourg, France, 2010.

[59] Svoboda, K. P.; Svoboda, T. G., Secretory structures of aromatic and medicinal plants: a review and atlas of micrographs, Microscopix, 2000. https://books.google.pt/books?id=mIhFAQAAIAAJ.

[60] Bakkali, F.; Averbeck, S.; Averbeck, D.; Idaomar, M., Biological effects of essential oils – a review. *Food Chem. Toxicol.*, 2008, *46* (*2*), 446–475.

[61] Figueiredo, A. C.; Barroso, J. G.; Pedro, L. G.; Scheffer, J. J. C., Factors affecting secondary metabolite production in plants: volatile components and essential oils. *Flavour Fragr. J.*, 2008, *23* (*4*), 213–226.

[62] Hüsnü, K.; Başer, C.; Demirci, F., Chemistry of essential oils, in: R. G. Berger (Ed.), Flavours and Fragrances, Springer Berlin Heidelberg, Berlin, Heidelberg, 2007: pp. 43–86.

[63] Rubiolo, P.; Sgorbini, B.; Liberto, E.; Cordero, C.; Bicchi, C., Essential oils and volatiles: sample preparation and analysis. A review. *Flavour Fragr. J.*, 2010, *25* (*5*), 282–290.

[64] Zuzarte, M.; Salgueiro, L., Essential oils chemistry, in: *Bioact. Essent. Oils Cancer*, Springer International Publishing, Cham, 2015: pp. 19–61.

[65] Cheng, S.; Fu, X.; Mei, X.; Zhou, Y.; Du, B.; Watanabe, N.; Yang, Z., Regulation of biosynthesis and emission of volatile phenylpropanoids/benzenoids in *Petunia*× *hybrida* flowers by multi-

factors of circadian clock, light, and temperature. *Plant Physiol. Biochem.*, 2016, *107* 1–8.

[66] Barbieri, C.; Borsotto, P., Essential oils: market and legislation, in: *Potential Essent. Oils*, InTech, 2018.

[67] Alves-Silva, J. M.; Monica, Z.; Carla, M.; Lígia, S.; Henrique, G.; Zuzarte, M.; Marques, C.; Salgueiro, L.; Girao, H., Protective effects of terpenes on the cardiovascular system: current advances and future perspectives. *Curr. Med. Chem.*, 2016, *23* (*40*), 1–1.

[68] Alves Silva, J. M.; Zuzarte, M.; Marques, C.; Girão, H.; Salgueiro, L., Protective effects of phenylpropanoids and phenylpropanoid-rich essential oils on the cardiovascular system. *Mini-Reviews Med. Chem.*, 2019, *19*.

[69] Andrade, T. de; Brasil, G.; Endringer, D.; da Nóbrega, F.; de Sousa, D., Cardiovascular activity of the chemical constituents of essential oils. *Molecules.*, 2017, *22* (*9*), 1539.

[70] Alves-Silva, J. M.; Barbeitos, J.; Marques, C.; Salgueiro, L.; Girão, H.; Zuzarte, M., Effects on the cardiovascular system of terpene-rich essential oils, in: A. Bjarke (Ed.), *Terpenes Biosynthesis, Appl. Res.*, 1st ed., Nova Science Publishers, Inc., New York, 2018: pp. 123–171.

[71] Giles, T. D.; Sander, G. E.; Nossaman, B.D.; Kadowitz, P.J., Impaired vasodilation in the pathogenesis of hypertension: focus on nitric oxide, endothelial-derived hyperpolarizing factors, and prostaglandins. *J. Clin. Hypertens.*, 2012, *14* (*4*), 198–205.

[72] Perera, R. K.; Fischer, T. H.; Wagner, M.; Dewenter, M.; Vettel, C.; Bork, N. I.; Maier, L. S.; Conti, M.; Wess, J.; El-Armouche, A.; Hasenfuß, G.; Nikolaev, V. O., Atropine augments cardiac contractility by inhibiting cAMP-specific phosphodiesterase type 4. *Sci. Rep.*, 2017, *7* (*1*), 15222.

[73] Alcayaga, J.; Del Rio, R.; Moya, E. A.; Freire, M.; Iturriaga, R., Effects of vagotomy on cardiovascular and heart rate variability alterations following chronic normobaric hypoxia in adult rabbits. *Biol. Res.*, 2018, *51* (*1*), 57.

[74] Li, P.; Gong, J. X.; Sun, W.; Zhou, B.; Kong, X. Q., Hexamethonium attenuates sympathetic activity and blood pressure in spontaneously hypertensive rats. *Mol. Med. Rep.*, 2015, *12* (*5*), 7116–7122.

[75] Kopincová, J.; Púzserová, A.; Bernátová, I., L-NAME in the cardiovascular system – nitric oxide synthase activator? *Pharmacol. Reports.*, 2012, *64* (*3*), 511–520.

[76] Ferreira, S. H.; Moncada, S.; Vane, J. R., Indomethacin and aspirin abolish prostaglandin release from the spleen. *Nat. New Biol.*, 1971, *231* (*25*), 237–239.

[77] Story, G. M.; Cruz-Orengo, L., Feel the burn. *Am. Sci.*, 2007, *95* (*4*), 326.

[78] Serrano-Martin, X.; Payares, G.; Mendoza-Leon, A., Glibenclamide, a blocker of K+ATP channels, shows antileishmanial activity in experimental murine cutaneous Leishmaniasis. *Antimicrob. Agents Chemother.*, 2006, *50* (*12*), 4214–4216.

[79] Armstrong, C. M., Interaction of tetraethylammonium ion derivatives with the potassium channels of giant axons. *J. Gen. Physiol.*, 1971, *58* (*4*), 413–437.

[80] McDonald, T. F.; Pelzer, S.; Trautwein, W.; Pelzer, D.J., Regulation and modulation of calcium channels in cardiac, skeletal, and smooth muscle cells. *Physiol. Rev.*, 1994, *74* (*2*), 365–507.

[81] Bigliani, M. C.; Rossetti, V.; Grondona, E.; Lo Presti, S.; Paglini, P. M.; Rivero, V.; Zunino, M. P.; Ponce, A. A.; Presti, S. Lo; Paglini, P. M.; Rivero, V.; Zunino, M. P.; Ponce, A. A., Chemical compositions and properties of *Schinus areira* L. essential oil on airway inflammation and cardiovascular system of mice and rabbits. *Food Chem. Toxicol.*, 2012, *50* (*7*), 2282–2288.

[82] Siqueira, R. J. B. de; Magalhães, P. J. C.; Leal-Cardoso, J. H.; Duarte, G. P.; Lahlou, S., Cardiovascular effects of the essential oil of *Croton zehntneri* leaves and its main constituents, anethole and estragole, in normotensive conscious rats. *Life Sci.*, 2006, *78* (*20*), 2365–72.

[83] Siqueira, R. J. B. de; Duarte, G. P.; Magalhães, P. J. C.; Lahlou, S., Cardiovascular effects of the essential oil of *Croton zehntneri* leaves in DOCA-salt hypertensive, conscious rats. *Nat. Prod. Commun.*,

2013, *8* (*8*), 1167–70. http://www.ncbi.nlm.nih.gov/pubmed/24079196.

[84] Siqueira, R. J. B. de; Leal-Cardoso, J.; Couture, R.; Lahlou, S., Role of capsaicin-sensitive sensory nerves in mediation of the cardiovascular effects of the essential oil of *Croton zehntneri* leaves in anaesthetized rats. *Clin. Exp. Pharmacol. Physiol.*, 2006, *33* (*3*), 238–47.

[85] Alves-Santos, T. R.; de Siqueira, R. J. B.; Duarte, G. P.; Lahlou, S., Cardiovascular effects of the essential oil of *Croton argyrophylloides* in normotensive rats: role of the autonomic nervous system. *Evidence-Based Complement. Altern. Med.*, 2016, *2016* 1–9.

[86] Interaminense, L. F. L.; Jucá, D. M.; Magalhães, P. J. C.; Leal-Cardoso, J. H.; Duarte, G. P.; Lahlou, S., Pharmacological evidence of calcium-channel blockade by essential oil of *Ocimum gratissimum* and its main constituent, eugenol, in isolated aortic rings from DOCA-salt hypertensive rats. *Fundam. Clin. Pharmacol.*, 2007, *21* (*5*), 497–506.

[87] Interaminense, L. F. L.; Leal-Cardoso, J. H.; Magalhães, P. J. C.; Duarte, G. P.; Lahlou, S., Enhanced hypotensive effects of the essential oil of *Ocimum gratissimum* leaves and its main constituent, eugenol, in DOCA-salt hypertensive conscious rats. *Planta Med.*, 2005, *71* (*4*), 376–8.

[88] Lahlou, S.; Interaminense Lde, F.; Leal-Cardoso, J. H.; Morais, S. M.; Duarte, G. P., Cardiovascular effects of the essential oil of *Ocimum gratissimum* leaves in rats: role of the autonomic nervous system. *Clin Exp Pharmacol Physiol.*, 2004, *31* (*4*), 219–225.

[89] Santos, M. R. V.; Carvalho, A. A.; Medeiros, I. A.; Alves, P. B.; Marchioro, M.; Antoniolli, A. R., Cardiovascular effects of *Hyptis fruticosa* essential oil in rats. *Fitoterapia.*, 2007, *78* (*3*), 186–91.

[90] Lahlou, S.; Carneiro-Leão, R. F. L.; Leal-Cardoso, J. H.; Toscano, C. F., Cardiovascular effects of the essential oil *Mentha x villosa* and its main constituent, piperitenone oxide, in normotensive anaesthetised rats: role of the autonomic nervous system. *Planta Med.*, 2001, *67* 638–643.

[91] Guedes, D. N.; Silva, D. F. F.; Barbosa-Filho, J. M. M.; Medeiros, I. A. de, Endothelium-dependent hypotensive and vasorelaxant effects of the essential oil from aerial parts of *Mentha x villosa* in rats. *Phytomedicine.*, 2004, *11* (*6*), 490–7.

[92] Lahlou, S.; Carneiro-Leão, R. F. L.; Leal-Cardoso, J. H., Cardiovascular effects of the essential oil of *Mentha x villosa* in DOCA-salt-hypertensive rats. *Phytomedicine.*, 2002, *9* (*8*), 715–20.

[93] Shiva Kumar, A.; Jeyaprakash, K.; Chellappan, D. R.; Murugan, R., Vasorelaxant and cardiovascular properties of the essential oil of *Pogostemon elsholtzioides. J. Ethnopharmacol.*, 2017, *199* (*May 2016*), 86–90.

[94] Siqueira, R. J. de; Rodrigues, K. M. S.; da Silva, M. T. B.; Correia Junior, C. A. B.; Duarte, G. P.; Magalhães, P. J. C.; dos Santos, A. A.; Maia, J. G. S.; da Cunha, P. J. S.; Lahlou, S., Linalool-rich rosewood oil induces vago-vagal bradycardic and depressor reflex in rats. *Phyther. Res.*, 2014, *28* (*1*), 42–8.

[95] Lahlou, S.; Magalhães, P. J. C.; Siqueira, R. J. B. de; Figueiredo, A. F.; Interaminense, L. F. L.; Maia, J. G. S.; Sousa, P. J. da C., Cardiovascular effects of the essential oil of *Aniba canelilla* bark in normotensive rats. *J. Cardiovasc. Pharmacol.*, 2005, *46* (*4*), 412–21.

[96] Menezes, I. A. C. de; Moreira, Í. J. A.; De Paula, J. W. A.; Blank, A. F.; Antoniolli, A. R.; Quintans-Júnior, L. J.; Santos, M. R. V.; Moreira, I. J. A.; De Paula, J. W. A.; Blank, A. F.; Antoniolli, A. R.; Quintans-Júnior, L. J.; Santos, M. R. V., Cardiovascular effects induced by *Cymbopogon winterianus* essential oil in rats: involvement of calcium channels and vagal pathway. *J. Pharm. Pharmacol.*, 2010, *62* (2), 215–21.

[97] Lahlou, S.; Galindo, C. A. B.; Leal-Cardoso, J. H.; Fonteles, M. C.; Duarte, G. P., Cardiovascular effects of the essential oil of *Alpinia zerumbet* leaves and its main constituent, terpinen-4-ol, in rats: role of the autonomic nervous system. *Planta Med.*, 2002, *68* (*12*), 1097–102.

[98] Lahlou, S.; Interaminense, L. F. L.; Leal-Cardoso, J. H.; Duarte, G. P., Antihypertensive effects of the essential oil of *Alpinia zerumbet*

and its main constituent, terpinen-4-ol, in DOCA-salt hypertensive conscious rats. *Fundam. Clin. Pharmacol.*, 2003, *17* (*3*), 323–330.

[99] Cunha, G. H. da; Moraes, M. O. de M.E. A. de M. O. de M. E. A. de; Fechine, F. V.; Frota Bezerra, F. A.; Silveira, E. R.; Canuto, K. M.; Moraes, M. O. de M. E. A. de M. O. de M. E. A. de, Vasorelaxant and antihypertensive effects of methanolic fraction of the essential oil of *Alpinia zerumbet*. *Vascul. Pharmacol.*, 2013, *58* (*5–6*), 337–345.

[100] França-Neto, A. de; Cardoso-Teixeira, A. C.; Medeiros, T. C.; Quinto-Farias, M. do S.; Sampaio, C. M. de S.; Coelho-de-Souza, A. N.; Lahlou, S.; Leal-Cardoso, J. H., Essential oil of *Croton argyrophylloides*: toxicological aspects and vasorelaxant activity in rats. *Nat. Prod. Commun.*, 2012, *7* (*10*), 1397–400. http://www.ncbi.nlm.nih.gov/pubmed/23157021.

[101] Magalhães, P. J. C.; Lahlou, S.; Jucá, D. M.; Coelho-De-Souza, L. N.; da Frota, P. T. T.; da Costa, A. M. G.; Leal-Cardoso, J. H., Vasorelaxation induced by the essential oil of *Croton nepetaefolius* and its constituents in rat aorta are partially mediated by the endothelium. *Fundam. Clin. Pharmacol.*, 2008, *22* (2), 169–177.

[102] Lahlou, S.; Leal-Cardoso, J. H.; Magalhães, P. J., Essential oil of *Croton nepetaefolius* decreases blood pressure through an action upon vascular smooth muscle: studies in DOCA-salt hypertensive rats. *Planta Med.*, 2000, *66* (2), 138–43.

[103] Martinsen, A.; Baccelli, C.; Navarro, I.; Abad, A.; Quetin-Leclercq, J. J.; Morel, N., Vascular activity of a natural diterpene isolated from *Croton zambesicus* and of a structurally similar synthetic trachylobane. *Vascul. Pharmacol.*, 2010, *52* (*1–2*), 63–69.

[104] Ballabeni, V.; Tognolini, M.; Bertoni, S.; Bruni, R.; Guerrini, A.; Rueda, G. M.; Barocelli, E., Antiplatelet and antithrombotic activities of essential oil from wild *Ocotea quixos* (Lam.) Kosterm. (Lauraceae) calices from Amazonian Ecuador. *Pharmacol. Res.*, 2007, *55* (*1*), 23–30.

[105] Pires, A. F.; Madeira, S. V. F.; Soares, P. M. G.; Montenegro, C. M.; Souza, E. P.; Resende, A. C.; Soares de Moura, R.; Assreuy, A. M. S.; Criddle, D. N., The role of endothelium in the vasorelaxant effects

of the essential oil of *Ocimum gratissimum* in aorta and mesenteric vascular bed of rats. *Can. J. Physiol. Pharmacol.*, 2012, *90* (*10*), 1380–5.

[106] Santos, B. A. A.; Roman-Campos, D.; Carvalho, M. S. S.; Miranda, F. M. F. M. F.; Carneiro, D. C. C.; Cavalcante, P. H. H.; Cândido, E. A. F. A. F.; Filho, L. X.; Cruz, J. S. S.; Gondim, A. N. S. N. S., Cardiodepressive effect elicited by the essential oil of *Alpinia speciosa* is related to L-type $Ca2^+$ current blockade. *Phytomedicine.*, 2011, *18* (*7*), 539–543.

[107] Pinto, N. V.; Assreuy, A. M. S.; Coelho-de-Souza, A. N.; Ceccatto, V. M.; Magalhães, P. J. C.; Lahlou, S.; Leal-Cardoso, J. H., Endothelium-dependent vasorelaxant effects of the essential oil from aerial parts of *Alpinia zerumbet* and its main constituent 1,8-cineole in rats. *Phytomedicine.*, 2009, *16* (*12*), 1151–1155.

[108] Tao, L.; Hu, H. S.; Shen, X. C., Endothelium-dependent vasodilatation effects of the essential oil from Fructus Alpiniae Zerumbet (EOFAZ) on rat thoracic aortic rings *in vitro*. *Phytomedicine.*, 2013, *20* (*5*), 387–393.

[109] Dib, I.; Fauconnier, M. L.; Sindic, M.; Belmekki, F.; Assaidi, A.; Berrabah, M.; Mekhfi, H.; Aziz, M.; Legssyer, A.; Bnouham, M.; Ziyyat, A., Chemical composition, vasorelaxant, antioxidant and antiplatelet effects of essential oil of *Artemisia campestris* L. from Oriental Morocco. *BMC Complement. Altern. Med.*, 2017, *17* (*1*), 82.

[110] Spadaro, F.; Costa, R.; Circosta, C.; Occhiuto, F., Volatile composition and biological activity of key lime *Citrus aurantifolia* essential oil. *Nat. Prod. Commun.*, 2012, *7* (*11*), 1523–6. http://www.ncbi.nlm.nih.gov/pubmed/23285822.

[111] Kang, P.; Suh, S. H.; Min, S. S.; Seol, G. H., The essential oil of *Citrus bergamia* Risso induces vasorelaxation of the mouse aorta by activating K(+) channels and inhibiting Ca(2+) influx. *J. Pharm. Pharmacol.*, 2013, *65* (*5*), 745–749.

[112] Kang, P.; Ryu, K. H.; Lee, J. M.; Kim, H. K.; Seol, G. H., Endothelium- and smooth muscle-dependent vasodilator effects of

Citrus aurantium L. var. *amara*: Focus on Ca2+ modulation. *Biomed. Pharmacother.*, 2016, *82* 467–471.

[113] Silva, F. S.; Menezes, P. M. N.; Sá, P. G. S. de; Oliveira, A. L. de S.; Souza, E. A. A.; Almeida, J. R. G. da S.; Lima, J. T. de; Uetanabaro, A. P. T.; Silva, T. R. dos S.; Peralta, E. D.; Lucchese, A. M., Chemical composition and pharmacological properties of the essential oils obtained seasonally from *Lippia thymoides*. *Pharm. Biol.*, 2016, *54* (*1*), 25–34.

[114] Pereira, S. L.; Marques, A. M.; Sudo, R. T.; Kaplan, M. A. C.; Zapata-Sudo, G., Vasodilator activity of the essential oil from aerial parts of *Pectis brevipedunculata* and its main constituent citral in rat aorta. *Molecules.*, 2013, *18* (*3*), 3072–85.

[115] Zadeh, G. S.; Panahi, N., Endothelium-independent vasorelaxant activity of *Trachyspermum ammi* essential oil on rat aorta. *Clin. Exp. Hypertens.*, 2017, *39* (*2*), 133–138.

[116] Correia, A. C. de; Ferreira, T. F.; Martins, I. R. R.; Macêdo, C. L.; S. Monteiro, F. de; Costa, V. C. O.; Tavares, J. F.; Silva, M.S.; Paredes-Gamero, E. J.; Buri, M. V.; Rigoni, V. L. S.; Nouailhetas, V. L. A.; Silva, B. A. Da, Essential oil from the leaves of *Xylopia langsdorfiana* (Annonaceae) as a possible spasmolytic agent. *Nat. Prod. Res.*, 2015, *29* (*10*), 980–984.

[117] Esmaeili, H.; Sharifi, M.; Esmailidehaj, M.; Rezvani, M.E.; Hafizibarjin, Z., Vasodilatory effect of asafoetida essential oil on rat aorta rings: The role of nitric oxide, prostacyclin, and calcium channels. *Phytomedicine.*, 2017, *36* (*January*), 88–94.

[118] Rasheed, H. M.; Khan, T.; Wahid, F.; Khan, R.; Shah, A. J., Chemical composition and vascular and intestinal smooth muscle relaxant effects of the essential oil from *Psidium guajava* fruit. *Pharm. Biol.*, 2016, *54* (*11*), 2679–2684.

[119] Interaminense, L. F. L.; Ramos-Alves, F. E. Dos; Siqueira, R. J. B. de; Xavier, F. E.; Duarte, G. P.; Magalhães, P. J. C.; Maia, J. G. S.; Sousa, P. J. D. C.; Lahlou, S., Vasorelaxant effects of 1-nitro-2-phenylethane, the main constituent of the essential oil of *Aniba*

canelilla, in superior mesenteric arteries from spontaneously hypertensive rats. *Eur. J. Pharm. Sci.*, 2013, *48 (4–5)*, 709–716.

[120] Cherkaoui-Tangi, K.; Israili, Z. H.; Lyoussi, B., Vasorelaxant effect of essential oil isolated from *Nigella sativa* L. seeds in rat aorta: proposed mechanism. *Pak. J. Pharm. Sci.*, 2016, *29 (1)*, 1–8. http://www.ncbi.nlm.nih.gov/pubmed/26826822 (accessed June 5, 2017).

[121] Rasheed, H. M.; Khan, T.; Wahid, F.; Khan, R.; Shah, A. J., Chemical composition and vasorelaxant and antispasmodic effects of essential oil from *Rosa indica* L. petals. *Evid. Based. Complement. Alternat. Med.*, 2015, *2015* 279247.

[122] Han, C.; Qi, J.; Gao, S.; Li, C.; Ma, Y.; Wang, J.; Bai, Y.; Zheng, X., Vasodilation effect of volatile oil from *Allium macrostemon* Bunge are mediated by PKA/NO pathway and its constituent dimethyl disulfide in isolated rat pulmonary arterials. *Fitoterapia.*, 2017, *120 (February)*, 52–57.

[123] Hur, M. H.; Lee, M. S.; Kim, C.; Ernst, E., Aromatherapy for treatment of hypertension: a systematic review. *J. Eval. Clin. Pract.*, 2012, *18 (1)*, 37–41.

[124] Jung, Y. J., Effects of aromatherapy on blood bressure, heart rate variability, and serum catecholamines in the pre-hypertension middle aged women, Seoul, 2007.

[125] Hwang, J. H., [The effects of the inhalation method using essential oils on blood pressure and stress responses of clients withessential hypertension]. *Taehan Kanho Hakhoe Chi.*, 2006, *36 (7)*, 1123–1134.

[126] Ma, S. C., Effects of aromatherapy for hypertension patients, Seoul, 2005.

[127] Jang, H. H., A clinical study on the effects of the aromatherapy for hypertension. *J. Orient Neuropsychiatry.*, 2002, *13 (1)*, 3–18.

[128] Basnyet, J., The effect of aromatherapy treatment on raised arterial blood pressure - pilot study. *Posit. Heal.*, 1999, *39* 20–23.

[129] Kim, I. H.; Kim, C.; Seong, K.; Hur, M. H.; Lim, H. M.; Lee, M. S., Essential oil inhalation on blood pressure and salivary cortisol levels

in prehypertensive and hypertensive subjects. *Evidence-Based Complement. Altern. Med.*, 2012, *984203*.

[130] Araujo, A. A. T. de, Essential oil of eucalyptus effect on cardiovascular responses. 2016,. https://clinicaltrials.gov/ct2/show/study/NCT02656004 (accessed January 26, 2020).

[131] Soares, M. C. M. S.; Damiani, C. E. N.; Moreira, C. M.; Stefanon, I.; Vassallo, D. V, Eucalyptol, an essential oil, reduces contractile activity in rat cardiac muscle. *Braz. J. Med. Biol. Res.*, 2005, *38* (*3*), 453–61.

[132] Soares, P. M. G.; Lima, R. F.; de Freitas Pires, A.; Souza, E. P.; Assreuy, A. M. S.; Criddle, D. N., Effects of anethole and structural analogues on the contractility of rat isolated aorta: involvement of voltage-dependent $Ca2^{+}$-channels. *Life Sci.*, 2007, *81* (*13*), 1085–93.

[133] Kundu, S.; Shabir, H.; Basir, S. F.; Khan, L. A., Inhibition of As(III) and Hg(II) caused aortic hypercontraction by eugenol, linalool and carvone. *J. Smooth Muscle Res.*, 2014, *50* (*Iii*), 93–102.

[134] Lahlou, S.; Interaminense, L. F.; Magalhaes, P. J.; Leal-Cardoso, J. H.; Duarte, G. P., Cardiovascular effects of eugenol, a phenolic compound present in many plant essential oils, in normotensive rats. *J Cardiovasc Pharmacol.*, 2004, *43* (*2*), 250–257.

[135] Lahlou, S.; Figueiredo, A. F.; Magalhães, P. J. C.; Leal-Cardoso, J. H., Cardiovascular effects of 1,8-cineole, a terpenoid oxide present in many plant essential oils, in normotensive rats. *Can. J. Physiol. Pharmacol.*, 2002, *80* (*12*), 1125–1131.

[136] Peixoto-Neves, D.; Silva-Alves, K. S.; Gomes, M. D. M.; Lima, F. C.; Lahlou, S.; Magalhães, P. J. C.; Ceccatto, V. M.; Coelho-de-Souza, A. N.; Leal-Cardoso, J. H., Vasorelaxant effects of the monoterpenic phenol isomers, carvacrol and thymol, on rat isolated aorta. *Fundam. Clin. Pharmacol.*, 2010, *24* (*3*), 341–50.

[137] Sensch, O.; Vierling, W.; Brandt, W.; Reiter, M., Effects of inhibition of calcium and potassium currents in guinea-pig cardiac contraction: comparison of beta-caryophyllene oxide, eugenol, and nifedipine. *Br. J. Pharmacol.*, 2000, *131* (*6*), 1089–96.

[138] Shabir, H.; Kundu, S.; Basir, S. F.; Khan, L. A., Modulation of Pb(II) caused aortal constriction by eugenol and carvacrol. *Biol. Trace Elem. Res.*, 2014, *161* (*1*), 116–122.

[139] Menezes-Filho, J. E. R. de; Gondim, A. N. S.; Cruz, J. S.; de Souza, A. A.; Santos, J. N. A. Dos; Conde-Garcia, E. A.; de Sousa, D. P.; Santos, M. S.; de Oliveira, E. D.; de Vasconcelos, C. M. L., Geraniol blocks calcium and potassium channels in the mammalian myocardium: useful effects to treat arrhythmias. *Basic Clin. Pharmacol. Toxicol.*, 2014, *115* (*6*), 534–44.

[140] Yanaga, A.; Goto, H.; Nakagawa, T.; Hikiami, H.; Shibahara, N.; Shimada, Y., Cinnamaldehyde induces endothelium-dependent and -independent vasorelaxant action on isolated rat aorta. *Biol. Pharm. Bull.*, 2006, *29* (*12*), 2415–8.

[141] Raffai, G.; Kim, B.; Park, S.; Khang, G.; Lee, D.; Vanhoutte, P. M., Cinnamaldehyde and cinnamaldehyde-containing micelles induce relaxation of isolated porcine coronary arteries: role of nitric oxide and calcium. *Int. J. Nanomedicine.*, 2014, *9* (*1*), 2557–66.

[142] Vasconcelos-Silva, A. A.; de Lima, F. J. B.; de Brito, T. S.; Lahlou, S.; Magalhães, P. J. C., Vasorelaxation induced by methyl cinnamate, the major constituent of the essential oil of *Ocimum micranthum*, in rat isolated aorta. *Clin. Exp. Pharmacol. Physiol.*, 2014, *41* (*10*), 755–762.

[143] Dantas, B. P. V.; Alves, Q. L.; de Assis, K. S.; Ribeiro, T. P.; de Almeida, M. M.; de Vasconcelos, A. P.; de Araújo, D. A. M.; de Andrade Braga, V.; de Medeiros, I. A.; Alencar, J. L.; Silva, D. F., Participation of the TRP channel in the cardiovascular effects induced by carvacrol in normotensive rat. *Vascul. Pharmacol.*, 2015, *67–69* 48–58.

[144] Magyar, J.; Szentandrássy, N.; Bányász, T.; Fülöp, L.; Varró, A.; Nánási, P. P., Effects of terpenoid phenol derivatives on calcium current in canine and human ventricular cardiomyocytes. *Eur. J. Pharmacol.*, 2004, *487* (*1–3*), 29–36.

[145] Earley, S.; Gonzales, A. L.; Garcia, Z. I., A dietary agonist of transient receptor potential cation channel V3 elicits endothelium-dependent vasodilation. *Mol. Pharmacol.*, 2010, *77* (*4*), 612–620.

[146] Aydin, Y.; Kutlay, Ö.; Ari, S.; Duman, S.; Uzuner, K.; Aydin, S., Hypotensive effects of carvacrol on the blood pressure of normotensive rats. *Planta Med.*, 2007, *73* (*13*), 1365–1371.

[147] Menezes, I. A. C.; Barreto, C. M. N.; Antoniolli, A. R.; Santos, M. R. V; de Sousa, D. P.; Antoniolli, Â. R.; Santos, M. R. V; de Sousa, D. P.; Antoniolli, A. R.; Santos, M. R. V; de Sousa, D. P., Hypotensive activity of terpenes found in essential oils. *Z. Naturforsch. C.*, 2010, *65* (*9–10*), 562–6.

[148] Bastos, J. F. A.; Moreira, Í. J. A.; Ribeiro, T. P.; Medeiros, I. A.; Antoniolli, A. R.; De Sousa, D. P.; Santos, M. R. V, Hypotensive and vasorelaxant effects of citronellol, a monoterpene alcohol, in rats. *Basic Clin. Pharmacol. Toxicol.*, 2010, *106* (*4*), 331–337.

[149] Anjos, P. J. C.; Lima, A. O.; Cunha, P. S.; De Sousa, D. P.; Onofre, A. S. C.; Ribeiro, T. P.; Medeiros, I. a; Antoniolli, A. R.; Quintans-Júnior, L. J.; Santosa, M. R. V, Cardiovascular effects induced by linalool in normotensive and hypertensive rats. *Zeitschrift Für Naturforschung. C A J. Biosci.*, 2013, *68* (*5–6*), 181–90. http://www.ncbi.nlm.nih.gov/pubmed/23923614.

[150] Höferl, M.; Krist, S.; Buchbauer, G., Chirality influences the effects of linalool on physiological parameters of stress. *Planta Med.*, 2006, *72* (*13*), 1188–1192.

[151] Johnson, C. D.; Melanaphy, D.; Purse, A.; Stokesberry, S. A.; Dickson, P.; Zholos, A. V, Transient receptor potential melastatin 8 channel involvement in the regulation of vascular tone. *Am. J. Physiol. - Hear. Circ. Physiol.*, 2009, *296* (*6*), H1868–H1877.

[152] Cheang, W. S.; Lam, M. Y.; Wong, W. T.; Tian, X. Y.; Lau, C. W.; Zhu, Z.; Yao, X.; Huang, Y., Menthol relaxes rat aortae, mesenteric and coronary arteries by inhibiting calcium influx. *Eur. J. Pharmacol.*, 2013, *702* (*1–3*), 79–84.

[153] Guedes, D. N.; Silva, D. F.; Barbosa-Filho, J. M.; Medeiros, I. A., Muscarinic agonist properties involved in the hypotensive and

vasorelaxant responses of rotundifolone in rats. *Planta Med.*, 2002, *68* (*8*), 700–704.

[154] Guedes, D. N.; Silva, D. F.; Barbosa-Filho, J. M.; Medeiros, I. A., Calcium antagonism and the vasorelaxation of the rat aorta induced by rotundifolone. *Brazilian J. Med. Biol. Res.*, 2004, *37* (*12*), 1881–1887.

[155] Maia-Joca, R. P. M.; Joca, H. C.; Ribeiro, F. J. P.; Nascimento, R. V. Do; Silva-Alves, K. S.; Cruz, J. S.; Coelho-De-Souza, A. N.; Leal-Cardoso, J. H., Investigation of terpinen-4-ol effects on vascular smooth muscle relaxation. *Life Sci.*, 2014, *115* (*1*), 52–58.

[156] Ribeiro, T. P.; Porto, D. L.; Menezes, C. P.; Antunes, A. A.; Silva, D. F.; De Souza, D. P.; Nakao, L. S.; Braga, V. A.; Medeiros, I. A., Unraveling the cardiovascular effects induced by α-terpineol: a role for the NO-cGMP pathway. *Clin. Exp. Pharmacol. Physiol.*, 2010, *37* (*8*), 811–816.

[157] Magyar, J.; Szentandrássy, N.; Bányász, T.; Fülöp, L.; Varró, A.; Nánási, P. P., Effects of thymol on calcium and potassium currents in canine and human ventricular cardiomyocytes. *Br. J. Pharmacol.*, 2002, *136* (2), 330–8.

[158] Szentandrássy, N.; Szigeti, G.; Szegedi, C.; Sárközi, S.; Magyar, J.; Bányász, T.; Csernoch, L.; Kovács, L.; Nánási, P. P.; Jóna, I., Effect of thymol on calcium handling in mammalian ventricular myocardium. *Life Sci.*, 2004, *74* (*7*), 909–921.

[159] Siqueira, R. J. B. de; Freire, W. B. S.; Vasconcelos-Silva, A. a.; Fonseca-Magalhães, P. a.; Lima, F. J. B.; Brito, T. S.; Mourão, L. T. C.; Ribeiro, R. a.; Lahlou, S.; Magalhães, P. J. C., *In-vitro* characterization of the pharmacological effects induced by (–)-α-bisabolol in rat smooth muscle preparations. *Can. J. Physiol. Pharmacol.*, 2012, *90* (*1*), 23–35.

[160] Siqueira, R. J. B. de; Ribeiro-Filho, H. V.; Freire, R. S.; Cosker, F.; Freire, W. B. S.; Vasconcelos-Silva, A. A.; Soares, M. A.; Lahlou, S.; Magalhães, P. J. C., (-)-α-Bisabolol inhibits preferentially electromechanical coupling on rat isolated arteries. *Vascul. Pharmacol.*, 2014, *63* (*1*), 37–45.

[161] Peixoto-Neves, D.; Wang, Q.; Leal-Cardoso, J. H.; Rossoni, L. V.; Jaggar, J. H., Eugenol dilates mesenteric arteries and reduces systemic BP by activating endothelial cell TRPV4 channels. *Br. J. Pharmacol.*, 2015, *172* (*14*), 3484–94.

[162] Lahlou, S.; Figueiredo, A. F.; Magalhães, P. J. C.; Leal-Cardoso, J. H.; Gloria, P. D., Cardiovascular effects of methyleugenol, a natural constituent of many plant essential oils, in normotensive rats. *Life Sci.*, 2004, *74* (*19*), 2401–2412.

[163] Siqueira, R. J. B. de; Macedo, F. I. B.; Interaminense, L. de F. L.; Duarte, G. P.; Magalhães, P. J. C.; Brito, T. S.; da Silva, J. K. R.; Maia, J. G. S.; Sousa, P. J. da C.; Leal-Cardoso, J. H.; Lahlou, S., 1-Nitro-2-phenylethane, the main constituent of the essential oil of *Aniba canelilla*, elicits a vago-vagal bradycardiac and depressor reflex in normotensive rats. *Eur. J. Pharmacol.*, 2010, *638* (*1–3*), 90–98.

[164] Arruda-Barbosa, L.; Rodrigues, K. M. S.; Souza-Neto, F. das C. V.; Duarte, G. P.; Borges, R. S.; Magalhães, P. J. C.; Lahlou, S., Vasorelaxant effects of 1-nitro-2-phenylethene in rat isolated aortic rings. *Vascul. Pharmacol.*, 2014, *63* (*2*), 55–62.

In: What to Know about Essential Oils
Editor: Malene M. Kjeldsen
ISBN: 978-1-53617-986-6

Chapter 2

PHARMACOLOGY OF ESSENTIAL OILS: CHEMICAL CONSTITUENTS, ANTI-INFLAMMATORY AND ANTI-NOCICEPTIVE ACTIVITIES OF ESSENTIAL OILS FROM NIGERIAN PLANTS

Opeyemi Nudewhenu Avoseh[1], Isiaka Ajani Ogunwande[2,*], Assumpta Ebere[1], Nasira Gbemisola Hassan[1], Do Ngoc Dai[3], Ascrizzi Roberta[4] and Flamini Guido[4]

[1]Department of Chemistry, Faculty of Science, Lagos State University, Lagos, Nigeria
[2]Foresight Institute of Research and Translation, Nigeria
[3]Faculty of Agriculture, Forestry and Fishery, Nghe An College of Economics, Vinh City, Nghe An Province, Vietnam
[4]Dipartimento di Farmacia, Università di Pisa, Italy

[*] Corresponding Author's Email: isiakaogunwande@gmail.com.

ABSTRACT

This study was designed to determine the chemical constituents and evaluate the anti-pain properties of the essential oils from *Thuja plicata* var. Excelsa Van den Berk (Cupressaceae), *Alstonia boonei* De Wild (Apocynaceae), *Curcuma longa* L. (Zingiberaceae) and *Allium sativum* L (Alliaceae). The essential oils were isolated using hydrodistillation method in an all glass Clevenger-type apparatus and characterized by gas chromatography (GC-FID) and gas chromatography-mass spectrometry (GC-MS). The hot plate method was used to determine the anti-nociceptive property while the anti-inflammatory activity was established by means of carrageenan induced and formalin models. The yields of the essential oils were 1.31%, 1.49%, 0.80% and 0.75% (v/w) respectively, calculated on a dry weight basis. The major constituents of T. plicata var. Excelsa were δ-3-carene (31.6%), α-pinene (20.3%), cedrol (7.3%) and β-caryophyllene (6.7%). Its carrageenan-induced inflammation study showed a high activity consistent with dose and time. Inflammatory mediators were significantly suppressed within the 1st to the 3rd h at a level of $p < 0.001$ by the 200 and 400 mg/kg. In addition, the activity of the 100 mg/kg rises steadily from $p > 0.05$ (non-significant) to $p < 0.001$ for the 1st to the 3rd h respectively. The oil only displayed a slight inhibition of heat latency activity at 90th and 120th min ($p < 0.05$) by the 400 mg/kg. The main constituents of *A. boonei* were cedrol (32.2%), α-humulene (18.9%), β-caryophyllene (17.2%) and α-pinene (13.4%). The hot plate model (maximal pain threshold) displayed significant activity ($p < 0.001$) for the 200 and 400 mg/kg within the 60th and the 90th min. Inflammation was significantly inhibited by all doses at the 3rd and 4th h. The 100 mg/kg of *A. boonei* essential oil displayed a steady activity at the 1st and 2nd h ($p < 0.01$) and increased at 3rd and 4th h ($p < 0.001$). 200 mg/kg of the essential oil also showed steady activity at the 3rd and 4th h ($p < 0.01$). The result showed that 400 mg/kg of the essential oil was significant at the 1st h ($p < 0.05$) but there was a total loss of activity at the 2nd h ($p > 0.05$) then it was highly significant at the 3rd and 4th h ($p < 0.001$).

Formalin model showed high inhibition (100% maximal) at the inflammatory phase than the neurogenic phase. The main constituents of the oil of C. *longa* were ar-tumerone (28.6%), β-atlantone (21.9%) and curlone (18.8%) while diallyl trisulfide (53.9%), diallyl disulfide (15.7%), diallyl tetrasulfide (11.7%), methylallyl trisulphide (9.2%) were the compounds identified in *A. sativum* oil. The essential oils of *A. sativum* and *C. longa* inhibited the proliferation of anti-nociceptors induced by hot plate method. There was prolonged activity ($p < 0.001$) independent of the time and the dose except for a reduced activity of the 400 mg/kg at the 90th min ($p < 0.001$ to $p < 0.05$) for *A. sativum.* The anti-inflammatory activity of the essential oils of *A. sativum* were only significant for the 100 mg/kg at the 2nd h ($p < 0.001$) and 3rd h ($p < 0.05$) of the analysis. Activity observed could be attributed to effect of absorption rate and inflammation mediators' modulation.

In conclusion, results in this study indicated that the essential oils could be considered as potential alternative source for amelioration of inflammation and pain disorders.

Keywords: *Thuja plicata* var. Excelsa, *Alstonia boonei*, *Curcuma longa*, *Allium sativum*, essential oil, anti-nociceptive activity, anti-inflammatory activity

INTRODUCTION

Thuja is a genus of coniferous trees in the Cupressaceae (*Cypress* family). *Thuja plicata* and its varieties are introduced to Nigeria. *Thuja plicata* var. Excelsa or Western red cedar is a gorgeous fast-growing, full-bodied conifer that can reach up to 35 feet tall with a 20 ft spread. Its bright green fan-like foliage emits an unmistakable aroma (Peng et al., 2008). Upright growing, the relatively openly branched tree with a pyramidal crown later becomes conical. The quite horizontal branches make the tree about 5 to 6 m wide. The bark is reddish brown, fibrous and flaky. The young twigs are green first, later turning reddish brown. Like the species, the lower branches can take root when they touch the ground and, seemingly form new trees. The scaly foliage is arranged in shingle form and glossy dark green, also in winter (Tsiri et al., 2009). *Thuja plicata* oils have demonstrated a number of biological actions such as antimicrobial (Jirovetz et al., 2006; Tsiri et al., 2009; Hudon et al., 2011; Puškárová et al., 2017), antifungal (Puškárová et al., 2017), cytotoxicity against HEL 12469 human embryo lung cells (Puškárová et al., 2017), insecticidal against woolly beech aphid, *Phyllaphis fagi*, and rice weevil, *Sitophilus oryzae* (Yazdgerdian et al., 2015), anti-inflammatory effects and beneficial action on human skin cells (Han and Parker, 2017). Considering the diversity of *Thuja* genus, with member mostly aromatic plants, the essential oils of *T. plicata* var. Excelsa has not been previously investigated. However, the compositions of essential oils from other varieties of *T. plicata* and its various cultivars were reported. A recent study showed α-thujone (52.1%-59.2%) and fenchone (10.1%-11.3%) were the major compounds in *T. plicata* cv "Fastigiata", "Kornik" and Zebrina" (Lis et al., 2019). The cone oil contained α-thujone (35.6%) and fenchone (24.0%). Likewise, α-thujone (54.13%) and fenchone (15.12%) were identified from sample in Egypt (Jirovetz et al., 2006). Quantitative amount of α-thujone (54.13%) in *T. plicata* and α-thujone (54.48%) in *T. plicata* var. gracialis were reported (Tsiri et al., 2009). High contents of α-thujone was also identified in mature tree (76.0%-77.5%) and young tree (73.16%) of *T. plicata* (Von Rudloff et al., 1988).

Alstonia boonei De Wild. (Apocynaceae) is a very large, deciduous, tropical-forest, which can reach 45 m in height and 3 m in girth, the bole being cylindrical and up to 27 m (89 ft) in height with high, narrow, deep-fluted buttresses. The leaves are borne in whorls at the nodes, the leaf shape is oblanceolate, with the apex rounded to acuminate and the lateral veins prominent and almost at right angles to the midrib. The flowers are yellowish-white and borne in lax terminal cymes. The fruits are pendulous, paired, slender follicles up to 16 cm (6.3 in) long, containing seeds bearing a tuft of silky, brown floss at either end to allow dispersal by the wind. The latex is white and abundant (Burkhill, 1985). It is native to tropical West Africa. The various ethnomedicinal, chemical, pharmacological, and toxicological properties of *A. boonei* were recently reviewed and the profile revealed that it is useful in the treatment and management of several illnesses (Adotey et al., 2012). These include antiplasmodial against Plasmodium falciparum with IC_{50} of 111.2 $\mu g.ml^{-1}$ (Ntalani et al., 2018), and *Plasmodium bergehei* (Iyiola et al., 2010), analgesic (Loretta et al., 2012), nematicidal against *Meloidogyne incognita* (Fabiyi et al., 2012), antihyperglycemic (Ya Nkono et al., 2014), antioxidant (Obiagwu et al., 2014; Ya Nkono et al., 2014), antimicrobial (Opoku and Akoto, 2014), insecticidal action towards *Sesamia calamistis* (Oigiangbe et al., 2007) and *Callosobruchus maculatus* (Ojo and Ogunleye, 2013). Iridoids isolated from *A. boonei* include boonein and loganin (Adotey et al., 2012). The triterpenoids isolated from *Alstonia boonei* include lupeol, ursolic acid, and β-amyrin (Adotey et al., 2012). The alkaloids of *A. boonei* include echitamine, echitamidine, voacangine and akuammidine, Nα-formylechitamidine, and Nα-formyl -12-methoxyechitamidine (Kucera et al., 1972; Oguakwu, 1984). Echitamine possess anticancer activities (Saraswathi et al., 1997). Two cardiac glycosides namely evomonoside and 3β-O-[5(3,4 -dihydroxy-5-methyltetrahydrofuran-2-yloxy)digitoxopyranosyl-2-yloxy]-5-en-14β-hydroxy-16β-acryloxydigitoxigenin were recently isolated from the plant (Attioua et al., 2018). Alstiboonine, recently isolated from *A. boonei* exhibited significant cytotoxicity to brine shrimps (Balogun et al., 2016). Alkaloids isolated from the plant possess insecticidal action against *Sesamia calamistis* (Oigiangbe et al., 2010). A previous study on its essential oil indicates that (*Z*)-9-octadecanoic acid (37.8%), hexadecanoic acid (22.8%) and octadecanoic acid (11.6%) were the main constituents of leaf essential oil while (*Z*)-9-octadecanoic acid (28.5%), hexadecanoic acid (15.0%), octadecanoic acid (12.7%) and methyl-(7*E*)-7-octadecanotae (11.7%) were abundant in the stem bark. However, methyl-(7*E*)-7-octadecanotae (27.0%), methyl linoleate (26.5%), methyl hexadecanoate (15.4%) and methyl octadecanoate (13.5%) occurred in the root oil (Moronkola et al., 2012). The essential oil was shown to displayed larvicidal activity against *Simulium yahense* (Ebigwai et al., 2012). The oil obtained from ethanolic extract was reported to contained 2,6-hexadecanoate (17.27%), 9-octadecanoic acid (15.4%), 1,2,3-propanetriyl ester (12.89%), octadecanoic acid (10.31%) and methyl ester octadecanoic acid (9.02%) as major compounds (Okwu and Ighodaro, 2010). The main constituents in the dichloromethane leaf extract analysed by GC-MS was eugenol (54.58%) while α-amyrin (32.25%) dominated the stem bark, with 1,2-benzenecarboxylic acid (49.2%) being abundant in the root (Babatunde, 2017).

Curcuma longa L. (Zingiberaceae) is a perennial, erect, glabrous herb 0.6-1 m high, forming dense clumps. Rhizome is stout and much branched with cylindrical, aromatic tubers (3 m across) and orange, orange-red or golden yellow inside with carrot-turmeric odour. The leaves are radical, distichous, entire and long sheathed. The leaf blade is green, oblong or elliptic, 30-50 cm long by 10-25 cm wide and glabrous. The flowers are not exserted beyond the bracts. The calyx is white and puberulent, and apex is unequally 3-toothed (Lim, 2016). *Curcuma longa*, commonly known as turmeric is native to southern Asia and some parts of Africa. The aromatic yellow powder from its mature rhizomes is extensively used for imparting colour and flavor to food. Several biological activities have been described to the volatile and non-volatile extracts of *C. longa*. Natural products from this plant also have analgesic, antibacterial, antifungal, anti-inflammatory, antioxidant and digestive properties (Lim, 2016)

Curcuma longa has curcumin (Francieli da Silva, et al. 2015; Schmidt et al., 2015), demethoxycurcumin and bisdemethoxycurcumin (Hwang et al., 2016) as its main phenolic compound. Curcumin has been shown to possess a variety of pharmacological activities, including antioxidant, anti-inflammatory, cancer chemopreventive, and neuroprotective activities. The polar fraction of essential oil of *C. longa* (Schmidt et al., 2015) contained ar-turmerone (40.1%), α-turmerone (21.8%) and curlone (+ *trans*-γ-atlantone, 14.3%), while ar-curcumene (36.7%) were found in the apolar fraction with ketone fraction made up of ar-turmerone (71.2%). A sample analysed from Nigeria showed turmerone (35.9%) as the major component (Oyemitan et al., 2017). Terpinolene and α-phellandrene were identified as the predominant constituents of leaf oil of a Nigerian grown *C. longa* (Oguntimehin et al., 1990) while the α-tumerone chemotype was reported from Southwest Nigeria (Ajaiyeoba et al., 2008). Another chemotype consisting of β-bisabolene (13.9%) was also reported from Nigeria (Usman et al., 2009). The major components of the rhizome oil (Ferreira et al., 2013) were ar-turmerone (33.2%), *α*-turmerone (23.5%) and *β*-turmerone (22.7%) while ar-turmerone (61.79%) and curlone (12.48%) were reported from sample anaysed in India (Liju et al., 2011). Large amount of α-turmerone (42.6%), β-turmerone (16.0%) and ar-turmerone (12.9%) were also reported (Avanço et al., 2017). Moreover, the major components of another sample from India (Gounder and Lingamallu, 2012) were ar-turmerone (21.0–30.3%), β-turmerone (26.5–33.5%) and ˇα-turmerone (18.9–21.1%). The compound, α-phellandrene (41.99%) represented the main constituent of the *C. longa* essential oil (Amanda et al., 2019). The representative compounds of *C. longa* oil (Hwang et al., 2016) were α-zingiberene (27.70–36.75%), ar-turmerone (19.54–32.24%) and β-sesquiphellandrene (13.14–18.23%). A recent analysis of the essential oil also revealed the presence of terpinolene (52.88%) and α-phellandrene (21.13%) as the major components (Kumar et al., 2018).

The essential oil exhibited stronger antifungal activity on *Aspergillus flavus* (Ferreira et al., 2013) and antimycotoxigenic activity towards *Fusarium verticillioides* (Avanço et al., 2017). Turmeric oil showed antioxidant action (Liju et al., 2011; Gounder and Lingamallu, 2012; Avanço et al., 2017), displayed significant reduction in paw thickness in carrageenan, dextran-induced acute inflammation, formalin-induced chronic inflammation and exhibited significant antinociceptive activity (Liju et al., 2011). Essential oil from ginger and turmeric rhizomes also exerts anti-inflammatory properties in Cd induced neurotoxicity (Akinyemi and Adeniyi, 2018). The oil exhibits significant anxiolytic, sedative and anticonvulsant activities in mice (Oyemitan et al., 2017), and larvicidal action towards *Anopheles garnbiae* (Ajaiyeoba et al., 2008). The essential oil has anti-arthritic effects (Funk et al., 2010), toxic against third instar larvae of *Cochliomyia macellaria* (Amanda et al., 2019) and produced anti-inflammatory effects by ameliorating the level of pro-inflammatory cytokines (TNF-α, IL-6, IL-1β) at protein and mRNA levels (Kumar et al., 2018). The oil has promising scolicidal effects against protoscoleces (Mahmoudvand et al., 2019). Climatic and genetic factors, harvesting time, soil type, fertilization, drying process, and period of storage can all affect the chemical composition of essential oils from *C. longa*. The composition and volatility of *C. longa* essential oils determine the characteristic smell of turmeric, whereas fixed phenolic compounds, such as the pigment curcumin, its derivatives and other substances, are responsible for the intense yellow color of the rhizomes.

Garlic (*Allium sativum* L., Amaryllidaceae) likely originated in Central Asia. The plant has been used as a flavoring agent and a traditional medicine since antiquity, and is now cultivated worldwide. *Allium sativum* has been used as a diaphoretic, diuretic, expectorant, and stimulant. Extracts of *A. sativum* have shown broad-spectrum antibacterial and antifungal activity and the plant has been used to treat tuberculosis, coughs, and colds (Satyal et al., 2017). There have been numerous investigations on the phytochemistry of garlic and its essential oil composition. Recently, the compositions of garlic essential oils from Spain (Satyal et al., 2017) obtained using three different distillation methods (Clevenger laboratory hydrodistillation, industrial steam distillation, and industrial hydrodistillation) were characterized by GC-MS. The oils were dominated by allyl polysulfides, including diallyl sulfide (1.9-9.5%), diallyl disulfide (20.8-27.9%), diallyl trisulfide (16.8-33.4%), allyl methyl disulfide (4.4-8.3%), and allyl methyl trisulfide (14.5-19.2%). In another report, diallyl disulfide (28.36%), dimethyl tetrasulfide (15.26%), trisulfide di-2-propenyl (10.41%), and tetrasulfide di-2-propenyl (9.67%) were the main compounds of oil isolated from Saudi Arabia (Mossah et al., 2017). The main components of the essential oil of *A. sativum* from China (Zhao et al., 2013) were diallyl trisulfide (50.43%) and diallyl disulfide (25.30%). Also, diallyl trisulfide (37.3–45.9%), diallyl disulfide (17.5–35.6%) and methyl allyl trisulfide (7.7–10.4%) were characterized as major compounds of garlic oil (Dziri et al., 2014). Other researchers have also identified 3-vinyl-4H-1,2-dithiin (31.89%), diallyl trisulfide (13.31%) and propyl allyl disulfide (13.89%) as major compounds of *A. sativum* oil (Rui et al., 2009). The main constituents of the garlic essential oil from Brazil (Malet et al., 2014) were diallyl trisulfide (38.81%), diallyl disulfide (25.23%), and methyl allyl trisulfide (12.52%). The Turkish sample of *A. sativum* (Üstüner et al., 2018) consisted mainly of diallyl trisulfide (33.40%), diallyl disulfide (20.80%) and allyl methyl trisulfide (19.20%). In addition, diallyl trisulfide (41.62%), diallyl disulfide (19.74%) and allyl methyl trisulfide (12.95%) were also observed as the main compounds from oil analysed in Camerron (Foe et al., 2016).

A study indicated that garlic essential oil may be useful for treatment of patients with inflammatory disease, especially gastric cancer (Rui et al., 2009). The essential oil was a potent antimicrobial agent against bacteria *Staphylococcus choleraesuis* and *P. aeruginosa* (Malet et al., 2014) and *Aspergillus versicolor* (Kocić-Tanackov et al., 2012). The essential oil of *A. sativum* was active against clinical isolates of *Candida* species (Alejandro et al., 2017). The oil possess strong insecticidal activity against adults of *Cacopsylla chinensis* (Zhao et al., 2013), *Reticuitermes speratus* (Park and

Shin, 2005) and *Callosobruchus maculates* (Douiri et al., 2013). The two main constituents, diallyl trisulfide and diallyl disulfide, exhibited strong acute toxicity against *C. chinensis* with LC_{50} values of 0.64 and 11.04 μg/adult, respectively (Zhao et al., 2013). *A. sativum* essential oil can be useful in the treatment of otitis external caused by *Ototecdes cynotis* infestation in cats and dogs (Yipel et al., 2016). The essential oil of *A. sativum* was effective as herbicides and fungicides and had 100% inhibition of the mycelial growth of *F. oxysporum* and *Verticilium dahlia* (Üstüner et al., 2018). The antiviral (Romeilah et al., 2016), antibacterial (Chekki et al., 2014; Mnayer et al., 2014), antioxidant (Chekki et al., 2014; Mnayer et al., 2014; Foe et al., 2016; Romeilah et al., 2016) and anti-inflammatory (Foe et al., 2016) potentials of the essential oil have been reported.

In continuation of our extensive research on the pharmacology of essential oils from Nigerian medicinal plants and herbs as they are made available (Avoseh et al., 2019; Ogunwande et al. 2019a; Ogunwande et al. 2019b), we report herein the compositions, anti-inflammatory and anti-nociceptive activities of *T. plicata* var. Excelsa, *A. boonei*, *C. longa* and *A. sativum* essential oils.

METHODS

Plants Collection

Mature leaves of *T. plicata* var. Excelsa, were collected from trees growing at Oluseyi Bus Stop, Eleyele Road, Ibadan, Nigeria, in April 2018. The sample was identified at National Forestry Proramme, Ibadan, with voucher number NFP 12306. The leaves of *A. boonei* were obtained from Ojo, Lagos, Nigeria (6.4619° N, 3.1579° E), in April 2018, while those of *C. longa* and *A. sativum* were purchased from Iyana-Iba Market Ojo, Lagos, in May 2017. Both *C. longa* and *A. sativum* were identified by Mr. Yebanji O.O at the University of Lagos herbarium under herbarium number LUH 7631 and LUH 7633 respectively.

Preparation of Samples

In this process, the plant samples were separately air-dried (22^{0}C) under laboratory shade for two weeks to reduce the moisture contents. Moreover, unwanted materials were also removed by handpicking. Afterwards, samples were pulverized to coarse powder using a locally made grinder.

Hydrodistillation Procedure

Known weight of air-dried and pulverized samples was used. Hydrodistillation was carried out separately with a Clevenger-type distillation unit designed according to the specification (British Pharmacopoeia, 1980). The time used for the distillation was 4 h and conducted at normal pressure. The distilled oils were collected into clean weighed sample bottles. The oils were kept under refrigeration (4°C) until the moment of analyses. All analyses were done in triplicate.

Gas Chromatography (GC) Analysis of the Oils

GC analysis was accomplished with a HP-5890 Series II instrument equipped with a HP-Wax and HP-5 capillary columns (both 30 m x 0.25 mm, 0.25 μm film thickness), working with the following temperature program: 60°C for 10 min, rising at 5°C/min to 220°C. The injector and detector temperatures were maintained at 250°C; carrier gas nitrogen (2 mL/min); detector dual, FID; split ratio 1:30. The volume injected was 0.5 μL. The relative amounts of individual components were calculated based on the GC peak area (FID response).

Gas Chromatography-Mass Spectrometry (GC/MS) Aanalysis of the Oils

GC-EIMS analysis was performed with a Varian CP-3800 gas-chromatograph equipped with a HP-5 capillary column (30 m x 0.25 mm; film thickness 0.25 µm) and a Varian Saturn 2000 ion trap mass detector. Analytical conditions: injector and transfer line temperature 220°C and 240°C, respectively; oven temperature programmed from 60°C-240°C at 3°C/min.; carrier gas helium at a flow rate of 1mL/min.; injection volume 0.2 µL (10% *n*-hexane solution); split ratio 1:30. Mass spectra were recorded at 70 eV. The acquisition mass range was m/z 30-300 at a scan rate of 1 scan/sec.

Identification of the Components of the Oils

Identification of the constituents of the essential oils was based on comparison of the retention times with those of authentic samples, comparing their linear indices relative to a series of *n*-alkanes. Further identifications were also made possible by the use of a homemade library of mass spectra built up from pure substances and components of known oils, and MS literature data as described previously (Avoseh et al., 2019; Ogunwande et al. 2019a; Ogunwande et al. 2019b). Moreover, the molecular weights of all the identified substances were confirmed by GC-CIMS, using MeOH as CI ionizing gas.

Bioloical Studies on Essential Oils

Drug and Chemicals

Carrageenan drug (Batch Number: SLBR0530V) of analytical grade was obtained from Sigma-Aldrich Chemical Co. (St Louis, MO, USA). Acetylsalicyclic salicylate injection (RX, Nigeria Ltd; Batch Number: MT2056) and Diclofenac Injection (FITZKING LINK LIMITED, Nigeria

Ltd; Batch Number: 180606) were purchased from Lagos State University Pharmacy.

Study Animals

Wistar rats (150-200 g) of both sexes were accommodated in the Biochemistry Department animal facility of Lagos State University, Ojo-Lagos. The animals were kept in a metal steel cage, where they had unrestricted supply to water and standard pellet food. They were acclimatized for two weeks before commencement of experiment. The animals were assigned at random to a group of 5 consisting of 6 animals per group:

Group 1- Control group (Saline solution); Group 2- Diclofenac treated group 100 mg/kg (Standard Group); Group 3- 100 mg/kg of essential oil; Group 4- 200 mg/kg of essential oil; and Group 5- 400 mg/kg of essential oil.

The rationale for selecting the studied doses was that animals of similar weight were grouped together to obtained average weight. The weight recorded was similar across the groups of animals. The dose was therefore determined from the weight of animals in the assigned group. Each essential oil was dissolved in a saline vehicle and administered to the animal in the order of 100, 200 and 400 mg/kg.

All experimental procedures were approved under the Lagos State University Research Ethical Clearance Committee (RECC) of the University (Approval no: 012/2018/LASU/BCH).

Toxicity Study

All the essential oils were tested for acute toxicity on the rats. Wistar rats were administered 500, 1000, 1500 and 2000 mg/kg of the essential oil per oral route. One group received normal saline that served as a negative control. The animals were observed for 12 h continuously for changes in their behavior. Mortality for the next 14 days was also noted as described in previous studies (Avoseh et al., 2019; Ogunwande et al. 2019a; Ogunwande et al. 2019b).

Carrageenan-Induced Paw Edema in Rats (Anti-Inflammatory Analysis)

Carrageenan induced rat paw edema experiment was carried out according to a modification form of an established procedure as described previously (Avoseh et al., 2019; Ogunwande et al. 2019a; Ogunwande et al. 2019b). Thirty Wistar rats (both sexes, 150-200 g each) divided into 6 animals in each groups. The animals were induced by subcutaneous injection of 0.1 mL of 1% freshly prepared carrageenan in saline in the right hind paw. In addition, 1mL of all other solutions was administered for all doses. Paw volume of the injected rats was measured every hour for four hours using a plethysmometer (Ugo Basile, Italy).

Formalin-Induced Anti-Inflammatory Test

Formalin assay is a model for both anti-nociceptive and anti-inflammation. The experiment was carried out using the method a modified method (Hunskar and Hole, 1987). The same grouping of animal applies for this test and the animals were also starved overnight to enable proper absorption of the sample. 1% formaldehyde was injected into the right hind paw of the rats. The time spent in licking and biting responses of the injected paw was taken as indicator of pain response. The time spent paw licking was counted from 0 to 5 min (first phase) and from 20 to 30 min (second phase). These phases represented neurogenic and inflammatory pain responses, respectively (Bars et al., 2001). Responses were measured for 5 min after formalin injection and 20-30 min after formalin injection. 0.5 mL of saline solution was administered orally to group 1 which is the control group, group 2 which is the standard group received 0.5 mL piroxicam and groups 3, 4 and 5 received 0.5 mL of 100, 200 and 400 mg/kg of the extract respectively, before injecting the 1% formaldehyde.

Hot Plate Test for Anti-Nociceptive Study

The experiment was carried out according to the method described previously (Avoseh et al., 2019; Ogunwande et al. 2019a; Ogunwande et al. 2019b). Thirty (30) mature Wistar rats of both sexes were randomly divided into 5 groups of equal rats. The animals were fasted for 12 h with provision of clean water *ad libitum*. Each mouse was placed upon the heated metal plate (Hot plate) maintained at the temperature of about 50-55 ^{0}C within the restraining glass cylinder. Group 1 mice received 10 mL/kg of saline solution and served as control. Group 2 mice received sodium salicylate (10 mg/kg (ASA) (standard control) and groups 3, 4 and 5 received 100, 200 and 400 mg/kg of each essential oil (p.o.). Animal response to the heat varies and such changes includes kicking of hind foot and jumping about, licking of foot, raising the foot, holding the foot tightly to its body or shaking of the foot. The reaction time was recorded 30, 60, 90 and 120 min after the administration of the treatments. The maximum reaction time was fixed at 30 s to prevent any injury to the tissues of the paws. If the reading exceeds 30 s, it would be considered as maximum analgesia.

Statistical Analysis

Repeated Measures Two way ANOVA Analysis using Bonferotti multiple comparisons post hoc test was performed using GraphPad Prism (version 7.02), San Diego CA, USA, www.graphPad.com) to compare activity between the control groups and rat treated with the test compounds and values were considered significant at $p < 0.05$ and above. Results were expressed as mean ± SEM (Avoseh et al., 2019; Ogunwande et al. 2019a; Ogunwande et al. 2019b).

RESULTS AND DISCUSSION

Chemical constituents of the essential oil of *T. plicata* var. Excelsa: The average yield of the light yellow essential oil was 1.31% (v/w), calculated on a dry weight basis. Table 1 indicates the chemical constituents present in *T. plicata* var. Excelsa, their percentages as well as linear retention indices on HP-5 column. A total of 46 compounds representing 99.9% of the total oil contents were identified by GC-MS. The main classes of compounds present in the leaf oil were monoterpene hydrocarbons (69.0%), sesquiterpene hydrocarbons (19.3%) and oxygenated sesquiterpenes (9.2%). The main constituents of the oil were the monoterpenes δ-3-carene (31.6%) and α-pinene (20.3%). Other significant constituents of the oil were cedrol (7.3%), β-caryophyllene (6.7%), terpinolene (6.4%) and α-humulene (5.6%). The compositions of essential oil of *T. plicata* var. Excelsa were markedly different from *T. plicata* and its various cultivars. α-Thujone and fenchone, the major compounds in *T. plicata* (Von Rudloff et al., 1988; Jirovetz et al., 2006) cultivar oils (Tsiri et al., 2009; Lis et al., 2019) were conspicuously absent in the present study.

Table 1. Chemical constituents of *Thuja plicata* var. Excelsa oil

Sr. No	Compounds[a]	RI[b]	RI[c]	Percent
1	(*E*)-3-Hexen-1-ol	853	851	0.2
2	Santolina triene	909	906	0.1
3	α-Thujene	931	921	0.6
4	α-Pinene	941	932	20.3
5	Camphene	954	946	3.3
6	Sabinene	976	968	1.1
7	β-Pinene	982	978	1.3
8	Myrcene	993	988	2.1
9	δ-3-Carene	1011	1008	31.6
10	Sylvestrene	1027	1022	0.3
11	Limonene	1032	1030	1.4
12	(*E*)-β-Ocimene	1052	1044	0.1
13	γ-Terpinene	1062	1056	0.4
14	Terpinolene	1088	1087	6.4
15	4-Terpineol	1178	1177	0.2
16	5-Isopropenyl-2-methyl-1-cyclopentene-1-carbaldehyde	1271	1269	0.5
17	Isobornyl acetate	1285	1285	0.2
18	Methyl myrtenate	1301	1301	0.2
19	1,2,6-Cyclononatriene	1309	1310	0.2
20	γ-Ionone	1340	1340	0.5
21	α-Terpinyl acetate	1352	1352	0.3
22	β-Bourbonene	1384	1383	0.1
23	β-Elemene	1392	1393	0.2
24	1,7-di-*epi*-β-Cedrene	1415	1413	0.9
25	β-Caryophyllene	1420	1419	6.7
26	*cis*-Thujopsene	1430	1430	0.2
27	α-Humulene	1456	1452	5.6
28	*cis*-Muurola-4(14),5-diene	1462	1460	0.1
29	α-Acoradiene	1463	1462	

Table 1. (Continued)

Sr. No	Compounds[a]	RI[b]	RI[c]	Percent
30	γ-Muurolene	1477	1477	2.5
31	β-Selinene	1485	1484	0.4
32	Viridiflorene	1493	1493	0.4
33	α-Muurolene	1498	1498	0.2
34	Germacrene A	1506	1505	0.2
35	*trans*-γ-Cadinene	1513	1513	0.7
36	δ-Cadinene	1524	1522	0.9
37	(*E*)-γ-Bisabolene	1535	1535	0.1
38	Caryophyllene oxide	1581	1581	0.5
39	Viridiflorol	1590	1590	0.8
40	Cedrol	1596	1600	7.3
41	Humulene epoxide II	1607	1606	0.2
42	α-Acorenol	1631	1632	0.1
43	β-Acorenol	1634	1636	0.1
44	*epi*-α-Cadinol	1640	1640	0.1
45	α-Cadinol	1654	1652	0.1
46	Nezukol	2126	2124	0.1
Total				**99.9**
Monoterpene hydrocarbons				**69.0**
Oxygenated monoterpenes				**1.4**
Sesquiterpene hydrocarbons				**19.3**
Oxygenated sesquiterpenes				**9.2**
Diterpenes				**0.1**
Non-terpene derivatives				**0.9**

[a] Elution order on HP-5MS column; [b] Retention indices on HP-5MS column; [c] Literature retention indices; Sr. No Serial number

Chemical constituents of *A. boonei*: The yield of the essential was 1.49% (v/w) calculated on a dry weight basis. Eight compounds representing 100% of the volatile contents were identified in the oil. The identity of the compounds, retention indices on HP-5 column and percentages could be seen in Table 2. These comprised of two monoterpene hydrocarbons (22.0%), four sesquiterpene hydrocarbons (43.4%) and two oxygenated sesquiterpenes (34.6%). No oxygenated monoterpene compound was identified in the oil sample. All the compounds were present in amount greater than 2%. The most abundant ones were cedrol (32.2%), α-humulene (18.9%), β-caryophyllene (17.2%) and α-pinene (13.4%).

Table 2. Chemical constituents of essential oil leaf of *Alstonia boonei*

Sr. No	Compounds[a]	LRI[b]	LRI[c]	*A. boonei*
1	α-Pinene	941	937	13.4
2	δ-3-Carene	1011	1008	8.6
3	β-Caryophyllene	1420	1419	17.2
4	α-Humulene	1456	1452	18.9
5	Germacrene D	1478	1478	3.9
6	δ-Cadinene	1524	1522	3.4
7	Viridiflorol	1590	1592	2.4
8	Cedrol	1596	1596	32.2
Total				**100**
Monoterpene hydrocarbons (Sr. No. 1,2)				**22.0**
Sesquiterpene hydrocarbons (Sr. No. 3-6)				**43. 4**
Oxygenated sesquiterpenes (Sr. No. 7, 8)				**34.6**

[a]Elution order on HP-5 column; [b]Retention indices on HP-5 column; [c]Literature retention indices (see experimental section)

The present oil compositions differed quantitatively and qualitatively from data reported previously for *A. boonei*. For example, terpenoids dominated the chemical constituents identified in the present oil sample against fatty acids identified previously in the oil (Moronkola et al., 2012) and ethanolic extract (Okwu and Ighodaro, 2010) as well as aromatic compounds present in the dichloromethane extract (Babatunde, 2017). Eugenol, an oxygenated monoterpene identified in the dichloromethane extract was not identified in the present study. It could be assumed that the variation in the oil contents may be due to method of analysis, environmental or climatic conditions between the points of study. Little literature information exists on the volatile compositions of other *Alstoonia* plants from other parts of the world. The flowers of *A. scholaris* analysed from Hanoi area, Vietnam (Dung et al., 2001) contained mainly oxygenated monoterpene compounds namely linalool (35.7%), *cis*- and *trans*-linalool oxides (14.7%) and α-terpineol (12.3%) while the principal component of the flower oil analysed in Bangladesh (Faridul et al., 2013) was 2-dodecyloxirane (31.83%). The differences in the chemical compounds identified in *A. boonei* and *A. scholaris* could be attributed to the different plant part being analysed.

Chemical constituents of *C. longa*: The essential oil was obtained in a yield of 0.80% (v/w) calculated on a dry weight basis. Twenty-seven compounds representing 96.5% of the oil content were identified in the oil. The dominant classes of compounds were oxygenated sesquiterpenes (69.3%) and monoterpenes hydrocarbons (11.4%). As seen in Table 3, the main constituents present in the oil were ar-tumerone (28.6%), β-atlantone (21.9%), curlone (18.8%) and 1,8-cineole (6.3%). The minor compounds include α-phellandrene (5.9%), ar-curcumene (2.3%), α-zingiberene (2.1%), β-sesquiphellandrene (2.0%), p-cymene (1.9%) and terpinolene (1.9%). The high content of ar-tumerone and curlone in the essential was consistent with data reported from previous investigated samples from other parts of the world (Liju et al., 2011; Gounder and Lingamallu, 2012; Schmidt et al., 2015; Oyemitan et al., 2017). However, β-atlantone, one of the main compounds of essential oil of *C. longa* in this study was found less in previous studies around the world. Moreover, some major compounds reported by previous studies were either absence or present in much lower quantity in the present oil sample. These include α-turmerone, β-turmerone and ar-curcumene (Ajaiyeoba et al., 2008; Ferreira et al., 2013; Schmidt et al., 2015; Avanço et al., 2017), β-bisabolene (Usman et al., 2009), α-zingiberene and β-sesquiphellandrene (Hwang et al., 2016) as well as terpinolene and α-phellandrene (Oguntimehin et al., 1990; Kumar et al., 2018)

Table 3. Compounds identified in the essential oil of *Curcuma longa*

Sr. No	Compounds[a]	LRI (Cal.)	LRI (Lit.)	Percent composition
1	(*E*)-3-Hexen-1-ol	853	851	0.3
2	Myrcene	993	988	0.2
3	α-Phellandrene	1006	1004	5.9
4	δ-3-Carene	1011	1008	0.1
5	α-Terpinene	1020	1020	0.2
6	p-Cymene	1028	1028	1.9
7	Limonene	1032	1030	0.6
8	1,8-Cineole	1034	1032	6.3
9	γ-Terpinene	1062	1056	0.3
10	Terpinolene	1088	1087	1.9
11	4-Terpineol	1178	1177	0.2

Sr. No	Compounds[a]	LRI (Cal.)	LRI (Lit.)	Percent composition
12	α-Terpineol	1191	1190	0.4
13	Cavacrol	1303	1305	0.2
14	4-Hydroxyl-3-methylacetophenone	1322	1322	0.1
15	β-Caryophyllene	1420	1419	0.5
16	(*Z*)-β-Farnesene	1444	1444	0.7
17	(*E*)-β-Farnesene	1460	1460	0.2
18	*allo*-Aromadendrene	1461	1461	0.1
19	γ-Curcumene	1481	1479	0.1
20	ar-Curcumene	1483	1481	2.3
21	α-Zingiberene	1496	1496	2.1
22	β-Bisabolene	1508	1505	0.5
23	β-Curcumene	1515	1515	0.1
24	β-Sesiquiphellandrene	1525	1525	2.0
25	ar-Tumerone	1666	1666	28.6
26	β-Atlantone	1667	1668	21.9
27	Curlone	1887	1886	18.8
Total				**96.8**
Monoterpene hydrocarbons (Sr. No. 2-10)				**11.1**
Oxygenated monoterpenes (Sr. No. 11-13)				**7.4**
Sesquiterpene hydrocarbons (Sr. No. 15-24)				**8.6**
Oxygenated sesquiterpenes (Sr. No. 25-27)				**69.3**
Non-terpene derivatives (Sr. No. 1, 14)				**0.4**

[a] Elution order on HP-5 column; LRI (Cal.), Calculated retention indices on HP-5 column; LRI (Lit.), Literature retention indices (see Experimental); Sr. No Serial number

Table 4. Chemical constituents of essential oil leaf of *Allium sativum*

Sr. No	Compounds[a]	LRI[b]	LRI[c]	Percentages
1	Diallyl sulphide	865	865	0.1
2	Methyl disulphide	919	920	0.1
3	Dimethyl trisulfide	974	976	0.1
4	Myrcene	993	988	0.1
5	Diallyl disulfide	1082	1082	15.7
6	(*Z*)-1-Propenylallyl disulphide	1098	1098	0.4
7	(*E*)-1-Propenylallyl disulphide	1102	1102	1.2
8	Methyl allyl trisulfide	1142	1144	9.2
9	3-Vinyl-1,2-dithiacyclohex-ene	1192	1191	0.1
10	2-Vinyl -1- 4H -1,3-dithiine	1207	1208	0.3
11	Dimethyl tetrasulphide	1208	1210	0.1
12	Nerol	1242	1244	0.3
13	Geranial	1270	1272	0.3

Table 4. (Continued)

Sr. No	Compounds[a]	LRI[b]	LRI[c]	Percentages
14	Diallyl trisulfide	1298	1296	53.9
15	Allyl propyl trisulfide	1306	1308	0.3
16	(Z)-1-Propenylallyl tetrasulphide	1328	1328	0.7
17	Diallyltetrasulfide	1539	1540	11.7
18	Dodecanoic acid	1570	1572	1.5
Total				**96.1**
Monoterpene hydrocarbons (Sr. No. 4)				**0.1**
Oxygenated monoterpenes (Sr. No. 12, 13)				**0.6**
Sulphur derivatives (Sr. No. 1-3, 5-8, 10, 11, 14-17)				**93.8**
Non-terpene derivatives (Sr. No. 9, 18)				**1.6**

[a]Elution order on HP-5 column; [b]Retention indices on HP-5 column; [c]Literature retention indices (see experimental section; Sr. No Serial number

Chemical constituents of *A. sativum*: The yield of the essential oil of *A. sativum* was 0.75% (v/w), calculated on a dry weight basis. Eighteen compounds representing 96.1% of the oil contents were identified (Table 4). Expectedly, sulphur derivatives (93.8%) were the most abundant class present in the oil. Monoterpenes and sesquiterpenes were less common (0.1%). The quantitatively significant constituents of the oil were diallyl trisulfide (53.9%), diallyl disulfide (15.7%), diallyl tetrasulfide (11.7%), methyl allyl trisulphide (9.2%). The oil compositions from this study show qualitative similarities with previously published reports on garlic oils from Egypt (Romeilah et al., 2010), Serbia (Kocić-Tanackov et al., 2012), Spain (Satyal et al., 2017), Cameroon (Foe et al., 2016), Turkey (Üstüner et al., 2018), Brazil (Malet et al., 2014), French (Mnayer et al., 2014), Tunisia (Chekki et al., 2014) and other parts of the world (Douiri et al. 2013; Dziri et al., 2014). The profile identified in this study was also different from China garlic (Zhao et al., 2013), Saudi Arabia (Mossah et al., 2017) and other parts of the world (Rui et al., 2009). These differences however attributed to the differences in the climatic and ecological conditions between the *A. sativum* from Nigeria and *A. sativum* from other parts of the world such as Asia and Europe.

Anti-Inflammatory, Anti-Nociceptive and Formalin Models

Pain related diseases have recently been on the rise due to low diagnosis or lack of scientific investigations. Recently, life threatening diseases such as cancer, tumor, ageing, atherosclerosis, etc. has been implicated to generate from pain or inflammatory markers (Chrysohoou et al., 2004; Nemat et al., 2009). Chronic inflammation and oxidative stress serves as a major cause of age-related diseases and cancer (Khansari et al., 2009). Several anti-inflammatory drugs have been developed in recent times ranging from Aspirin, Ibuprofen, Naproxen, celoxib and indomethacin (NSAID's- Non-steroidal anti-inflammatory Drugs). However, reports have shown that these drugs can interfere with bone healing, by having effect on the coagulation and angiogenesis (Lisowska et al., 2018). Therefore the use of alternative drugs with better potency and devoid of healing interference, addiction and other side effects is imperative. The use of natural products most especially from plant origin has been since primitive times. They are easy to source, available everywhere and easily processed.

In this report, we investigated the anti-inflammatory and anti-nociceptive properties of *T. plicata* var. Excelsa, *A. boonei*, *C. longa* and *A. sativum.* Inflammation processes involves synthesis and liberation of certain pro-inflammatory mediators. These mediators increases inflammation and thereby reduce healing time. Carragenaan induced model was used because it enables the realease of inflammatory and proinflammatory mediator including prostaglandins, leukotrienes, histamine and several cytokines. This model is considered to be a biphasic model. The early stage (1-2 h) contributes to the release of histamine, bradykinin, and serotonin which facilitate the increased synthesis of prostangladins (PGs) from surrounding tissues of the injured site. The late phase (3-4 h) is characterized by the increased level of PG mediated by the elevated modulation of leukotrienes and bradykinin. During this phase the cyclo-oxygenase-2 converts arachidonic acid into PGs which is a key factor of inflammation regulation (Ogunwande et al., 2019b).

The antinociceptive assay which involves the hot-plate model is used to evaluate the analgesia effect of plant extract and most especially the effect of opioid drugs on the spinal cord. The hot plate test was carried out to ascertain either the peripheral or the central acting effect with response of cerebral cortex or spinal cord integration of the essential oils (IASP, 1979). Owing to the new interest for natural products like EOs as alternative drugs and their major constituents, it is important to develop a better understanding of their antinociceptive action for new applications in human health.

The formalin-induced test is a pain model used to analyze both the analgesic and anti-inflammatory properties simultaneously. The initial phase is linked to the stimulation of nociceptors and principal afferent fibers by the formalin, triggering the liberation of bradykinin and tachykinins which occurs for 5 min (Correa and Calixo, 1993). The latter phase is accompanied by the discharge of inflammation facilitators such as prostaglandins, cytokines, histamine, nitric oxide (NO) and serotonin. In addition, these phases are inhibited by different classes of drugs. Opioid drugs inhibit the early phase and non-steroidal, anti-inflammatory drugs (NSAIDs) and opioid drugs inhibit the latter phase (Loretta et al., 2012).

Anti-Inflammatory Activity of *T. plicata* var. Excelsa

The essential oil of *T. plicata* var. Excelsa (TPEO) on subjection to anti-inflammatory evaluation using carrageenan-induced inflammation model displayed activity as shown in Figure 1. Carrageenan-induced inflammation study of the extracts showed a high activity consistent with dose and time. Inflammatory mediators were significantly suppressed within the 1st to the 3rd h at a level of $p < 0.001$ by the 200 and 400 mg/kg. In addition, the activity of the 100 mg/kg rises steadily from $p > 0.05$ (non-significant) to $p < 0.001$ for the 1st to the 3rd h respectively.

Essential oils activities declined considerably at the 4th h as most extract were non-significant. These activities could be attributed to the high rate of the absorption within the 1st to the 3rd h and also it's potential to suppress the inflammatory mediators within the latter and late phase of the carrageenan-induced model.

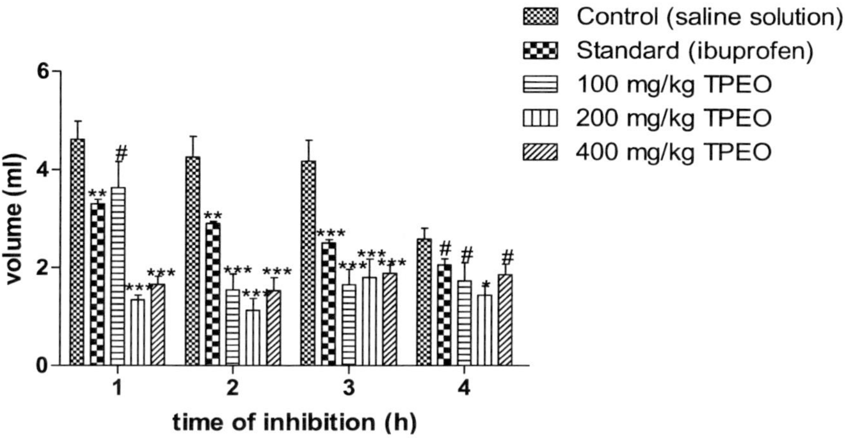

Figure 1. Effect of TPEO on Carragenan-induced inflammation. Control, Standard, and TPEO represent 1 mL saline solution, 100 mg/kg of Diclofenac injection and 100, 200 and 400 mg/kg of essential oils of TPEO respectively. *$p < 0.05$, **$p < 0.01$, *** $p < 0.001$, # = non-significant statistically compared to control.

In previous reports, a related species, *T. plicata* significantly inhibited the expression of vascular cell adhesion molecule 1 (VCAM-1), intracellular cell adhesion molecule 1 (ICAM-1), interferon gamma-induced protein 10 (IP-10), interferon-inducible T-cell chemoattractant (I-TAC), monokine induced by interferon gamma (MIG), and macrophage colony-stimulating factor (M-CSF). By this *T. plicata* essential oil significantly inhibited critical inflammation- and tissue remodeling-related proteins and genes in human dermal fibroblasts (Han and Parker, 2017). Also ethanolic extract of *T. occidentalis* leaves showed significant ($p < 0.05$) analgesic and anti-inflammatory activity in dose dependent manner (Janadri and Yogesh, 2016). The anti-inflammatory activities of several essential oils from Nigeria have been widely reported (Avoseh et al., 2019; Ogunwande et al., 2019a; Ogunwande et al., 2019b). Such activities are attributed to the synergistic effects of the oil components or that of the main components present (Miguel, 2010). The syngeristic effects of some minor compounds of the essential should also be taken into consideration (Ounwande et al., 2019b). In this study, α-pinene and δ-3-carene were the major components and are very common components of most plant. *Salvia* essential oils from South

Africa contains high amounts of α-pinene and it succesfuly inhibited the proliferations of 5-lipoxygenase (Kamatou et al., 2006). The essential oils of leaves and rhizomes of *Alpinia murdochii*, *Alpinia scabra* and leaves of *Alpinia pahangensis* with high content of α-pinene were also good 5-lipoxynease inhibitors. The ability of oils from *Torreya nucifera* to possess COX-2 selective inhibitor having significant inhibitory effects on PGE2 production was attributed to the presence of δ-3-carene and α-pinene (Yoon et al., 2009). Other anti-inflammatory activities of α-pinene was reported from the oil of *Juniperus oxycedrus* which showed a great inhibition of IL-1-induced NO production in the human chondrocytic cell line C-28/12 and also reduced markedly IL-1-induced IκBα degradation and phosphorylation, NF-κB-DNA binding activity and NO production (Neves et al., 2010). The main constituents of the oil of *Ugni myricoides*, α-pinene, significantly reduced inflammation and neuropathic pain (Him et al., 2008).

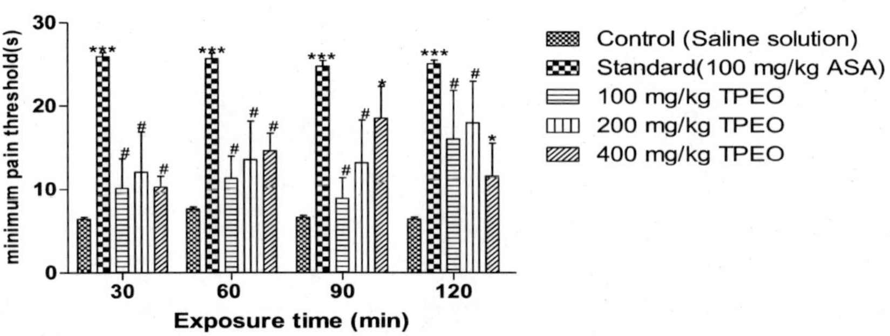

Figure 2. Effect of TPEO on Hot Plate model. Control, Standard, and TPEO represent 1 mL saline solution, 100 mg/kg of Peroxicam injection and 100, 200 and 400 mg/kg of TPEO respectively. *$p < 0.05$, **$p < 0.01$, *** $p < 0.001$, # = non-significant statistically compared to control.

Anti-Nociceptive Activities *T. plicata* var. Excelsa

Figure 2 shows the analgesic activity of TPEO using hot plate test. To assess the centrally-mediated nociceptive effects of the essential oils through the use of thermal stimuli where the latency of nociceptive reaction were initiated by heat sensation; hot plate model was adopted. In this study, animal response to heat was assessed by paw licking, shaking and jumping measured at 30, 60, 90 and 120 min following administration. The results indicated that the longer the response time, the higher the analgesia properties of the essential oil.

The analgesic activities of the oils were considerably low as displayed in Figure 2. TPEO displayed a very low heat latency activity. Doses activities were non-significant ($p > 0.05$) except for a slight inhibition at 90th and 120th min ($p < 0.05$) by the 400 mg/kg.

The antinociceptive activities of several doses of *T. plicata* var. Excelsa are as shown in Figure 2. The activites was very low at minimum doses of 100 to 200 mg/kg of essential oils. Volatile oils have become a central remedy for nociception due to their high permeability through skin vessels. Nociceptive tests may use chemical, electrical, mechanical, or thermal stimuli (Bars et al., 2001). The hot-plate test is commonly used to investigate nociception and analgesia in rodents. Earlier reports of the analgesic properties of *T. plicata* is limited, however, the essential oils component reported in this study are perfect candidates for pain remediation (Shah et al., 2001). For instance, the essential oils of *Teucrium stocksianum* at doses of 20, 40, 80 and 160 mg/kg i.p. significantly reduced pain by inhibiting the synthesis of prostaglandins, PGE2 and then PGF2 and free arachidonic acid (Derardt et al., 1980)

Anti-Nociceptive Activity of *A. boonei*

A. boonei has been used traditionally for the treatment of pain related conditions. In this report, we investigated its anti-nociceptive and anti-inflammatory properties. A thermal nociceptive model such as hot plate test was carried out to elucidate the central analgesic activity of the essential oil. Several reports have indicated that essential oils and its component acts by inhibiting the formation and/or liberation of the mediators in the paw tissue. The results of the analgesic activity of *A. boonei* essential oil (ABGH) using the hot plate test are shown in Figure 3. The results showed that there was no significant difference on the thermal stimulus in the rats treated with the normal saline throughout the 90 min observation. In comparison to the saline treated animals, significant increase in the reaction to thermal pain was detectable in 100 and 400 mg/kg of the essential oil. The 100 and 400 mg/kg of the essential oil were highly significant with a value of $p < 0.001$ at 60th and 90th min.

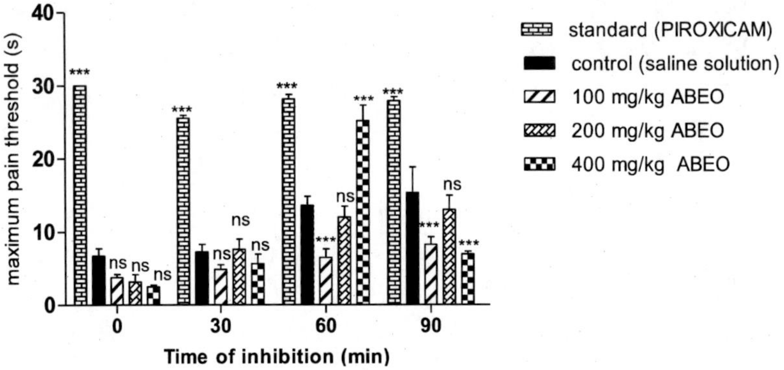

Figure 3. Effect of ABGH on heat induced pain. Control, Standard and ABGH represent 0.5 ml saline solution, 5 mg/kg of piroxicam injection and 100, 200 and 400 mg/kg of essential oils of *A. boonei* respectively. $^{*}p < 0.05$, $^{**}p < 0.01$, $^{***}p < 0.001$ statistically compared to control.

Anti-Inflammatory Activity of *A. boonei*

Intraplantar injection of carrageenan in rats resulted in a time dependent increase in paw volume (Figure 4). However, treatment with *A. boonei* essential oil (ABGH) reduced the paw edema in a dose dependent manner at 1, 2, 3 and 4 h after an injection of carrageenan. The significant activities of the different doses of the essential oils were inconsistent. The 100 mg/kg of ABGH displayed a steady activity at the 1st and 2nd h ($p < 0.01$) and increased at 3rd and 4th h ($p < 0.001$). 200 mg/kg of the essential oil also showed steady activity at the 3rd and 4th h ($p < 0.01$). The result showed that 400 mg/kg of the essential oil was significant at the 1st h ($p < 0.05$) but there was a total loss of activity at the 2nd h ($p > 0.05$) then it was highly significant at the 3rd and 4th h ($p < 0.001$). The reference drug (ibuprofen) caused a significant inhibition of post carrageenan edema.

The results of this study showed that the essential oil of *A. boonei* suppressed the rat hind paw edema induced by intraplantar injection on carrageenan, signifying marked anti-acute inflammatory efficiency. There is significant inhibition of histamine and serotonin at the first hour by all the dose concentration used except 200 mg/kg. Prostaglandins and other cytokines were inhibited by all the dose concentration at the 3rd and 4th h. The methanolic extract of *A. boonei* stem bark inhibited inflammation to a significant value of $p<0.05$ when induced by carrageenan oedema and cotton pellet assays in rats (Kweifio-Okai, 1991).

Cedrol, a sesquiterpenoid occurring in higher percentage in the studied oil sample has been reported as an excellent anti-inflammatory agent (Hyeon-Uk et al., 2014). Our results confirmed previous findings that *A. boonei* exhibits anti-inflammatory effect.

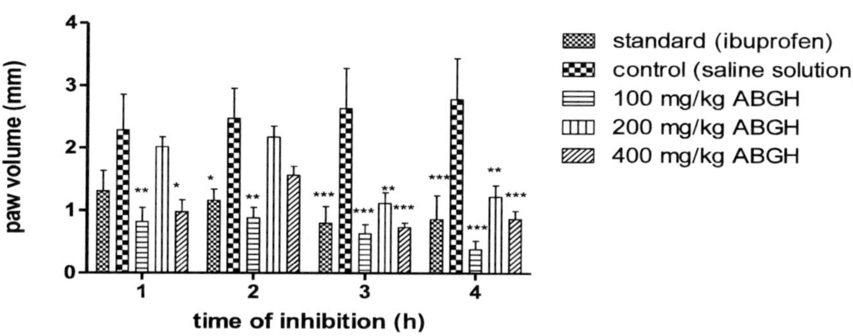

Figure 4. Effect of ABGH on carrageenan- induced inflammation. Control, Standard and ABGH represent 0.5 ml saline solution, 12.5 mg/kg of aspirin injection and 100, 200 and 400 mg/kg of essential oils of *A. boonei* respectively. $^{*}p < 0.05$, $^{**}p < 0.01$, $^{***}p < 0.001$ statistically compared to control.

Formalin Assay on *A. boonei*

Formalin assay is a model of both anti-nociceptive and anti-inflammation (Hunskar and Hole, 1987). For this study, the essential oil showed high inhibition in the inflammatory phase than the neurogenic phase as shown in Table 5. The methanolic extract of *A. boonei* had earlier shown the inhibition of both phases with more pronounced inhibition at the inflammatory phase (Loretta et al., 2012).

Table 5. Results of formalin induced nociceptive of *A. boonei*

Treatment	Dose (mg/kg)	Neuroenic phase		Inflammatory phase	
		No. of licks	Inhibition (%)	No. of licks	Inhibition
Control (Saline)		23.5 ± 1.62		7.50 ± 0.60	
Standard (Piroxicam)		12.5 ± 1.74	46.81	16.5 ± 2.83	100
A. boonei	100	28.83 ± 2.61	22.69	11.67 ± 1.05	55.56
A. boonei	200	35.33 ± 5.12	50.35	11.83 ± 1.43	57.78
A. boonei	400	23.33 ± 2.99	60.71	15.67 ± 0.91	100

Mean ± SEM for the 6 rats

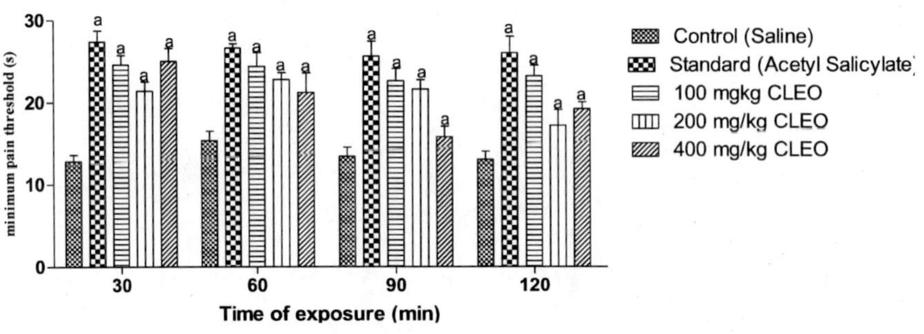

Figure 5. Effect of *C. Longa* on heat induced pain. Control, Standard, and *C. longa* represent 1 mL saline solution, 100 mg/kg of Aspirin injection and 100, 200 and 400 mg of *C. longa* respectively. [a] $P < 0.001$ statistically compared to control.

As expected, aspirin used as the piroxicam drug significantly inhibited the first phase (83%) and second phase (73%) of the test which is expected for a non-steroidal drug. The essential oil of *A. boonei* exhibited high activity at the inflammatory phase with 100% at a dose level of 400 mg/kg.

Anti-Nociceptive Activities of *C. longa*

Turmeric is widely used in therapeutic preparations against several infectios and diseases such as anorexia, rhinitis, herpes zoster, acne, cough, urinary tract diseases, diabetic wounds, hepatic disorder, rheumatism and sinusitis (Devaraj et al., 2010). The herb contains curcumin as the active ingredient, which is a yellow coloured phenolic pigment obtained from the powdered rhizome of *C. longa*. In the present study, the essential oils displayed high inhibitions that are independednt on dose or duration of exposure. The 100-400 mg/kg of the essential oil significantly ($p < 0.001$) increases the heat latency of the Wistar rats (Figure 5). This activity was very fundamental due to the components and ethnopharmacological applications of the plant.

Specialised cell pain receptors comprising of transduction, conduction, transmission processes which are initiated by by activation of pain receptors are called nociceptors (Pinheiro et al., 2011). They conduct and transmit pain from site of effect to the brain and vice versa. The ability of plant extracts to prolong this process increases its chance as an anti-pain drug. Ethanolic extract of *C. longa* collected from India significantly increases heat latency for the 100-400 mg/kg extracts evaluated (Zhu et al., 2014; Jogdand and Bhattacharje, 2017).

Anti-Inflammatory Activity of *A. sativum*

The complex biochemistry of garlic makes it possible for variations in processing to yield different preparations with differences in final composition and compound proportion. Anti-inflammatory activities of *A. sativum* essential oil (ASEO) in this study were only significant for the 100 mg/kg at the 2nd h ($p < 0.001$) and 3rd h ($p < 0.05$) of the analysis as shown in Figure 6. This shows that the essential oils can have maximum activity at low concentration and also within a short period of contact. In addition, it can significantly inhibit inflammation mediators produced within the 1st phase while showing less activities for those of latter stages. The GC-MS analysis in Table 4 showed the presence of high amounts of diallyl disulfide. This component has already been reported to inhibit inflammation by several mechanisms such as modulation of cytokine secretion (Spelman et al., 2006), inhibition of transcription factor NF-κB, a master regulator, and inhibiting the transcription of several cytokine genes involved in proinflammatory responses, such as TNF-α, interleukin-1beta (IL-1β), IL-6, MCP-1, and IL-12 (Fu et al., 2015)

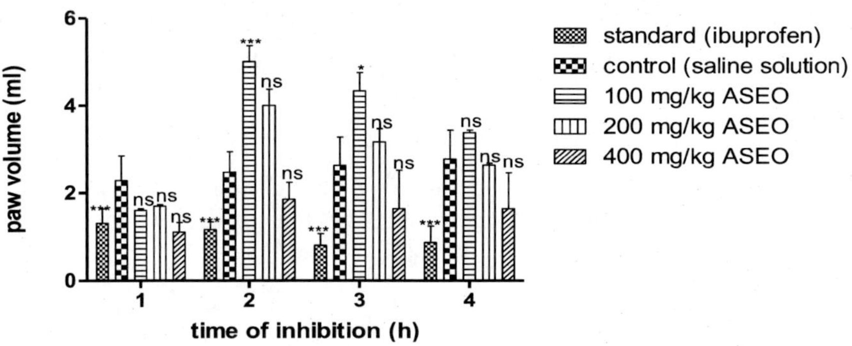

Figure 6. Effect of *A. sativum* on carrageenan- induced inflammation. Control, Standard and ASEO represent 0.5 ml saline solution, 12.5 mg/kg of aspirin injection and 100, 200 and 400 mg/kg of essential oils of *A. sativum* respectively. $^{*}p < 0.05$, $^{**}p < 0.01$, $^{***}p < 0.001$ statistically compared to control.

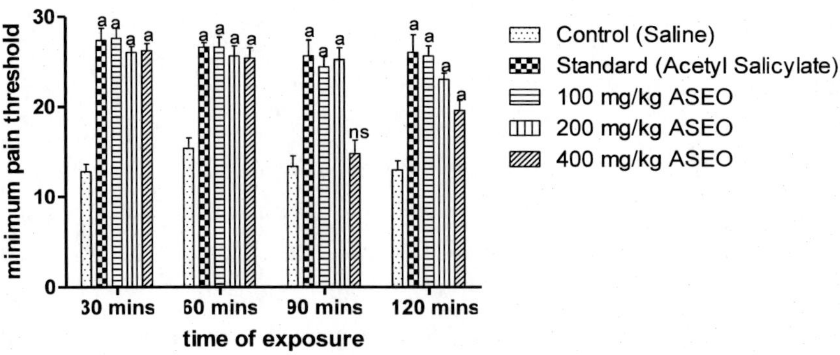

Figure 7. Effect of *A. sativum* on heat induced pain. Control, Standard, and *A. sativum* represent 1 mL saline solution, 100 mg/kg of Aspirin injection and 100, 200 and 400 mg/kg of *A. sativum* respectively. $^{a}P < 0.001$, ns-non-significant statistically compared to control.

Analysis performed on four anti-inflammatory sulfur containing compounds from garlic indicated that sulfur compounds inhibited the production of nitric oxide (NO) and prostaglandin E_2 (PGE_2) and the expression of the pro-inflammatory cytokines tumor necrosis factor-α, interleukin-1β, and interleukin-6 in lipopolysaccharide (LPS)-activated macrophages. Therefore, in this study, the inflammation inhibition observed could be linked to the presence of sulphur compounds in the essential oils.

Anti-Nociceptive Activities of *A. sativum*

Nociceptive activities or transmission in neuropathic pain inhibition is a fundamental mechanism in the activities of analgesics. Both opioids and non-opiods (e.g., NSAIDs) acts in such a way to ameliorate the progressive proliferation of pain. Deprivation of substance P or glycine or glutamate from the nerve endings can results in analgesia. Preliminary investigation has revealed that garlic successfully decrease Glutamate levels. Components such ajoene, allicin and dially sulphur found in oil are high anti-pain drugs (Nasri et al., 2012).

The result obtained in the hot plate antinociceptive assay showed that the essential oils of *A. sativum* at 100, 200 and 400 mg/kg significantly prolonged the heat latency capacity ($p < 0.001$) of the Wistar rats at all reaction time except for the 90th minute where activity was non-significant for the 400 mg/kg as shown in Figure 7. This exceptional result agrees with previous studies on the analgesics and antinocieptive properties of *A. sativum*. A previous study (Keiss et al., 2003) investigated the cytokine modulation capacity of *A. sativum*; the result shows that garlic powder extracts (GPE) and single garlic metabolites significantly modulate lipopolysaccharide (LPS)-induced cytokine levels in human whole blood. This activity was due to the presence of diallydisulfide. Generally, the activity of garlic reported herein can be mainly due to the sulfur componenets present in the essential oils. However, synergistic interactions can also be another reason for the effect. Allium sativa is a perfect candidate for mediating central analgesia and depicts the ability of the plant extract to act as opioid antagonist.

Conclusion

Analgesic and anti-inflammatory drugs have varied effects on pain and inflammation. Their mode of application, preparation and doses becomes imperative for effective activity. The flora of Nigeria, West Africa has been one of the untapped resources due to lack of focus on its chemical and medicinal importance. *Alstonia boonei*, *T. plicata* var. Excelsa, *A. sativum* and *C. longa* in this study had shown to be very effective source of anti-inflammatory and antinoniceptive agents. Mechanistic interpretation of the modes of activities of these plant materials will further establish their usefulness. In addition, molecular level analysis of active or more abundant essential oil components with cytokines and pain mediators is highly recommended for further studies.

References

Adotey, JP; Kwaku, Adukpo GE. Etornam, Yaw O. Boahen; Frederick A. Armah "A Review of the Ethnobotany and Pharmacological Importance of *Alstonia boonei* De Wild (Apocynaceae)." *ISRN Pharmacology*, vol. 2012, (July 2012), Article ID: 587160. Doi: 10.5402/2012/587160.

Ajaiyeoba O. Edith, Sarna, W; Essien E. Emmanuel, Olayemi, IO; Ekundayo Olusegun, Walker M. Tameka; Setzer, N. William. "Larvicidal Activity of Turmerone-rich Essential Oils of *Curcuma longa* Leaf and Rhizome from Nigeria on *Anopheles gambiae*". *Pharmaceutical Biology*, vol. 46, no. 4 (October 2008), 279-282.

Akinyemi Ayodele Jacob; Philip Adeyemi Adeniyi. "Effect of Essential Oils from Ginger (*Zingiber officinale*) and Turmeric (*Curcuma longa*) Rhizomes on Some Inflammatory Biomarkers in Cadmium Induced

Neurotoxicity in Rats". *Journal of Toxicology*, vol. 2018, Article ID 4109491 (2018): 7 pages. Doi: org/10.1155/2018/4109491.

Alejandro Mendoza-Juache, Saray Aranda-Romo, Bermeo-Escalona, R. Josué, Araceli Gómez-Hernández, Amaury Pozos-Guillén, and Luis Octavio Sánchez-Vargas. "The Essential Oil of *Allium sativum* as an Alternative Agent against *Candida* Isolated from Dental Prostheses". *Revista Iberoamericana de Micologia*, vol. 34, no. 3, (June 2017), 158-164.

Amanda Chaaban, Gomes E. Nunes, Richardi V. Sobrinho, Martins Carlos E. Nogueira, Brum J. Sperotto, Navarro-Silva M. Antônio, Deschamps Cícero, and Molento M. Beltrão. "Essential Oil from *Curcuma longa* Leaves: Can an Overlooked by Product from Turmeric Industry be Effective for *Myiasis* Control?" *Industrial Crops and Products*, vol. 312, (June 2019), 352-364.

Attioua Barthélemy Koffi, Vincent Assamoi Adiko, Harisolo Rhamiarantsoa, Faustin Aka Kabran, Ahmont Landry Claude Kablan, Philomène Akoua Kouassi, Timothée Aboua Okpekon, and Leon Atoutou Djakoure. "A New Cardiac Glycoside from *Alstonia boonei* (Apocynaceae)." *International Journal of Chemical Studies*, vol. 6, no. 4, (July-August 2018), 238-242.

Avanço G. Brado, Flavio D. Ferreira, Natália S. Bomfim, Paula Andréia de Souza Rodrigues dos Santos, Rosane Marina Peralta, Tatiane Brugnari, Carlos A. Mallmann, Benício A. de Abreu Filho, Jane MG. Mikcha; Miguel Machinski Jr. "*Curcuma longa* L. Essential Oil Composition, Antioxidant Effect, and Effect on *Fusarium verticillioides* and Fumonisin Production." *Food Control*, vol. 73, Part B (March 2017), 806-813.

Avoseh N. Opeyemi, Ogunwande A. Isiaka, Lawal O. Adejumobi, Atabo John, Roberta Ascrizzi; Guido Flamini. "Anti inflammatory and Anti-nociceptive Activities of Essential Oil of *Waltherica indica*." *Boletín Latinoamericano y del Caribe de Plantas Medicinales y Aromáticas*, vol. 18, no. 6, (December 2019), 566-576.

Babatunde, O. “GC-MS Analysis of Leaf, Stem-bark and Root Extracts of *Alstonia boonei*.” *African Journal of Pharmacy and Pharmacology*, vol. 11, no. 46, (December 2017), 577-581.

Balogun S. Olaoye, Ajayi S. Olukayode; Agberotimi J. Bukola. “A Cytotoxic Indole Alkaloid from *Alstonia boonei.” Journal of Biologically Active Products from Nature*, vol. 6, no. 6, (December 2016), 347-351.

Bars D. Lers, Gozariu, M; Cadden, SW. “Animal Models of Nociception.” *Pharmacological Reviews*, vol. 53, no. 4, (December 2001), 597-652.

Burkhill, HM. “*The Useful Plants of Tropical West Africa*” (Families A-D), 2nd Edition, Royal Botanic Gardens Kew vol.1. 1985), pp. 138-140.

Chekki Raja Zouari, Snoussi Ahmed, Hamrouni Imen; Bouzouita Nabiha. “Chemical Composition, Antibacterial and Antioxidant Activities of Tunisian garlic (*Allium sativum*) Essential Oil and Ethanol Extract.” *Mediterranean Journal of Chemistry*, vol. 3, no 4, (August 2014), 947-956.

Chrysohoou, C; Pitsavos, C; Panaglotakos, DB; Skoumas, John; Stefanadis, C. “Association between Prehypertension Status and Inflammatory Markers Related to Atherosclerotic Disease”. *American Journal of Hypertension*, vol. 17, no. 7, (July 2004), 568-573.

Correa, CR; Calixto, JB. “Evidence of Participation of B1 and B2 Kinase Receptors in Formalin-induced Nociceptive Response in the Mouse.” *British Journal of Pharmacology*, vol. 110, no. 1, (January 1993), 193-198.

Derardt, R; Jougney, S; Delevalcee, F; Falhourt, M. “Release of Prostaglandins E and F in an Algogenic Reaction and its Inhibition.” *European Journal of Pharmacology*, vol. 61, no. 1, (January 1980), 17-24.

Devaraj, S; Esfahani, AS; Ismail, S; Ramanathan, S; Yam, MF. “Evaluation of the Antinociceptive Activity and Acute Oral Toxicity of Standardized Ethanolic Extract of the Rhizome of *Curcuma xanthorrhiza* Roxb.” *Molecules,* vol. 15, no. 4, (April 2010), 2925-2934.

Douiri Lalla Fatima, Boughdad Ahmed, Assobhei Omar, Moumni Mohieddine. “Chemical Composition and Biological Activity of *Allium sativum* Essential Oils against *Callosobruchus maculatus*." *IOSR Journal of Environmental Science, Toxicology and Food Technology*, vol. 3, no. 1, (January 2013), 30-36. DOI: 10.9790/2402-0313036.

Dung N. Xuan, Pham H. Ngoc, Do D. Rang, Nguyen T. Nhan, Naja Klinkby, Piet Leclercq. "Chemical Composition of the Volatile Concentrate from the Flowers of Vietnamese *Alstonia scholaris* (L.) R. Br., *Apocynaceae*." *Journal of Essential Oil Research*, vol. 13, no. 2, (April 2001), 424-426.

Dziri Salma, Hervé Casabianca, Belgacem Hanchi, Karim Hosni. "Composition of Garlic Essential Oil (*Allium sativum* L.) as Influenced by Drying Method". *Journal of Essential Oil Research*, vol. 26, no. 2, (March 2014), 91-96.

Ebigwai, JK; Ilondu, EM; Markson, AA; Ekeleme, E. "*In vitro* Evaluation of the Essential Oil Extract of Six Plant Species and Ivermectin on the Microfilaria Larva of *Simulium yahense*." *Research Journal of Medicinal Plants*, vol. 6, (December 2012), 461-465.

Fabiyi O. Adenike, Atolani O. Olatunji, Ademola Gabriel. "Nematicidal Activity of *Alstonia boonei* and *Bridelia ferruginea* Leaves." *Albanian Journal of Agricultural Sciences*, vol. 11, no. 2, (June 2012), 105-114.

Faridul Islam, Islam Sahidul, Nandi C. Numa, Mohammed A. Satter. "Essential oil Composition from the Flowers of *Alstonia scholaris* of Bangladesh." *International Food Research Journal*, vol. 20, no. 6, (December 2013), 3185-3188.

Ferreira F. Dias, Simone AG. Mossini, Francine MD. Ferreira, Carla Cristina Arrotéia, Christiane L. da Costa, Celso V. Nakamura, Miguel M. Junior. "The Inhibitory Effects of *Curcuma longa* L. Essential Oil and Curcumin on *Aspergillus flavus* Link Growth and Morphology." *Scientific World Journal.*, Vol. 2013, (2013), 343804. doi: 10.1155/ 2013/343804

Foe Florentine MC. Ndoye, Tatiana FK. Tchinang, Ascencion M. Nyegue, Jean-Pierre Abdou, Abel JG. Yaya, Alembert T. Tchinda, Jean-Louis O. Essane, Francois-Xavier Etoa. "Chemical Composition, *in vitro* antioxidant and Anti inflammatory Properties of Essential Oils of Four Dietary and Medicinal Plants from Camerron". *BMC Complementary and Alternative Medicine*, vol. 16, (April 2016), 17-34. doi:10.1186/ s12906-0116-1098y.

Francieli da Silva Gislaine, Lilian Wunsch Rocha, Nara Lins, Meira Quintão. Chapter 10 – "Nutraceuticals, Dietary Supplements, and Functional Foods as Alternatives for the Relief of Neuropathic Pain." In Bioactive Nutraceuticals and Dietary Supplements in Neurological and Brain Disease-Prevention and Therapy (Eds. Watson R.R, and Preedy, VR), Academic Press, (2015), 87-93.

Fu, E; Tsai, MC; Chin, YT; Tu, HP; Fu, MM; Chian, CY. "The Effects of Diallyl Sulfide upon Porphyromonas gingivalis Lipopolysaccharide Stimulated Proinflammatory Cytokine Expressions and Nuclear Factor Kappa B Activation in Human Gingival Fibroblasts". *Journal of Periodontal Research*, vol. 50, no 3, (June 2015), 380-388.

Funk L. Janet, Frye B. Jennifer, Oyarzo N. Janice, Zhang Hua-Ping, Timmermann N. Barbara "Anti-Arthritic Effects and Toxicity of the Essential Oils of Turmeric (*Curcuma longa* L.)." *Journal of Agricultural and Food Chemistry*, vol. 58, no. 2, (December 2010), 842-849.

Gounder Dhanalakshmi Kutti, Jaganmohanrao Lingamallu. "Comparison of Chemical Composition and Antioxidant Potential of Volatile Oil from Fresh, Dried and Cured Turmeric (*Curcuma longa*) Rhizomes." *Industrial Crops and Products*, vol. 38, (July 2012), 124-131

Han Xuesheng, Tory L. Parker. "Arborvitae (*Thuja plicata*) "Essential Oil Significantly Inhibited Critical Inflammation and Tissue Remodeling-related Proteins and Genes in Human Dermal Fibroblasts." *Biochimie Open*, vol. 4, no. 6, (June 2017), 56-60.

Him Aydin, Ozbek Hanefi, Turel Idris, Oner Ahmet Cihat. "Anti-nociciceptive Activity of Alpha-Pinene and Fenchone." *Pharmocology Online*, vol. 3, (January 2008), 363-369.

Hwang Kyu-Won, Daniel Son, Hyeong-Wook Jo, Chun Hwan-Kim, Ki Cheol-Seong, Joon-Kwan Moon. "Levels of Curcuminoid and Essential Oil Compositions in Turmerics (*Curcuma longa* L.) Grown in Korea." *Applied Biological Chemistry*, vol. 59, (January 2016), 209-215.

Hudson James, Michael Kuo, Selvarani Vimalanathan. "The Antimicrobial Properties of Cedar Leaf (*Thuja plicata*) Oil; A Safe and Efficient Decontamination Agent for Buildings." *International Journal of Environmental Research and Public Health*, vol. 8, no. 12, (December 2011), 4477-4487.

Hunskaar, S; Hole, K. "The Formalin Test in Mice: Dissociation Between Inflammatory and Non-inflammatory Pain." *Pain*, vol. 30, no. 1, (January 1987), 103-114.

Hyeon-Uk, J; Soon-Sang, K; Tae, YK; Hyun, K; Hye-Suk, L. "Inhibitory Effects of Cedrol, Cedrene and Thujopsene on Cytochrome P450 Enzyme Activities in Human Liver Microsomes." *Journal of Toxicology and Environmental Health*, vol. 77, no. 1, (January 2014), 22-24.

International Association for the Study of Pain. IASP Pain Terminology, (1979), Accessed January 21, 2020.

Iyiola, OA; Tijani, AY; Lateef, KM. "Antimalarial Activity of Ethanolic Stem Bark Extract of *Alstonia boonei* in Mice." *Asian Journal of Biological Sciences*, vol. 4, no. 3, (June 2011), 235-243.

Janadri Suresh, Yogesh HS. Gowda. "Evaluation of Analgesic and Anti-inflammatory Activity of *Thuja occidentalis* Leaves in Chemically Induced Animal Models." *Advanced Pharmaceutical Journal*, vol. 1, no. 1, (March-April 2016), 26-30.

Jirovetz, L; Buchbauer, G; Denkova, Z; Slavchev, A; Stoyanova, A; Schmidt, Erich. "Chemical Composition, Antimicrobial Activities and Odor Descriptions of Various *Salvia* sp. and *Thuja* sp. Essential Oils." *Nutrition*, vol. 30, no. 4, (August 2006), 152-159.

Jogdand Sangita, Jagruti Bhattacharjee. "Evaluation of Analgesic Activity of Turmeric (*Curcuma longa* Linn.) in Wister rats." *International Journal of Basic Clinical Pharmacology*, vol. 6, no. 3, (March 2017), 568-571.

Kamatou PP. Guy, van Zyl RL; van Vuuren, SF; Viljoen, AM; Figueiredo, AC; Barroso, JG; Pedro, LG; Tilney, PM. "Chemical Composition, Leaf Trichome Types and Biological Activities of the Essential Oils of Four Related *Salvia* Species Indigenous to Southern Africa." *Journal of Essential Oil Research*, vol. 18, no. 1, (February 2006), 72-79.

Keiss Hans-Peter, Verena M. Dirsch, Thomas Hartung, Thomas Haffner, Laurence Trueman, Jacques Auger, Rémi Kahane, Angelika M. Vollmar. "Garlic (*Allium sativum* L.) Modulates Cytokine Expression in Lipopolysaccharide-Activated Human Blood Thereby Inhibiting NF-κB Activity." *The Journal of Nutrition*, vol. 133, no. 7, (July 2003), 2171-2175.

Kocić-Tanackov Suncica, Dimić Gordana, Lević Jelena, Tanackov Ilija, Tepić Aleksandra, Vujičić Biserka, Gvozdanović-Varga Jelica. "Effects of onion (*Allium cepa* L.) and garlic (*Allium sativum* L.) Essential Oils on the *Aspergillus versicolor* Growth and Sterigmatocystin Production". *Journal of Food Sciece*, vol. 77, no. 5, (April 2012), 278-184. doi: 10.1111/j.1750 3841.2012.02662.x.

Kumar Anant, Karishma Agarwal, Monika Singh, Archana Saxena, Pankaj Yadav, Anil K. Maurya, Anju Yadav, Sudeep Tandon, Debabrata Chanda, Dnyaneshwar U. Bawankule." Essential Oil from Waste Leaves of *Curcuma longa* L. Alleviates Skin Inflammation." *Inflammopharmacology*, vol. 26, no. 5, (October 2018), 1245-1255.

Kweifio-Okai, G. "Anti-inflammatory Activity of a Ghanaian Antiarthritic Herbal Preparation." *Journal of Ethnopharmacology*, vol. 33, no. 3, (July 1991), 263-267.

Liju B. Vijayastelter, Kottarapat Jeena, Ramadasan Kuttan. "An Evaluation of Antioxidant, Anti-inflammatory, and Anti-nociceptive Activities of Essential Oil from *Curcuma longa* L." *Indian Journal of Pharmacology*, vol. 43, no. 5, (September-October 2011), 526-531.

Lim, TK. "*Curcuma longa*". In: Edible Medicinal and Non Medicinal Plants. Springer, *Cham*, (2016), pp. 241-362.

Lis Anna, Agnes Swaczyna, Agnieszka Krajewska, Karolina Mellor. "Chemical Composition of the Essential Oils from Twigs, Leaves, and Cones of *Thuja plicata* and its Cultivar varieties "Fastigiata", "Kornik," and "Zebrina." *Natural Product Communications*, vol. 14, no. 7, (July 2019), 1-10.

Lisowska Barbara, Kosson Dariusz, Domaracka Karolina. "Positives and Negatives of Nonsteroidal Anti-inflammatory Drugs in Bone Healing:

the Effects of These Drugs on Bone Repair". *Drug Design Development and Therapy*, vol. 12, (June 2018), 1809-1814.

Loretta O. Iniaghe, Stephen O. Okpo, Jacob E. Olung, Eguae A. Agharese. "Analgesic Effect of Methanol Leaf Extract of *Alstonia boonei* De Wild (Apocynaceae)". *Tropical Journal of Pharmaceutical Research*, vol. 11, no. 5 (October 2012): 793-798.

Mahmoudvand Hossein, Mahbobeh Pakravanan, Mohammad Reza Aflatoonian, Amal Khudair Khalaf, Massumeh Niazi, Seyyed Reza Mirbadie, Amir T. Kareshk, Mehrdad Khatami. "Efficacy and Safety of *Curcuma longa* Essential Oil to Inactivate Hydatid Cyst Protoscoleces". *BMC Complementary and Alternative Medicine*, vol. 19, (July 2019), 187. Doi: 10.118/s129060195273.

Mallet, ACT; Cardoso, MG; Souza, PE; Machado, SMF; Andrade, MA; Nelson, DL; Piccoli, RH; Pereira, CG. "Chemical Characterization of the *Allium sativum* and *Origanum vulgare* Essential Oils and their Inhibition Effect on the Growth of some Food Pathogens.". *Revista Brasileira de Plantas Medicinais*, vol. 16, no. 4, (October-December 2014), 804-811.

Miguel Maria Graça. "Antioxidant and Anti-Inflammatory Activities of Essential Oils: A Short Review." *Molecules*, vol. 15, no. 12, (December 2010), 9252-9287.

Mnayer Dima, Fabiano-Tixier Anne-Sylvie, Petitcolas Emmanuel, Hamieh Tayssir, Nehme Nancy, Ferrant Christie, Fernandez Xavier, Chemat Farid. "Chemical Composition, Antibacterial and Antioxidant Activities of Six Essetial Oils from the Alliaceae Family". *Molecules*, vol. 19, no. 12, (December 2014), 20034-20053. Doi: 10.3390/ molecules191220034.

Moronkola O. Dorcas, Kunle O. Funke. "Essential oil Compositions of Leaf, Stem bark and Root of *Alsonia boonei* De Wild (Apocyanaceae)." *International Journal of Biology and Pharmacy Research*, vol. 3, no. 1, (February 2012), 51-60.

Mossah Abdeltawab, Afia I. Sahar, Samia MM. Mohafeash, Badawi A. Abou-Awad. "Formulation and Characterization of Garlic (*Allium sativum* L.) Essential Oil nanoemulsion and its Acaricidal Activity on

Eriophyid Olive Mites (Acari: Eriophyidae)." *Environmental Science and Pollution Research International*, vol. 25, no. 3 (November 2017: 10526-10537.

Nasri Sima, Anoush Mahdieh, Khatami Nares. "Evaluation of Analgesic and Anti-inflammatory Effects of Fresh Onion Juice in Experimental animals." *African Journal of Pharmacy and Pharmacology*, vol. 6, no. 23, (June 2012), 1679-1684.

Nemat, K; Yadollah, S; Mahmoudi, M. "Chronic Inflammation and Oxidative Stress as a Major Cause of Age-related Diseases and Cancer". *Recent Patents on Inflammation and Allergy Drug Discover.* vol. 3, no 1, (March 2009), 73-80.

Neves, A; Rosa, S; Gonçalves, J; Rufino, A; Judas, F; Salgueiro, L; Lopes, MC; Cavaleiro, C; Mendes, AF. "Screening of Five Essential Oils for Identification of Potential Inhibitors of IL-1-induced NF-κB Activation and NO Production in Human Chondrocytes: Characterization of the Inhibitory Activity of α-pinene." *Planta Medica*, vol. 76, no. 3, (February 2010), 303-308.

Ntalani Hermeline, Mon-Sang CA. Bouanga, Gelase FN. Ntandou, Dieudonné Mumba Ngoyi, Papy Mandoko Nkoli, Ange Landela, Pascal Robin Ongoka, and Jean-Maurille Ouamba. "Phytochemical Study, Antiplasmodial Activity and Acute Toxicity of the Aqueous Extract of the Stem Bark of *Alstonia boonei* De Wild." *Advancement in Medicinal Plant Research*, vol. 6, no. 3 (January 2018), 33-39.

Obiagwu M. Oluebubechukwu, Chibueze P. Ihekwereme, Lotanna D. Ajaghaku, Basden FC. Okoye. "The Useful Medicinal Properties of the Root-Bark Extract of *Alstonia boonei* (Apocynaceae) May Be Connected to Antioxidant Activity." *ISRN Pharmacology*, vol. 2014, (2014), Article ID 741478, Doi: http://dx.doi.org/10.1155/2014/741478.

Oguakwa JU. "N-α-formylechitamidine, an Alkaloid from *Alstonia boonei*." *Phytochemistry*, vol. 23, no. 11, (November 1984), 2708, 2709.

Oguntimehin, BO; Weyerstah, P; Marschall-Weyerstah, H. "Essential Oil of *Curcuma longa* L." Leaves. *Flavour and Fragrance Journal*, vol. 5, no. 5, (March 1990), 89-90.

Ogunwande A. Isiaka, Avoseh N. Opeyemi, Olasunkanmi N. Kazeem, Lawal O. Adejumobi, Ascrizzi Roberta, Guido Flamini. "Chemical Composition, Anti-nociceptive and Anti-inflammatory Activities of Essential Oil of *Bougainvillea glabra*". *Journal of Ethnopharmacology.*, vol. 232, (February 2019a), 188-192.

Ogunwande A. Isiaka, Avoseh N. Opeyemi, Igile O. Daniel, Lawal O. Adejumobi, Ascrizzi Roberta, Guido Flamini. "Chemical Constituents, Anti-nociceptive and Anti-inflammatory Activities of Essential Oil of *Phyllanthus muellerianus*". *Natural Product Communications.*, vol. 14, no. 7, (July 2019b), 1-7.

Oigiangbe O. Nathaniel, Igbinosa I. Benjamin, Tamo Manuele. "Insecticidal Activity of the Medicinal Plant, *Alstonia boonei* De Wild, against *Sesamia calamistis* Hampson." *Journal of Zhejiang University. Science. B*, vol. 8, no. 10, (October 2007), 752-755.

Oigiangbe O. Nathaniel, Igbinosa I. Benjamin, Tamo Manuele. "Insecticidal Properties of an Alkaloid from *Alstonia boonei* De Wild." *Journal of Biopesticides*, vol. 3, no. 1, (January 2010), 265-270.

Ojo O. Durojaye, Rachael F. Ogunleye. "Comparative Effectiveness of the Powders of some Underutilized Botanicals for the Control of *Callosobruchus maculatus* (Coleoptera: Bruchidae)." *Journal of Plant Diseases and Protection*, vol. 120, no. 5/6, (December 2013), 227-232

Okwu E. Donaatus, Ighodaro U. Benson. "GC-MS Evaluation of Bioactive Compounds and Antibacterial Activity of the Oil Fraction from the Leaves of *Alstonia boonei* De Wild." *Der Pharma Chemica*, vol. 2, no. 1, (2010), 261-262.

Opoku Francis, Osei Akoto. "Antimicrobial and Phytochemical Properties of Alstonia Boonei Extracts." *Organic Chemistry Current Research*, vol. 4, no. 1, (January 2014), 137-140.

Oyemitan A. Idris, Christianah A. Elusiyan, Ayoola O. Onifade, Moses A. Akanmu, Adebola O. Oyedeji, Armando G. McDonald. "Neuropharmacological Profile and Chemical Analysis of Fresh Rhizome Essential Oil of *Curcuma longa* (Turmeric) Cultivated in Southwest Nigeria." *Toxicoloy Reports*, vol. 4, (2017), 391-398.

Park Il-Kwon, Sang-Chul Shin. "Fumigant Activity of Plant Essential Oils and Components from Garlic (*Allium sativum*) and Clove Bud (*Eugenia caryophyllata*) Oils against the Japanese Termite (*Reticulitermes speratus* Kolbe)." *Journal of Agriculture and Food Chemistry*, vol. 53, no 11, (April 2005), 4388-4392.

Peng, D; Wang, XQ. "Reticulate Evolution in *Thuja* Inferred from Multiple Gene Sequences: Implications for the Study of Biogeographical Disjunction Between Eastern Asia and North America." *Molecular Phylogenetics and Evolution*, vol. 47, no. (June 2008), 1190-1202.

Puškárová Andrea, Mária Bučková, Lucia Kraková, Domenico Pangallo, Katarína Kozics. "The Antibacterial and Antifungal Activity of Six Essential Oils and Their Cytogenotoxicity to Human HEL 12469 Cells." *Scientific Reports*, vol. 7, no. 8211, (August 2017), 8211. DOI:10.1038/s41598-017-08673-9.

Romeilah M. Ramy, Fayed A. Sayed; Ghada I. Mahmoud. "Chemical Compositions, Antiviral and Antioxidant Activities of Seven Essential Oils." *Journal of Applied Science Research*, vol. 6, no 1, (January 2010), 50-62.

Rui, Li; Chen, WC; Wang, WP; Tian, WY; Zhang, XG. "Extraction of Essential Oils from Garlic (*Allium sativum*) using Ligarine as Solvent and its Immunity Activity in Gastric Cancer Rat". *Medicinaal Chemistry Research*, vol. 19, no. 9, (December 2009), 1092-1105.

Satyal Prabodh, Jonathan D. Craft, Noura S. Dosoky; William N. Setzer. "The Chemical Compositions of the Volatile Oils of Garlic (*Allium sativum*) and Wild Garlic (*Allium vineale*)." *Foods*, vol. 6, no. 8, (August 2017), 63-74. Doi: 10.3390/foods6080063.

Saraswathi, V; Mathuram, V; Subramanian, S; Govindasamy, S. "Modulation of the Impaired Drug Metabolism in Sarcoma-180 Bearing Mice by Echitamine Chloride." *Cancer Biochemistry Biophysics*, vol. 17, no. 1-2, (July 1999), 79-88.

Schmidt Erich, Boris Ryabchenko, Juergen Wanner, Walter Jäger; Leopold Jirovetz. "Cytotoxic Active Constituents of Essential Oils of *Curcuma longa* and *Curcuma zanthorrhiza*." *Natural Product Communications*, vol. 10, no. 1, (January 2015), 139-141.

Shah, SMM; Ullah, F; Shah, SMH; Zahoor, M; Sadiq, A. "Analysis of Chemical Constituents and Antinociceptive Potential of Essential Oil of *Teucrium Stocksianum* bioss Collected from the North West of Pakistan." *BMC Complementary Alternative Medicine*, vol. 12, (2012), 244.

Spelman, K; Burns, JJ; Nichols, D; Winters, N; Ottersberg, S; Tenborg, M. "Modulation of Cytokine Expression by Traditional Medicines: a Review of Herbal Immunomodulators." *Alternative Medicine Review*, vol. 11, no. 2, (June 2006), 128-150.

Usman A. Lamidi, Hamid, AA; George, OC; Ameen, OM; Muhammad, NO; Zubair, MF; Lawal, A. "Chemical Composition of Rhizome Essential Oil of *Curcuma longa* L. growing in North Central Nigeria." *World Journal of Chemistry*, vol. 4, no. 2, (July-December 2009), 178-181.

Üstüner Tamer, Saban Kordali; Ayse U. Bozhüyük. "Herbicidal and Fungicidal Effects of *Cuminum cyminum*, *Mentha longifolia* and *Allium sativum* Essential Oils on Some Weeds and Fungi." *Record of Natural Products*, vol. 12, no. 6, (November-December 2018), 619-629.

Tsiri, D; Graikou, K; Pobłocka-Olech, L; Krauze-Baranowska, M; Spyropoulos, C; Chinou, I. "Chemosystematic Value of the Essential Oil Composition of *Thuja* species Cultivated in Poland-Antimicrobial Activity." *Molecules*, vol. 14, no. 11, (November 2009), 4707-4715. Doi: 10.3390/molecules14114707.

Von Rudloff Ernst. "Gas-liquid Chromatography of Terpenes VI. The Volatile Oil of *Thuja plicata* Donn." *Phytochemistry*, vol. 1, no. 3, (September 1962), 195-202.

Von Rudloff Ernst, Lapp S. Martin, Yeh C. Francis. "Chemosystematics Study of *Thuja plicata*: Multivariate Analysis of Leaf Oil Terpene Composition." *Biochemical Systematics and Ecology*, vol. 16, no. 2, (January 1988), 119-125.

Ya Nkono BL. Nkono, Selestin D. Sokeng, Dzeufiet DP. Désiré; Pierre Kamtchouing. "Antihyperglycemic and Antioxidant Properties of *Alstonia boonei* De Wild. (Apocynaceae) Stem Bark Aqueous Extract in Dexamethasone-Induced Hyperglycemic Rats." *International*

Journal of Experimental Diabetes Research, vol. 3, no. 3, (January 2014), 27-35.

Yazdgerdian R. Aurash, Yasmin Akhtar; Murray B. Isman. "Insecticidal Effects of Essential Oils against Woolly Beech Aphid, *Phyllaphis fagi* (Hemiptera: Aphididae) and Rice Weevil, *Sitophilus oryzae* (Coleoptera: Curculionidae)." *Journal of Entomology and Zoology Studies*, vol. 3, no. 3, (March 2015), 265-271.

Yipel Fulya Altinok, Abuzer Acar; Mustafa Yipel. "Effect of Some Essential oils (*Allium sativum* L., *Origanum majorana* L.) and Ozonated Olive Oil on the Treatment of Ear Mites (*Otodectes cynotis*) in Cats." *Turkish Journal of Veterinary and Animal Sciences*, vol. 40, no. 6, (December 2016), 782-787.

Yoon, WJ; Kim, SS; Oh, TH; Lee, NH; Hyun, CG. "*Torreya nucifera* Essential Oil Inhibits Skin Pathogen Growth and Lipopolysaccharide-induced Inflammatory Effects." *International Journal of Pharmacology*, vol. 5, no. 1, (February 2009), 37, 43.

Zhao Na-Na, Hang Zhang, Xue Chang-Zhang, Xiao Bing-Luan, Cheng Zhou, Qi Zhi-Liu, Wang Peng-Shi; Zhi Long-Liu. "Evaluation of Acute Toxicity of Essential Oil of Garlic (*Allium sativum*) and Its Selected Major Constituent Compounds against Overwintering *Cacopsylla chinensis* (Hemiptera: Psyllidae)". *Journal of Economic Entomology*, vol. 106, no. 3, (June 2013), 1349-1354. Doi: https://doi.org/10.1603/EC12191.

Zhu, Q; Sun, Y; Yun, X; Yuntao, O; Zhang, W; Jun-Xu, L. "Antinociceptive Effects of Curcumin in a Rat Model of Postoperative Pain." *Scientific Reports*, vol. 4, (2014), 4932.

Reviewed by:

Dr. Emmanuel Essien, Associate Professor, Department of Chemistry, University of Uyo, AKwa Ibom State, Nigeria

In: What to Know about Essential Oils ISBN: 978-1-53617-986-6
Editor: Malene M. Kjeldsen

Chapter 3

BIOLOGICAL POTENTIALS OF ESSENTIAL OIL: ANTIMICROBIAL ACTIVITY, LARVICIDAL EFFICACY AND CHEMICAL COMPOSITIONS OF ESSENTIAL OILS FROM *ALPINIA MALACCENSIS* (ZINGIBERACEAE) FROM VIETNAM

***Do Ngoc Dai*[1,*]*, Le Thi Huong*[2]*, Nguyen Huy Hung*[3]*, Hoang Van Chinh*[4] *and Isiaka A. Ogunwande*[5,*]

[1]Faculty of Agriculture, Forestry and Fishery, Nghe An College of Economics, Vinh City, Nghe An Province, Vietnam

[2]School of Natural Science Education, Vinh University, Vinh City, Nghệ An Province, Vietnam

[3]Center for Advanced Chemistry, Institute of Research and Development, Duy Tan University, Da Nang, Vietnam

[4]Facculty of Science and Natural, Hong Duc University, Thanh Hoa Province, Vietnam

[5]Foresight Institute of Research and Translation, Ibadan, Nigeria

[*] Corresponding Author's Email: daidn23@gmail.com and isiakaogunwande@gmail.com.

ABSTRACT

The chemical compositions, antimicrobial activity and mosquito larvicidal action of essential oils from the leaves, pseudo-stem, rhizome and fruits of *Alpinia malaccensis* grown in Vietnam are being reported. The essential oils were obtained by hydrodistillation of the different parts of the plant using Clevenger-type apparatus. The oils were separately analysed using gas chromatography-flame ionization detector (GC-FID) and gas chromatography coupled with mass spectrometry (GC-MS). The Minimum inhibitory concentration (MIC) values of the antimicrobial activity of the essential oils were determined by the micro-dilution broth susceptibility assay using eight standardized American Type Culture Collection (ATCC) strains. The mortality rate and larvicidal activity of the essential oils against fourth-instar larvae of *Aedes albopictus* and *Culex quinquefasciatus* were evaluated according to World Health Organization protocol. The yields of the essential oils were 0.23%, 0.19%, 0.25% and 0.40% (v/w), for the leaf, pseudo-stem, rhizome and fruit of the plant respectively, calculated on dry weight basis. The main constituents of the leaf oil were β-eudesmol (33.3%), β-pinene (22.5%) and δ-cadinene (8.9%). The quantitatively significant compounds of the pseudo-stem oil were β-pinene (40.8%), τ-muurolol (10.7%), α-phellandrene (9.1%) and β-phellandrene (9.1%). However, β-pinene (24.3%), β-phellandrene (16.7%), benzyl salicylate (8.9%) and farnesol (8.1%) were the most abundant compounds in the rhziome oil. Moreover, the principal constituents in the fruit oil were methyl cinnamate (16.5%), germacrene D (16.4%) and δ-cadinene (11.8%).

The results of antimicrobial study indicated that the studied essential oil samples exhbited potent and varying activity towards the tested microorganisms with MIC vaues ≤ 50.0 μg/mL. The pseudo-stem and fruits of *A. malaccensis* inhibited the growth of *Escherichia coli* (ATCC 25922; MIC 50 μg/mL) and *Saccharomyces cerevisiae* (ATCC 16404; MIC < 50 μg/mL). Only the fruit essential oil displayed microbial action against *Pseudomonas aeruginosa* (ATCC 25923; MIC < 50 μg/mL). Essential oils from fruits and rhizome exhibited antimicrobial activity on *Staphylococcus aureus* subsp. *aureus* (ATCC 11632; MIC < 50 μg/mL). The leaf, pseudo-stem and fruit oils also showed activity against *Aspergillus niger* (ATCC 9763; MIC 50 μg/mL). Only the rhizome oil displayed potential antimicrobial action against *Fusarium oxysporum* (ATCC 48112; MIC 50 μg/mL). However, all the oil samples did not inhibited the growth of *Bacillus subtilis* (ATCC 11774) and *Candida albicans* (ATCC 10231). All the tested essential oils displayed mortality (100%) against the mosquito vectors. In addition, the essential showed potential larvicidal action with reasonable minimum lethal concentrations

(LC_{50} and LC_{90}) values at 24 h and 48 h comparable with established standards.

In conclusion, the antimicrobial and larvicidal activities of essential oils from different parts of *A. malaccensis* revealed that the oils could be considered as a potentially alternative source for developing novel formulation for controlling diseases.

Keywords: *Alpinia malaccensis,* essential oil, monoterpenes, sesquiterpenes, antimicrobial activity, larvicidal activity

INTRODUCTION

Vietnam is among one of the biodiversity rich countries in the world. The country occupies the eastern and southern part of the Indo-Chinese peninsula in Southeast Asia. Vietnam covers an area 3,31,123 km^2 (north to south length of 1,650 km) along with south China sea coast, China in the north and Laos and Cambodia are in the west with 63 provinces (Hanh et al., 2014). The genus *Alpinia* is the largest, most widespread and taxonomically complex genus under family Zingiberaceae with 230 species occurring throughout the tropical and subtropical Asia (Sri Lanka and the Western Ghats of India to China, Japan, all of Southeast Asia, the Pacific as far as Fiji, Samoa, and the Caroline Islands, and Australia as far south as northern New South Wales (Smith, 1990). The genus is one of the important medicinal plants in Vietnam, which has a greater role in day to day life of Vietnamese people. Many species are traditionally used in folk remedies to treat diseases. Juice obtained from boiled rhizomes of *A. malaccensis* was used to treat intestinal diseases and crushed rhizomes used to treat scabies (Hanh et al., 2014). The leaf extracts was shown to possess antimicrobial (Habsah et al., 2000), antioxidant (Habsah et al., 2000; Sahoo et al., 2012) and potent cytotoxic (Thu et al., 2010) activities. Phytochemical investigation has led to the isolation of 5,6-dehydrokawain, coronarin E, coronarin A, (E)-8(17), 12-labdadiene-15,16-dial, hedyforrestin B, cardamonin, pinocembrin and alpinetin (Nuchnipa & Suksamrarn, 2008). Essential oils have also been extracted from various parts of the plant grown in Vietnam. Earlier report revealed the abundance of β-Pinene (56.0%) and α-pinene (10.3%) in the leaf oil while β-pinene (46.0%), β-phellandrene (12.1%) and α-pinene (9.8%) were the major compounds in the pseudo-stem (Huong et al., 2015). The main constituents in the root oil were β-pinene (31.7%) and β-phellandrene (12.9%) while methyl cinnamate (27.8%), β-pinene (18.5%) and β-phellandrene (12.9%) were the most prominent compounds in the fruit oil (Huong et al., 2015). The antioxidant, antimicrobial and locomotor inhibitory activities of the oils had also been established (Muchtaridi et al., 2013; Sahoo et al., 2014).

Vietnam is classified as a hyperendemic dengue country. Cases of dengue fever epidemics have increased in frequency over the year. Dengue fever and other related diseases are transmitted by mosquitoes such as *Aedes albopictus, Aedes aegypti* and *Culex quinquefasciatus* (Hung et al., 2019). Chemical controls of these vectors have negative impact on the environment and humans in addition to being expensive. Thus, efforts are on in searching for alternative natural insecticides from plants with little or no side effects.

The purpose of this research was to determine the killing power (mortality) and larvicidal activity of the leaf, pseudo-stem, rhizome and fruits essential oil of *A. maaccensis* against the fourth-instant larvae of *Ae. albopictus, Ae. aegypti* and *Cx quinquefasciatus*. In addition, the effect of the essential oils on some microorganism was also determined. This is in continuation of our extensive research aimed at sourcing for biologically active products to combat the spread of the vector mosquitoes and microorganisms (Ban et al., 2019; Hung et al., 2019).

METHODS

Plants Collection

The leaves, pseudo-stem, rhizome, fruits of *A. malaccensis* were collected from Xuân Thái Commune, Bến En, National Park, Thanh Hoa, Vietnam, in August 2018. Botanical identification was achieved by Dr. Dai.

A voucher specimen NTC 291 was deposited at the Botany Museum, Vinh University, Vietnam.

Preparation of Samples

In the course of preparation for hydrodisitillation process, the leaves, pseudo-stem, rhizome and fruits of *A. malaccensis* were air-dried (22^0C) under laboratory shade for two weeks to reduce the moisture contents. Moreover, unwanted materials were also removed by handpicking. Afterwards, samples were pulverized to coarse powder using a locally made grinder.

Hydrodistillation Procedure

Air-dried and pulverized (2000 g each) leaves, pseudo-stem, rhizomes and fruits of *A. malaccensis* were separately subjected to hydrodistillation for 3 h using Clevenger-type apparatus according to established specification (Vietnamese Pharmacopeia, 1990) at different time. Known weight of samples was separately and carefully introduced into a 5 L flask and distilled water was added until it covers the sample completely. Essential oils were obtained hydrodistillation which was carried out in an all glass Clevenger-type distillation unit designed according to established protocol (Vietnamese Pharmacopoeia, 1990). The distillation time was 3 h and conducted at normal pressure. The volatile oils which distilled over water were collected by running through the tap in the receiver arm of the apparatus into clean and previously weighed sample bottles. The oils were kept under refrigeration (4^oC) until the moment of analyses as described previously (Ban et al., 2019).

Gas Chromatography (GC) Analysis

Gas chromatography (GC) analysis was performed on an Agilent Technologies HP 6890 Plus Gas chromatograph equipped with a FID and fitted with HP-5MS column (30 m x 0.25 mm, film thickness 0.25 μm, Agilent Technology). The analytical conditions were: carrier gas He (1 mL/min), injector temperature at 250°C, detector temperature 260°C, column temperature programmed from 40°C (2 min hold) to 220°C (10 min hold) at 4°C/min. Samples were injected by splitting and the split ratio was 10:1. The volume of diluted oil in hexane (1: 10) injected was 1.0 μL. Inlet pressure was 6.1 kPa. Each analysis was performed in triplicate. The relative amounts of individual components were determined on normalized percentages.

Gas Chromatography-Mass Spectrometry (GC/MS) Experiment

An Agilent Technologies HP 6890N Plus Chromatograph fitted with capillary HP-5 MS column (30 m x 0.25 mm, film thickness 0.25 μm) and interfaced with a mass spectrometer HP 5973 MSD was used for this experiment, under the same conditions as those used for gas chromatography analysis as described previously (Ban et al., 2019). The GC conditions were the same as described above with He (1 mL/min) as carrier gas. The MS conditions were as follows: ionization voltage 70eV; emission current 40 mA; acquisitions scan mass range of 35-350 amu at a sampling rate of 1.0 scan/s.

Identification of the Components of the Oils

The identification of constituents from the GC/MS spectra of Z.*nitens* and *Z. castaneum* was performed on the basis of retention indices (RI) determined with reference to a homologous series of *n*-alkanes (C_4-C_{40}), under identical experimental conditions. In some cases, co-injection with known compounds or standards (Sigma-Aldrich, St. Louis, MO, USA) under the same GC conditions was employed. The mass spectral (MS) fragmentation patterns were checked with those of other essential oils of known composition (NIST, 2011) and with those in the literature as described previously (Ban et al., 2019).

Larvicidal Activity

Rearing of Mosquito Larvae

Adults of *Culex quinquefasciatus, Aedes aegypti* and *Aedes albopictus* were collected in Hoa Khanh Nam ward, Lien Chieu district, Da Nang city (16°03'14.9"N, 108°09'31.2"E). Adult mosquitoes were maintained in entomological cages (40 x 40 x 40 cm) and fed a 10% sucrose solution and were allowed to blood feed on mice. Eggs hatching were induced with tap water. Larvae were reared in plastic trays (24×35×5 cm). The larvae were fed on dog biscuits and yeast powder in the 3:1 ratio. All stages were held at 25 ± 2°C, 65–75% relative humidity, and a 12:12 h light:dark cycle at the Center for Entomology and Parasitology Research, Duy Tan University.

Larvicidal Test

Larvicidal activity of the essential oils from *A. malaccensis* was evaluated according to established method (WHO, 2005) with slight modifications. For the assay, aliquots of the essential oils from both samples dissolved in EtOH (1% stock solution) was placed in a 200-mL beaker and added to water that contained 20 larvae (fourth instar). With each experiment, a set of controls using EtOH was also run for comparison. Mortality was recorded after 24 h and again after 48 h of exposure during which no nutritional supplement was added. The experiments were carried out 25 ± 2°C. The larvicidal test was conducted with four replicates using four concentrations (100, 50, 25 and 12.5 μg/mL).

The mortality rate was calculated according to the formula

Mc = (Mo)/(Mt) × 100

Mo = number of larvae dead in the treated groups, Mt = number of larvae introduced and Mc = calculated mortality

Antimicrobial Activity Assay

Test Microbes

Eight standardized ATCC strains from laboratory stock cultures were used in the evaluation of the antimicrobial activity of the oil samples. The Gram negative strains were *Escherichia coli* (ATCC 25922) and *Pseudomonas aeruginosa* (ATCC 25923). The Gram positive strains were *Bacillus subtilis* (ATCC 11774), *Staphylococcus aureus* subsp. *aureus* (ATCC 11632), *Aspergillus niger* (ATCC 9763) and *Fusarium oxysporum* (ATCC 48112). Two strains of yeast, *Candida albicans* (ATCC 10231) and *Saccharomyces cerevisiae* (ATCC 16404) were also used for the experiment. Testing media included Mueller-Hinton Agar (MHA) used for bacteria and Sabouraud Agar (SA) used for fungi.

Microdilution Broth Susceptibility Assay

The minimum inhibitory Concentration (MIC) values were measured by the microdilution broth susceptibility assay (Vlietnick, 1999). For the assays, the essential oil was diluted with DMSO and loaded into the microtiter plate with each of the microbial strains. The plate was then incubated overnight at 37°C. One hundred microlitre of microbial culture of an approximate inoculums size of 1.0 x 10^6 CFU/mL was added to all well and incubated at 37°C for 24 h. The last row, containing only the serial dilutions of sample without microorganisms, was used as a negative control. Sterile distilled water and DMSO served as a positive control. The MIC values were determined as the lowest concentration of the test sample that completely inhibits the growth of microorganisms.

Statistical Analysis

The data obtained were subjected to log-probit analysis (Finney 2009) to obtain LC_{50} values, LC_{90} values, 95% confidence limits, and chi square values using XLSTAT v. 2018.5 (Addinsoft, Paris, France). Statistical analysis of the differences between mean values obtained for experimental groups were calculated as a mean of standard deviation (SD) of four independent measurements using Microsoft excel program 2003.

RESULTS AND DISCUSSION

Chemical Constituents of the Essential Oil

The yields of the essential oils were 0.23%, 0.19%, 0.25% and 0.40% (v/w), for the leaf, pseudo-stem, rhizome and fruit respectively, calculated on a dry weight basis. The fruit sample produced larger quantity of essential oils than other parts of the plant. The identities, retention indices and percent compositions of the oils are shown in Table 1. A total of 25, 25, 41 and 26 compounds that represented 99.1, 96.2, 93.4and 94.4% of the oils were identified in the leaf, pseudo-stem, rhizome and fruit essential oils respectively. The main classes of terpenoids identified in the leaf oil were hydrocarbon monoterpenes (43.3%), hydrocarbon sesquiterpenes (15.0%) and oxygenated sesquiterpenoids (35.7%). The major constituents of the leaf oil were β-eudesmol (33.3%), β-pinene (22.5%) and δ-cadinene (8.9%). There are significant amount of α-pinene (5.7%), camphene (5.3%) and γ-cadinene (4.0%). The abundance of β-pinene revealed that the oil was of β-pinene chemotype. This was similar to the β-pinene chemotype earlier reported for the leaf essential oil of the plant grown in Vietnam (Huong et al., 2015) and Indonesia (Muchtaridi et al., 2013). However, essential oil from this work contained lower amount of α-pinene and higher quantity of β-eudesmol compared to the leaf oils of the Vietnamese and Indonesian grown plants. Meanwhile, the leaf oil contained low amount of methyl cinnamate which compared favourably with the leaf oil of the Vietnamian grown plant (Huong et al., 2015). In the same vein, hydrocarbon monoterpenes (73.6%), and oxygenated sesquiterpenoids (16.1%) were the most abundant classes of terpenoids present in the pseudo-stem oil. The pseudo-stem oil was predominated by β-pinene (40.8%), τ-muurolol (10.7%), α-phellandrene (9.1%), β-phellandrene (9.1%) and α-pinene (7.2%). Other notable compounds in the oil includes; α-phellandrene (7.1%), α-pinene (6.9%) and methyl cinnamate (6.0%). This compositional pattern of the pseudo-stem differs from the result obtained from the oils of the Indonesian (Muchtaridi et al., 2013) and Malaysian grown plants (Nor et al., 2005) that were predominated by methyl cinnamate, 1,8-cineole, α-pinene and β-pinene. In addition, the stem oil from this work contained lower amount of methyl cinnamate and 1,8-cineole was not detected when compared to the other oils from the literature. Interestingly, the high amount of τ-muurolol in the oil is noteworthy as this compound has not been reported before as a major compound in the pseudo-stem oil of *A. malaccensis*.

Hydrocarbon monoterpenenes (64.2%), and oxygenated sesquiterpenes (18.4%) were the major classes of terpenoids in the rhizome essential oil with predominant of β-pinene (24.3%), β-phellandrene (16.7%), benzyl salicylate (8.9%) and farnesol (8.1%) (Table 1). In the earlier reports, compounds such as 1,8-cineole found in the oil of the Bangladesh grown sample (Bhuiyan et al., 2010) and *p*-cymene and sabinene in the oil of the Indian grown sample (Gaj et al., 2010; Sahoo et al., 2014) were not detected in this oil. (*E*)-cinnamate and o-cymene that were the main constituents of the essential oils from the rhizome of Malaysian and Bangladesh grown *A. malaccencis* (Sirat et al., 2011; Bhuiyan et al., 2010) were detected in much lower quantities in this study. However, the higher amounts of α-phellandrene and β-pinene in the rhizome oil had been reported previously (Bhuiyan et al., 2010; Sahoo et al., 2014). However, the fruit oil was devoid of any oxygenated sesquiterpene compounds. The main class of compounds identified in the oil were hydrocarbon monoterpenes (15.4%), oxygenated monoterpenoids (16.0%) and hydrocarbon sesquiterpenes (62.6%). Moreover, the most abundant constituents in the fruit oil were; methyl cinnamate (16.5%), germacrene D (16.4%) and δ-cadinene (11.8%). Other prominent constituents in the oil were benzyl acetate (7.3%) and limonene (5.3%). The higher quantity of methyl cinnamate in the oil confers similarity with previous report (Huong et al., 2015). The previous study (Huong et al., 2015) contained higher amounts of β-pinene and β-phellandrene, while the proportion of germacrene D and δ-cadinene are higher than in the previous study.

Table 1. Chemical Composition of essential oils from different parts of *A. malaccensis*

Sr. No	Compounds [a]	RI b	RI c	Percent composition (%)			
				Leaf	Pseudo-stem	Rhizome	Fruit
1	α-Thujene	930	921	-	0.4	0.3	-
2	α-Pinene	939	932	5.7	7.2	6.9	0.6
3	Camphene	953	946	5.3	1.6	2.0	-
4	Sabinene	976	964	-	-	-	2.7
5	β-Pinene	980	978	22.5	40.8	24.3	3.0
6	β-Myrcene	990	988	0.5	1.5	1.6	0.9
7	α-Phellandrene	1006	1004	1.3	9.1	7.1	-
8	δ-3-Carene	1011	1008	4.5	-	0.1	-
9	α-Terpinene	1017	1014	-	0.7	0.5	-
10	o-Cymene	1024	1022	3.0	1.3	1.2	-
11	β-Phellandrene	1028	1026	-	9.1	16.7	-
12	Limonene	1032	1030	-	-	-	5.3
13	1,8-Cineole	1034	1032	-	-	-	0.8
15	(E)-β-Ocimene	1052	1044	-	0.5	1.6	-
16	γ-Terpinene	1061	1056	0.5	1.0	1.0	1.5
17	α-Terpinolene	1090	1089	-	0.6	0.8	-
18	Linalool	1100	100	-	-	0.1	-
19	*allo*-Ocimene	1128	1128	-	-	0.1	1.4
20	Camphor	1145	1145	2.1	0.6	0.4	-
21	Benzyl acetate	1162	1160	-	-	-	7.3
22	Pinocarvone	1165	1164	-	-	-	3.2
23	Borneol	1167	1167	0.9	-	0.2	2.0
24	Terpinene-4-ol	1177	1177	0.4	0.7	0.4	1.3
25	α-Terpineol	1189	1189	-	-	0.3	1.8
26	α-Fenchyl aceate	1222	1220	-	-	0.4	-
27	(*Z*)-Citral	1318	1318	-	0.4	0.1	-
28	Bicycloelemene	1327	1337	-	-	-	1.5
29	β-Citronellol	1344	1340	-	0.7	-	-
30	Linalyl propionate	1346	1345	-	0.9	-	-
31	α-Cubebene	1351	1345	-	-	-	1.1
32	α-Copaene	1377	1374	-	-	-	1.3
33	Methyl cinnamate	1379	1378	0.8	1.9	6.0	16.5

Table 1. (Continued)

Sr. No	Compounds [a]	RI b	RI c	Percent composition (%)			
				Leaf	Pseudo-stem	Rhizome	Fruit
34	β-Elemene	1391	1389	-	-	0.4	2.5
35	β-Caryophyllene	1419	1417	0.3	-	0.3	0.9
36	α-Bergamotene	1435	1435	-	-	-	1.5
37	γ-Elemene	1437	1437	-	-	0.1	-
38	α-Guaiene	1440	1440	-	-	-	1.5
39	Aromadendrene	1441	1441	-	-	-	3.8
40	α-Humulene	1454	1452	-	-	0.2	-
41	γ-Gurjunene	1477	1477	-	-	0.5	-
42	Germacrene D	1485	1484	-	-	-	16.4
43	β-Selinene	1486	1486	-	-	0.3	2.3
44	Zingiberene	1494	1493	1.0	-	0.5	-
45	Bicyclogermacrene	1500	1500	0.4	-	-	1.5
46	β-Bisabolene	1506	1503	0.4	-	0.4	-
47	(*E,E*)-α-Farnesene	1508	1505	-	-	0.1	-
48	2,4-bis(1,1-dimethylethyl)-Phenol	1513	1513	0.5	0.4	0.4	-
49	δ-Cadinene	1525	1522	8.9	-	-	11.8
50	γ-Cadinene	1541	1539	4.0	-	-	-
51	β-Sesquiphellandrene	1543	1541	-	-	0.3	-
52	(*E*)-Nerolidol	1563	1561	0.9	0.9	0.3	-
53	Spathulenol	1578	1577	0.5	0.5	-	-
54	2,6-di-t-Butyl-4-ethylene-2,5-cyclohexadiene-1-one	1583	1579	-	-	0.4	-
55	Caryophyllene oxide	1583	1581	0.7	0.4	0.1	-
56	Viridiflorol	1593	1593	-	2.6	-	-
57	Guaiol	1601	1600	0.3	1.9	-	-
58	τ-Muurolol	1646	1644	-	10.7	-	-
59	β-Eudesmol	1651	1650	33.3	-	-	-
60	α-Bisabolol	1662	1662	-	-	0.2	-
61	Bulnesol	1672	1672	-	-	0.3	-
62	Farnesol [d]	1718	1718	-	-	8.1	-
63	Benzyl benzoate	1760	1760	-	-	0.2	-
64	Benzyl salicylate	1866	1866	-	-	8.9	-
65	Phytol	2125	2119	0.4	-	-	-
Total				99.1	96.2	93.4	94.4
Monoterpene hydrocarbons				42.3	73.6	64.2	15.4
Oxygenated monoterpenes				4.2	5.2	7.2	16.0
Sesquiterpene hydrocarbons				15.0	0.9	2.8	62.6
Oxygenated sesquiterpenes				35.7	16.1	18.4	-
Diterpenes				0.4	-	-	-
Non-terpenes				0.5	0.4	0.8	-

[a] Elution order on HP-5MS column; [b] Retention indices on HP-5MS column; [c] Literature retention indices; [d] Correct isomer not identified; Sr. No, Serial Number; - Not identified.

Mortality of the Essential Oils Against Vector Mosquitoes

The leaf oil of *A. malaccensis* also exhibited 100% mortality against *Ae. albopictus* (concentration, 100 μg/mL) at both testing periods of 24 h and 48 h. However, the oil displayed much more potent mortality (100%) against *Ae. aegypti* at a much lower concentrations of 25 μg/mL (48 h) and 50 μg/mL (24 h and 48 h) as seen in Table 2. On the other hand, the rhizome oil achieved the same mortality rate only against *Cx. quinquefasciatus* at concentration of 100 μg/mL over the same test periods of 24 h and 48 h. The leaf oil was more toxic towards *Ae. aegypti* than *A. albopictus*. The rate of susceptibility of the vectors towards the rhizome oil of *A. malaccensis* was *Ae. aegypti* > *Cx. quinquefasciatus* > *Ae. albopictus.* There was no mortality in the EtOH used as control for all the tested oil samples. The percentage mortality was dependent on the concentration of the tested oil samples. Thus, higher inhibition of mosquito larvae was observed as concentration increases.

Mosquito Larvicidal Tests

From Table 2, *A. malaccensis* the leaf oil displayed significant larvicidal activity against *Ae. albopictus* with LC_{50} of 33.43 μg/mL (24 h) and 32.52 μg/mL (48 h). However, LC_{90} values of 73.46 μg/mL and 65.50 μg/mL were also recorded respectively at 24 h and 48 h. On the other hand, the leaf essential oil also exhibited greater potent larvicidal action towards *Ae. aegypti* with LC_{50} values of 11.90 μg/mL and LC_{90} 25.65 μg/mL at 24 h, while LC_{50} values of 9.70 μg/mL and LC_{90} of 19.42 μg/mL were obtained at 48 h. Moreover, the rhizome oil sample also showed potential larvicides towards *Cx. quinquefasciatus* with LC_{50} values of 24.58 μg/mL and LC_{90} of 82.45 μg/mL at 24 h. At 48 h test period, however, the oil exhibited larvicidal activity with LC_{50} values of 11.66 μg/mL and LC_{90} of 22.70 μg/mL. Permethrin, the standard drug used as control displayed larvicidal activity at much lower values. These findings showed that the concentrations of test substances affected degree of toxicity and mortality rates.

Overall results in this study showed that essential oils hydrodisitlled from the leaf and rhizome of *A. malaccensis* exhibited good mortality and larvicidal activity on *Ae. albopictus, Ae. aegypti* and *Cx. quinquefasciatus* larvae. The observed larvicidal action of *A. malaccensis* in this study was comparable with findings from essential oils of other *Alpinia* plants in particular and essential oils from other plants in general, analysed for their larvicidal activity from Vietnam and other parts of the world. The rhizome oil of *A. galanga* displayed larvicidal action among others against *Ae. albopictus* (Cotchakaew & Soonwera, 2019). The leaf of *A. speciosa* showed larvicidal action against *Ae. aegypti* larvae with LC_{50} of 1.18 µL/mL (Freitas et al., 2010). Oils from flowers of *A. purpurata* presented potent larvicidal activities against 4th instar *Ae. aegypti* with LC_{50} values of 80.7 and 71.5 ppm, respectively (Santos et al., 2012). The flower essential oil of *A. nigra* was active at 125 ppm (Goshi et al., 2014). Essential oil from *A. zerumbet* flowers exhibited repellent activity, irritating action and toxic activity against the mosquito *Ae. Aegypti* (de Souza et al., 2014). The essential oil of *Z. collinsii* from Vietnam displayed larvicidal action against *Ae. albopictus* (LC_{50} = 25.51 µg/mL; LC_{90} = 40.22 µg/mL) and *Cx. quinquefasciatus* (LC_{50} = 50.11 µg/mL and LC_{90} = 71.53 µg/mL) after 24 h (Huong et al., 2020a). *Zingiber zerumbet* oil showed potent larvicidal activity against *Cx. quinquefasciatus* with LC_{50} of 33.28 µg/mL and 21.81 µg/mL respectively after 24 h and 48 h test period. Moreover, the oil exhibited significant larvicidal action against *Ae. albopictus* within the 24 h and 48 h tested period having LC_{50} of 55.75 µg/mL and 36.22 µg/mL respectively (Huong et al., 2019). The 24 h mosquito larvicidal activity of the rhizome oil of *Z. montanum* from Vietnam (Huong et al., 2020b) was *Ae. albopictus* (LC_{50} = 35.17 µg/mL; LC_{90} = 56.02 µg/mL), *Ae. aegypti* (LC_{50} = 32.20 µg/mL; LC_{90} = 45.64 µg/mL) and *Cx. quinquefasciatus* (LC_{50} = 31.12 µg/mL; LC_{90} = 52.25 µg/mL). Likewise, *Z. cernuum* was toxic towards *Ae. aegypti* (LC_{50} = 44.88 µg/mL), *Ae. albopictus* (LC_{50} = 55.84 µg/mL) and *Cx. quinquefasciatus* (LC_{50} = 48.44 µg/mL) after 24 h (*Rajeswary* et al., 2018). *Zingiber officinale* was shown to have larvicidal activity against *Cx.*

quinquefasciatus with a LC_{50} value of 50.78 ppm (Pushpanathan et al., 2008). The essential oils from the rhizome of *Z. nimmonii* demonstrated significant larvicidal activity against *Ae. aegypti* and *Cx. quinquefasciatus*, with LC_{50} values of 37.6 and 48.1 μg/mL, respectively. The leaf essential oil of *Manglietia dandyi* showed larvicidal potential against *Ae. albopictus* with minimum lethal concentrations LC_{50} values of 29.57 μg/mL (24 h) and 29.02 μg/mL (Ban et al., 2020). The leaf essential oil of *Vitex gardineriana* demonstrated high larvicidal activity against *Ae. aegypti* with LC_{50} value of 28.0 μg/mL (Pereira et al., 2018).

Since the WHO has not established a standard criterion for determining the larvicidal activity of natural products, several authors (Komalamisra et al., 2005; Kiran et al., 2006; Magalhães et al., 2010) have developed individual criteria to characterize the potency of mosquito larvicides developed from natural products. For example, Komalamisra et al. (2005) considered products showing $LC_{50} \leq 50$ mg/L to be active, 50 mg/L $< LC_{50} \leq 100$ mg/L to be moderately active, 100 mg/L $< LC_{50} \leq 750$ mg/L to be effective, and $LC_{50} > 750$ mg/L to be inactive. It should be stressed that these criteria must be directly correlated with the time of exposure and the origin of larvae, which are variables that can alter the LC_{50} values. The results obtained in this study showed that the essential oil of *A. malaccensis* rhizome had promising effects, according to the criterion established previously (Magalhães et al., 2010), exhibiting larvicidal activity against *Ae. albopictus, Ae. aegypti* and *Cx. quinquefasciatus* larvae and stands as a promising tool to manage the phenomenon of insecticides resistant vectors in malaria endemic regions.

The variations in toxicity of essential oils against different species of mosquitoes are common, due to qualitative and quantitative variations of chemical constituents. The larvacidal activity of *A. malaccensis* was likely caused by the wide variety of phytochemicals and volatile composites present in the oil. The observed mosquito larvicidal activity of the leaf and rhizome essential oils may be due to the synergistic actions of the major compounds or some minor compounds present in the oil. Interestingly, the active larvicidal activity of some compounds in this work, including,

Table 2. Percentage mortality and larvicidal action of *A. malaccensis* essential oils

	Leaf essential oil				Rhizome essential oil	
	Ae. albopictus		*Ae. aegypti*		*Cx. quinquefasciatus*	
	24 h	**48 h**	**24 h**	**48 h**	**24 h**	**48 h**
	Mortality (%) [a]					
Concentration (μg/mL)						
12.5	3.75 ±	5.0 ±	37.5 ±	52.5 ±	5.0±	8.75 ±
25	25.0 ± 1.546	25.0± 1.909	96.25 ±	100 ± 0.000	38.73 ±	75.0 ±
50	91.3 ±	93.7 ±	100± 0.000	100 ± 0.000	91.25 ±	96.25 ±
100	100 ± 0.000	100 ± 0.000	100± 0.000	100 ± 0.000	100 ± 0.000	100 ± 0.000
	Minimum lethal concentration (μg/mL)					
Parameters						
LC_{50}	33.43 (27.493 - 49.264)	32.52 (27.284 - 46.397)	11.90 (10.410 -14.353)	9.78 (8.768-11.140)	24.58 (20.140-33.772)	11.66 (10.503-12.928)
LC_{90}	73.46 (49.695 - 175.269)	65.50 (46.052 - 147.128)	25.65 (19.751-40.198)	19.42 (16.019-26.184)	82.45 (52.786-192.523	22.70 (19.658-27.729)
Regression equation	Y = -6.374+ 4.215x	y = -5.713 + 3.748x	Y = -4.132+ 3.842x	Y = -4.264+4.305x	Y = -3.390+ 2.438x	y = -4.724 + 4.428x
X^2	4.821	4.994	6.919	8.055	6.054	9.671
P	0.000	0.000	0.000	0.000	0.000	0.000

[a] (n = 4); There was no mortality in the EtOH controls.

α-pinene, β-pinene, sabinene, limonene, p-cymene, 1,8-cineole, terpinen-4-ol, β-caryophyllene, bicyclogermacrene and germacrene D (Fries et al., 2010; Tabanca et al., 2014; Wafaa et al., 2017) have been documented and reported. The isolation and purification of active compound which could be responsible for the larvicidal activity against mosquito vectors of would be an important step in the development of novel mosquitocidal agents. Production of larvicides from the locally available plants could be a new acceptable alternative to employ which may lead to decreasing dependence on imported synthetic insecticides and be beneficial for developing countries such as Vietnam.

Antimicrobial Test

The results of antimicrobial study indicated that the studied essential oil samples exhbited potent and varying activity towards the tested microorganisms with MIC vaues ≤ 50.0 μg/mL. The pseudo-stem and fruits of *A. malaccensis* inhibited the growth of *E. coli* (MIC 50 μg/mL) and *S. cerevisiae* (MIC < 50 μg/mL). Only the fruit essential oil displayed microbial action against *P. aeruginosa* (MIC < 50 μg/mL). Essential oil from fruits and rhizome exhibited antimicrobial activity on *S. aureus* subsp. *aureus* (MIC < 50 μg/mL). The leaf, pseudo-stem and fruit essential oils also showed activity against *A. niger* (MIC 50 μg/mL). Only the rhizome essential oil displayed potential antimicrobial action against *F. oxysporum* (MIC 50 μg/mL). However, all the oil samples did not inhibited the growth of *B. subtilis* and *C. albicans*. In this test experiment, activity was presumed to occur with MIC ≤ 50 μg/mL while MIC > 50 μg/mL is considered inactive towards the tested microorganism. The observed antimicrobial activity of essential oils from *A. malaccensis* was consistent with a previous report (Sahoo et al., 2014). The antimicrobial actions of the studied oil samples of *A. malaccensis* support the notion that several *Alpinia* essential oils possess antimicrobial activity.

Table 3. Antimicrobial action of *A. malaccensis* essential oils

Microorganisms	MIC µg/mL			
	Leaves	Rhizomes	Pseudo-stem	Fruits
E. coli	-	-	50	50
P. aeruginosa	-	-	-	<50
B. subtilis	-	-	-	-
S. aureus subsp. *aureus*	-	< 50	-	50
Niger	50	-	50	50
F. oxysporum	-	50	-	-
S. cerevisiae	-	-	<50	<50
C. albicans	-	-	-	-

- Not active, MIC > 50 µg/mL.

The oils from unripe and ripe fruits of *A. mutica* showed antimicrobial activity against *B. subtilis* (MIC of 2.50 and 1.25 mg/mL respectively) and *S. aureus* with MIC of 2.50 mg/mL (Ibrahim et al., 2014). However, both oil samples showed no activity against the pathognes *E. coli, P. aeruginosa* and *C. albicans*. The oils of *A. latibaris*, both unripe and ripe, showed inhibition towards *S. aurues* and *B. subtilis* with MIC values between 2.50 mg/mL and 5.0 mg/mL (Ibrahim et al., 2014). Also, the leaf oils of *A. rafflesiana* were active against *E. coli* (MIC 15.6 µg/mL) and *S. aureus* (MIC 7.81 µg/mL) (Jusoh et al., 2013). The rhizome oil of *A. pahangensis* inhibited several strains of *S. aureus* with MIC values between 0.08 and 0.31 µg/µL as well as *C. albicans* and *C. galabrata* with MIC of 1.25 and 2.50 µg/µL respectively (Awang et al., 2011). The oil of *A. galangal* was found to moderately inhibit (MIC values from 1.1-2.2 µg/mL) the growth of *B. subtilis, S. aureus* var. *aureus, Proteus vulgaris, E. coli, A. niger* and *C. albicans* (Yusoff et al., 2011). Also, *A. ligulata* exhibited antimicrobial property against *S. aureus* var. *aureus* and *E. coli* (MIC 3.2 µg/mL) and *A. nieuwenhuizii* inhibited the growth of *E. coli* and *S. aureus* var. *aureus* with MIC of 3.2 and 2.0 µg/mL respectively (Yusoff et al., 2011). The rhizome of *A. galangal* was most active towards *Salmonella typhi* (Eff & Rahayu, 2016). The observed *antimicrobial activity* of *A. malaccensi essential oils* can be related to the compounds present in it. For example, essential oil constituents such as α-pinene, β-pinene, sabinene, 1,8-cineole, terpinen-4-

ol, β-caryophyllene, bicyclogermacrene and germacrene were previously reported to inhibit significantly the growth and cell viability of potential infectious of broad spectrum microorganisms (Yob et al., 2011).

REFERENCES

Awang Khadihaj, Halijah Ibrahim, Devi R. Syamsir, Mastura Mohtar, Ali M. Rasadah, and Mohammad N. Azah. "Chemical Constituents and Antimicrobial Activity of the Leaf and Rhizome Oils of *Alpinia pahangensis* Ridl., and Endemic Wild Ginger from Penninsular Malaysia." *Chemistry and Biodiversity,* vol. 8, no. 4 (April 2011): 668-673.

Ban H. Pham, Dinh D. Le, Huong T. Le, Hoi M. Than, Hung H. Nguyen, Dai D. Ngoc, and Ogunwande A. Isiaka. "Mosquito larvicidal activity on *Aedes albopictus* and constituents of essential oils from *Manglietia dandyi* (Gagnep.) dandy." *Records of Natural Product,* vol. 15 (2020, in press).

Bhuiyan M.N. Islam, Jasim U. Chowdhury, Jaripa Begum, and Nemai C. Nandi. "Essential Oils Analysis of The Rhizomes of *Alpinia conchigera* Griff. and Leaves of *Alpinia malaccensis* (Burm. f.) Roscoe from Bangladesh." *African Journal of Plant Science*, vol. 4, no. 6 (May 2010): 197-201. Doi: 0AE9EEA11766.

Cotchakaew Nuttavich, and Mayura Soonwera. "Toxicity of Several Botanical Essential Oils and Their Combinations Against Females of *Aedes albopictus* (Skuse) and *Anopheles minimus* (Theobald): Oviposition Deterrent, Ovividal and Adulticidal Efficacies." *Asian Pacific Journal of Tropical Biomedicine*, vol. 9, no. 1 (2019): 29-39. DOI: 10.4103/2221-1691.250267.

de Souza de A. Thamiris, Marcio B.P. Lopes, Aline de S. Ramos, José L.P. Ferreira, Jefferson Rocha de A. Silva, Margareth M.C. Queiroz, de Lima A.G. Kátia, and Ana C.F. Amaral. "*Alpinia* Essential Oils and Their Major Components Against *Rhodnius nasutus*, a Vector of Chagas

Disease." *The Scientific World Journal*, vol. 2018 (2018): Article ID 2393858, 6 pages https://doi.org/10.1155/2018/2393858.

Eff R.Y. Aprilita, and Rahayu S. Teguh. "Antibacterial Effects of Essential Oil from Galangarhizome, *Alpinia galangal* (Linn.) on Pierreon Rat (*Ratus Norvegicus* L.) Infected by *Salmonella typhi*." *Asian Journal of Pharmaceutical and Clinical Research,* vol. 9, no. 7 (August 2016): 189-193. https://innovareca.in/journal/index.php/ajpcr/article/view/12879.

Finnih D. *Probit Analysis*; Reissue, Ed, Cambridge University Press, UK (2009).

Freitas P. Flávia, Silvério P. Freitas, Gloria C.S. Lemos, Ivo J.C. Vieira, Geraldo A. Gravina, and Francisco J.A. Lemos. "Comparative Larvicidal Activity of Essential Oils from Three Medicinal Plants Against *Aedes aegypti* L." *Chemistry and Biodiversity*, vol. 7, no. 11 (November 2010): 2801-2807.

Ghosh Sudipta, Temel Ozek, Nurhayat Tabanca, Abbas Ali, Junaidur Rehman, Ikhlas A. Khan, and Latha Rangan. "Chemical Composition and Bioactivity Studies of *Alpinia nigra* Essential Oils." *Industrial Crops and Products*, vol. 53 (February 2014): 111-119, https://doi.org/10.1016/j.indcrop.2013.12.026.

Habsah Mohamad, Amran Mohidin, Mackeen M. Mohamed, Lajis H. Nordin, Kikuzaki Hiroe, Nakatani Nobuji, Abdul Rahman Ahmad, Ghafar A, Ali M. Aied. "Screening of Zingiberaceae Extracts for Antimicrobial and Antioxidant activities." *Journal of Ethnopharmacology,* vol. 72, no. 3 (October 2000): 403-410. DOI:10.1016/s0378-8741(00)00223-3.

Hanh N. Phuong, Nguyen Q. Binh, and Bhupendra S. Adhikari Distribution of *Alpinia* (*Zingiberaceae*) and Their Use Pattern in Vietnam." *Journal of Biodiversity and Endangered Species,* vol. 2, no. 2 (March 2014): 121. doi:10.4172/2332-2543.1000121.

Hung H. Nguyen, Satyal P, Hieu H.V, Chuong N.H.H, Dai N. Do, Huong T. Le, Tai T.A, Setzer N. William. "Mosquito Larvicidal Activity of The Essential Oils of *Erechtites* Species Growing Wild in Vietnam." *Insects*, vol. 10, no. 2 (February 2019): 47-57.

Huong T. Le, Huong T. Trinh, Huong T.T. Nguyen, Hung N. Hung, Dat T.T. Pham, Luong X. Nguo, and Ogunwande A. Isiaka. "Mosquito Larvicidal Activities of The Essential Oil of *Zingiber collinsii* Against *Aedes albopictus* and *Culex quinquefasciatus*." *Journal of Oleo Science,* vol. 69. No. 2 (February 2020a in press).

Huong T. Le, Chinh H.V., An N.T.G., Viet N.T., Hung H. Nguyen, Thuong T.H. Nguyen, and Ogunwande A. Isiaka. "*Zingiber zerumbet* Rhizome Essential Oil: Chemical Constituents, Antimicrobial and Larvicidal Activities." *European Journal of Medicinal Plants,* vol. 30, no. 4 (December 2019): 1-12.

Huong T. Le, Huong T. Trinh, Huong T.T. Nguyen, Hung N. Hung, Dat T.T. Pham, Luong X. Nguo, and Ogunwande A. Isiaka. "Chemical Composition and Larvicidal Activity of Essential Oils from *Zingiber montanum* Against Three Mosquito Vector." *BLACPMA* (2020b in press).

Ibrahim Halijah, Yasodha Sivasothy, Devi R. Syamsir, Noor H. Nagoor, Natasha Jamil, and Khalijah Awang. "Essential Oil Composition and Antimicrobial Activities of Two Closely Related species, *Alpinia mutica* Roxb. and *Alpinia latilabris* Ridl. From Peninsular Malaysia." *The Scientific World Journal,* vol. 2014 (2014): Article ID 430831, 6 pages http://dx.doi.org/10.1155/2014/430831

Jusoh Shariha, Hasnah M. Sirat, and Ahmad Farediah. "Essential Oils of *Alpinia rafflesiana* and Their Antimicrobial Activities." *Natural Product Communication*, vol. 8, no. 9 (September 2013): 1317-1320. https://doi.org/10.1177/1934578X130080093 3.

Kiran S. Ravi, Bhavani K, Devi P.Sita, Rajeswara B.R. Rao, and Reddy K. Janardhan. "Composition and Larvicidal Activity of Leaves and Stem Essential Oils of *Chloroxylon swietenia* DC Against *Aedes aegypti* and *Anopheles stephensi*.'' *Bioresources Technology, vol. 97, no. 18 (December 2006): 2481-2484:* https://doi.org/10.1016/j.biortech. 2005.10.003.

Komalamisra Narumon, Yuwadee Trongtokit, Yupha Rongsriyam, and Chamnarn Apiwathnasorn. "Screening for Larvicidal Activity in Some Thai Plants Against Four Mosquito Vector Species.'' *Southeast Asian*

Journal of Tropical Medicine and Public Health, vol. 36, no. 6 (November 2005): 1412-1422.

Pereira Jose P. Evaristo, Horlando C. Silva, Carlos L. Holanda, Jane E.S.A. de Menezes, Sonia Maria C. Siqueeira, Tigressa Helena S. Rodrigues, Raquel Oliveira S. Fontenelle, do Vale J.C. Parcelli, da Silva T. Priscilla, Maria P. Gilvandete Santiao, and Helcio S. Santos. "Chemical Composition, Cytotoxicity and Larvicidal activity against *Aedes aegypti* of Essential Oils from *Vitex gardineriana* Schauer." *Boletin Latinoamericano y del Caribe de Plantas Medicinales y Aromaticas.* vol. 17, no. 3 (May 2018): 302-309. http://www.revistas.usach.cl/ojs/indes.php/blacpma/article.view 3501.

Pushpanathan Thambusamy, Arulsamy Jebanesan, and Marimuthu Govindarajan. "The Essential oil of *Zingiber officinalis* Linn (Zingiberaceae) as A Mosquito Larvicidal and Repellent Agent Against the Filarial Vector *Culex quinquefasciatus* Say (Diptera: Culicidae)." *Parasitology Research,* vol. 102, no. 6 (May 2008): 1289-1291, https://doi.org/10.1007/s00436-008-0907-6.

Magalhães Lyege, da Paz M. Lima, Marcia O.M. Marques, Facanali Roselaine, da Silva Pinto A. Christiana, and Wanderli Pedro Tade. "Chemical Composition and Larvicidal Activity Against *Aedes aegypti* Larvae of Essential Oils from Four *Guarea* Species." *Molecules.* vol. 15, no. 8 (2010): 5734-5741; https://doi.org/10.3390/molecules 15085734.

Muchtaridi Muchtaridi, Ida Musfiroh, Anas Subarnas, Ikhsan Rambia, Hokcu Suganda, and Enas M. Nasrudin. "Chemical Composition and Locomotors Activity of Essential Oils from the Rhizome, Stem and Leaf of *Alpinia malaccencis* (Burm F.) of Indonesian Spices." *Journal of Applied Pharmaceutical Sciences*, vol. 4, no. 1 (January 2014): 52-56.

National Institute of Science and Technology. Chemistry Web Book Data. Data from Nist Standard Reference Database 69 (2011).

Nor M.A. Azan, Sam Y.Y., Mailina J, and Chua L.S.L. "(*E*)-Methyl cinnamate: The Major Component of Essential Oils of A*lpinia malaccensis* var. *nobilis*." *Journal of Tropical Forest Science,* vol. 17, no. 4 (October 2005): 631-633. https://www.jstor.org/stable/23616599?seq=1.

Nuchnipa Nuntanwong, and Suksamrarn Apichart. "Chemical Constituents of The Rhizomes of *Alpinia malaccensis*." *Biochemical Systematics and Ecology,* vol. 36, no. 8 (August 2008): 661-664. DOI:10.1016/j.bse.2008.04.003.

Raj Gopan, Pradeep D.P., Yusuf C. Ali, Mathew Dan, and Sabulal Baby. "Chemical Profiles of Volatiles in Four *Alpinia* Species From Kerala, South India." *Journal of Essential Oil* Research, vol. 25, no. 2 (March 2013): 97-102. https://doi.org/10.1080/10412905.2012.751058

Rajeswary Mohan, Marimuthu Govindarajan, Naiyf S. Alharbi, Shine Kadaikunnan, Jamal M. Khaled, and Giovanni Benelli. *"Zingiber cernuum (Zingiberaceae) Essential Oil as Effective Larvicide and Oviposition Deterrent on Six Mosquito Vectors, With Little Non-target Toxicity on Four Aquatic Mosquito Predators." Environmental Science and Pollution Research*. vol. 25, no. 11 (April 2018): 10307-10316. *doi:* 10.1007/s11356 -017-9093-3.

Sahoo Suprava, Ghosh Goutam, Nayak Sanghamitra. "Evaluation of *in vitro* Antioxidant Activity of Leaf Extract of *Alpinia malaccensis*." *Journal of Medicinal Plant Research*. vol. 6, no. 23 (June 2012): 4032-4038. DOI: 10.5897/JMPR12.374.

Sahoo Suprava, Shikha Singh, and Sanghamitra Nayak. "Chemical Composition, Antioxidant and Antimicrobial Activity of Essential Oil and Extract of *Alpinia malaccensis* Roscoe (Zingiberaceae)." *International Journal of Pharmacy and Pharmaceutical Sciences*, vol. 6, no. 7, (July 2014): 183-188. https://innovareacademics.in/journals/index.php/ijpps/article/view/1716.

Santos K.N. Geanne, Kamilla A. Dutra, Rosângela A. Barros, Claudio A.G.da Câmara, Diana D. Lira, Norma B. Gusmão, and Daniela M.A.F. Navarro. "Essential Oils from *Alpinia purpurata* (Zingiberaceae): Chemical Composition, Oviposition Deterrence, Larvicidal and Antibacterial Activity." *Industrial Crops and Product*, vol. 10, no. 40 (November 2012): 254-260. https://doi.org/10.1016/j.indcrop.2012.03.020.

Sirat M. Hasnah, Basar Norazah, and Jani A. Nor. “Chemical Compositions of The Rhizome Oils of two *Alpinia* Species of Malaysia.” *Natural Product Research*, vol. 25, no. 10, (June 2011):982-986. https://doi.org/10.1080/14786419.2010.529079.

Smith R.M. “*Alpinia* (Zingiberaceae): A Proposed New Infrageneric Classification.” *Edinburgh Journal of Botany,* vol. 47, no. 1 (March 1990): 1-75. https://doi.org/10/1017S0960428600000314.

Tabanca Nurhayat, Gao Zen-Ping, Demirci Betul, Techen Natascha, Wedge E. David, Ali Abbas, and Sampson J. Blair. et al., “Molecular and Phytochemical Investigation of *Angelica dahurica* and *Angelica pubescentis* Essential Oils and Their Biological Activity Against *Aedes aegypti, Stephanitis pyrioides*, and *Colletotrichum* Species.” *Journal of Agricultural and Food Chemistry*. vol. 62, no. 35 (September 2014): 8848-8857. https://doi.org/10.1021/jf5024752.

Thu N. Bich, Trinh N. Trung, Do T. Ha, Nguyen M. Khoi, Tran V. Hung, Tran T. Hien, Yim Namhui, and Ki H. Bae. “Screening of Vietnamese medicinal plants for cytotoxic activity.” *Natural Product Science* vol.16, no. 1 (March 2010): 43-49.

Vietnamese Pharmacopoeia. Medical Publishing House, Hanoi, Vietnam (2009).

Vlietinck A.J. “Screening Methods for Detection and Evaluation of Biological Activity of Plant Preparation.” L. Bohlin et al. (eds.), Bioassay Methods in Natural Product Research and Drug Development. Kluwer academic publishers, USA, pp. 37-52 (1999).

Wafaa M. Hikal, Rowida S. Baeshen, and Hussein A.H. Said-Al Ahl. “Botanical Insecticide as Simple Extractives for Pest Control.’’ *Cogent Biology* vol. 3 (November 2017): 1404274, https://doi.org/10.108/23312 025.2017.1404274.

WHO. “Guidelines for Laboratory and Field Testing of Mosquito Larvicides.” WHO/CDS/WHOPES/GCDPP, Geneva, Switzerland (2005).

Yob N.J, Jofrry S. Mohammad, Affandi M.M.R. Mohammad, The L. Kek, Salleh M.Z., and Zakaria Z.A. “*Zingiber zerumbet* (L.) Smith: A Review of Its Ethnomedicinal, Chemical, and Pharmacological Uses.’’

Evidence-Based Complementary and Alternative Medicine. vol. 2011, (2011): Article ID 543216, 12 pages, http://dx.doi.org/10.1155/2011/543216.

Yusoff M. Mashitah, Halijah Ibrahim, and Nurulhusna A. Hamid. "Chemical Characterization and Antimicrobial Activity of Rhziome Essential Oils of very Closely Allied Zingiberacae species Endemic to Borneo: *Alpinia* ligulata K.Schum and *Alpinia nieuwenhuizii* Val." *Chemistry and Biodiversity,* vol. 8, no. 5 (May 2011): 917-923.

Reviewed by Dr. Ismaeel Ridwan Olanrewaju, Department of Chemistry, University of Ilorin, Kwara State, Nigeria

In: What to Know about Essential Oils
Editor: Malene M. Kjeldsen
ISBN: 978-1-53617-986-6

Chapter 4

ESSENTIAL OILS: THERAPEUTIC EFFECTS AS ANTHELMINTICS

Akinsola A. Akande and Sherifat A. Aboaba*
Department of Chemistry, University of Ibadan, Ibadan, Nigeria

ABSTRACT

The rate at which ignorance of hygiene and sanitary practices is being neglected in the suburban and rural areas of developing regions of the world never seem to reduce. Lack of adequate sanitation and health facilities together with deficiency in educating these rural dwellers on how to maintain proper hygiene has made the prevalence and impact of helminthiasis on public health and animal production a great socio-economic problem. Often associated with these problems are conditions such as anaemia, malnutrition, vitamin deficiencies, poor cognitive ability, less intellectual and mental development which are prominent in underage children and pregnant women. Animal health care and husbandry has also been hit as a result of this inadequate hygiene and sanitary practices which thus pose great challenge in food production. Most of the domestic animals serve as primary host to infectious helminths (worms) from which they are transmitted into humans. However, many naturally occurring secondary

* Corresponding Author's Email: saboaba@gmail.com; sa.aboaba@mail.ui.edu.ng.

metabolites (phytochemicals) of plants such as terpenoids from essential oils, alkaloids, flavonoids, glycosides and tannins have been explored as leads to develop medicines for a disease-free and healthy society. Plant essential oils are ingredients present in formulations used ethno-medicinally, pharmaceutically, in food and cosmetic industries due to their potential bioactive and therapeutic activities against a wide spectrum of pathogenic organisms. Results from many reported researches as well as from our research findings, using the essential oils of plants from the Fabaceae species, showed the efficacy of some of these plant constituents as anthelmintics against various test organisms. The essential oils explored from plants of choice premised on their ethnobotanical survey in the treatment of one or more gastrointestinal troubles (GIT). The different essential oils studied demonstrated varying inhibitory activities (*in vitro* and *in vivo*) against different classes of helminth parasites (nematodes, cestodes, trematodes) and annelids which could be a lead to developing potent anthelmintics. As a result of these findings, the discovery of natural plant constituents should be kept on-going.

Keywords: phytochemicals, helminthiasis, terpenoids, hygiene

INTRODUCTION

Helminthiasis (known as parasitic worm infection) is caused by a group of pathogenic macro-organisms reported to infect more than two (2) billion of the world's population. It is ranked among the most important neglected tropical diseases (NTDs) of the world, with the most significant morbidity attributable to human soil-transmitted helminth (STH) infections [1, 2]. The rate at which ignorance of hygiene and sanitary practices in the suburban and rural areas of developing nations of the world is being neglected never seem to reduce. About 40% of world's population ($\approx$ 2.5 billion people) lack adequate sanitation habit and good health facilities [3]. Negligence in instilling hygiene education and failure to continuously emphasis on the importance of proper usage of health facilities by suburban and rural dwellers could increase this statistics.

Helminthiasis is one of the major diseases of veterinary animals and humans in countries with poor socioeconomic status. Among the seventeen NTDs, over 1.4 billion people are infected with one or more of schistosomiasis, lymphatic filariasis, onchocerciasis, trachoma and the three soil-transmitted helminth infections (hookworm, ascariasis and trichuriasis), own to be the most common afflictions of the world's poorest people [4].

A vast number of medicinal plant species are rich in bioactive components called secondary metabolites (Phytochemicals) such as terpenes/terpenoids from essential oils (EOs), alkaloids, flavonoids, glycosides, phenolics, poly-phenols, coumarins and tannins. They are important ingredients present in formulations used ethno-medicinally, pharmaceutically, esthetically as well as in food and cosmetic industries for their pharmacological properties [5, 6]. Among these bioactive components, EOs have been applied in folkloric medicine since ancient times. Many of the common EO constituents obtained from medicinal herbs, plant parts such as the leaves, stems and roots, have been a major source of lead compound(s) to develop medicines for a disease-free and healthy society [7] and are still widely used till today.

Prevalence and Burden of Helminth Infections

Helminths are invertebrates, classified based on the external and internal morphology of their egg, larval and adult stages. They are elongated, flat (platy helminths) or cylindrical (round worms) in shape. Many often live in the gastrointestinal tract of their host while many may burrow into other organs to induce physiological damages. In order to really understand the epidemiology and pathogenesis of helminth diseases, as well as diagnose and treat hosts harboring these parasites, the different stages in relation to their growth and development must be well understood. The three major pathogenic groups are the nematodes (roundworms), cestodes (tapeworms) and trematodes (flukes). Clinically relevant groups are identified according to their general external shape and the host organ they inhabit [8].

Worm infection (Helminthiasis) is often asymptomatic [9] and rarely causes death, but the burden of infection on the host's nutritional status and the overall well-being vis-à-vis morbidity or mortality [10, 11] cannot be over emphasised. Its impact on child's growth and development include malnutrition, vitamin deficiencies, stunted growth, poor cognitive ability, poor iron status and anemia as well as less intellectual and mental development [12, 13]. Infected pregnant women usually suffer from iron deficiency anemia which often contributes to maternal-fetal consequences such as premature birth, risk of giving birth to low birth-weight babies, impaired lactation and are highly susceptible to death during childbirth [4, 14].

Malnourished hosts living in endemic communities are regularly exposed to polyparasitism (i.e., simultaneous infection with multiple parasite species). When there is an overlap of malnutrition with poverty and endemicity, the true effect of these infections is obscured [15, 16, 17, 18] and in some cases directly and/or indirectly, infections increase the susceptibility and severity of host to malaria, HIV/AIDS and tuberculosis [4, 13, 19, 20, 21, 22, 23]. Reports have revealed helminth co-infection with these associated diseases to be on the rise [24, 25, 26, 27, 28, 29].

Routine efforts, predominantly periodic administration of drugs (preventive chemotherapy) as anthelmintics, to reduce morbidity by deworming (decreasing worm burden) hosts have been relied upon to control these pathogenic parasites. However, due to frequent, repeated and indiscriminate usage of drugs such as Albendazole, Mebendazole, Praziquantel and Piperazine citrate, there has been diminished efficacy and reduced effectiveness of periodic deworming [30, 31], resulting in emergence, re-emergence [32, 33] and gradual wide spread of anthelmintic resistance. Thus, the uprising of treatment failures in humans [15, 34] and the increase in nematode populations resistant to virtually all anthelmintic classes among species of veterinary importance [35, 36] is evident. Therefore, there is the need to continually research for newer formulations.

Essential Oil Constituents' Formation and Classification

The term essential oil (EO) can be used to describe a complex mixture of volatile organic components secreted in specialised cells of different parts of a plant and contribute to its flavour and fragrance. They are a class of secondary metabolites which consist mainly organic compounds based on isoprene (2-methylbuta-1,3-diene) units [37]. These compounds are derived by a hypothetical linkage of isoprene units in a head to tail manner to the terpenes/terpenoids. This form of linkage, referred to as 'isoprene rule', has helped in a rational classification established based on the number of isoprene units incorporated in the basic molecular skeleton – a concept of divisibility into units (by head-to-tail union). Such classification often include the mono-, sesqui-, di-, tri-, tetra- and polyterpenes/ terpenoids (i.e., 2, 3, 4, 6, 8 and several isoprene units respectively) [5].

In general, mono- and sesquiterpenes/terpenoids are the most prevailing complex class of components found in essential oils [38, 39]. They are found in form of acids, alcohols, aldehydes, esters, furans, phenols ketones, lactones, oxides and peroxides [37, 40]. The degradation/decomposition products of higher terpenoids and lipids [41] however, do occur.

Table 1. Classes of some naturally occurring terpenes/terpenoids

Class of terpenoids	Isoprene units	No. of carbon atoms	Examples
Hemiterpenoids	1	5	Isovaleric acid
Monoterpenoids	2	10	Limonene, camphor
Sesquiterpenoids	3	15	α-farnesene, nerolidol
Diterpenoids	4	20	Retinal, Abietic acid
Triterpenoids	6	30	Lanosterol, Ursolic acid
Tetraterpenoids	8	40	β-carotene
Polyterpenoids	Several units	>40	Natural rubber

Biosynthetically, terpenoid essential oils are believed to originate from the mevalonic acid (MVA) pathway (Figure 1) [42, 43] and the non-mevalonic acid (also known as the methyl-erythritol phosphate (MEP)) pathway [44, 45], via polymerisation and derivatisation of 5-membered isoprene-like alkenes – isopentenyl diphosphate (IPP) and its isomer, dimethylallylpyrophosphate (DMAPP) – both known to be the basic building blocks of terpenes and terpenoids. There is an overlap in the two pathways both producing IPP and DMAPP. The MVA pathway occurs mainly in plants' cytoplasm, endoplasmic reticulum and mitochondria to predominantly produce the sesquiterpenes, sterols and ubiquinones, while the MEP pathway occurs in the plastids of plant cells responsible for the synthesis of the hemi-, mono-, diterpenes and higher terpenes/terpenoids (not found in essential oils) such as the carotenoids and the phytols of chlorophyll [5, 46, 47, 48].

The precursor for all monoterpenoids is geranyl pyrophosphate, which in nature exists as incipient carbocation held in enzyme active sites. Some monoterpenoids originating from a series of geranyl carbocation reactions are geraniol (found in rose, lemon and *Monarda fistulosa* EOs), myrcene, limonene (occur majorly in citrus EOs), α-pinene, β-pinene, carene (major constituents of turpentine), borneol, camphor (commonly extracted from the woods of *Cinnamomum camphora*) and fenchone (highest concentrations in the essential oil of *Foeniculum vulgare*) [49, 50]. Others are 1,8-cineole (a common constituent of eucalyptus and cajeput EOs), carvone (the (*R*)-(–)-enantiomer provides the characteristic odour of spearmint while the (*S*)-(+)-enantiomer is found in caraway) and menthofuran (occurs in mint oils) [41, 50].

Farnesyl pyrophosphate is the precursor for all the sesquiterpenoids. Heterolysis of the bond between carbon and oxygen of the phosphate leads to many sesquiterpenoids via nascent farnesyl carbocation. Examples include farnesol (an important rose flower EO component), nerolidol, β-caryophyllene (common in cloves EO), α-humulene (found in hops EO) and α-bisabolol (lavender and rosemary oil constituents) [41, 50, 51].

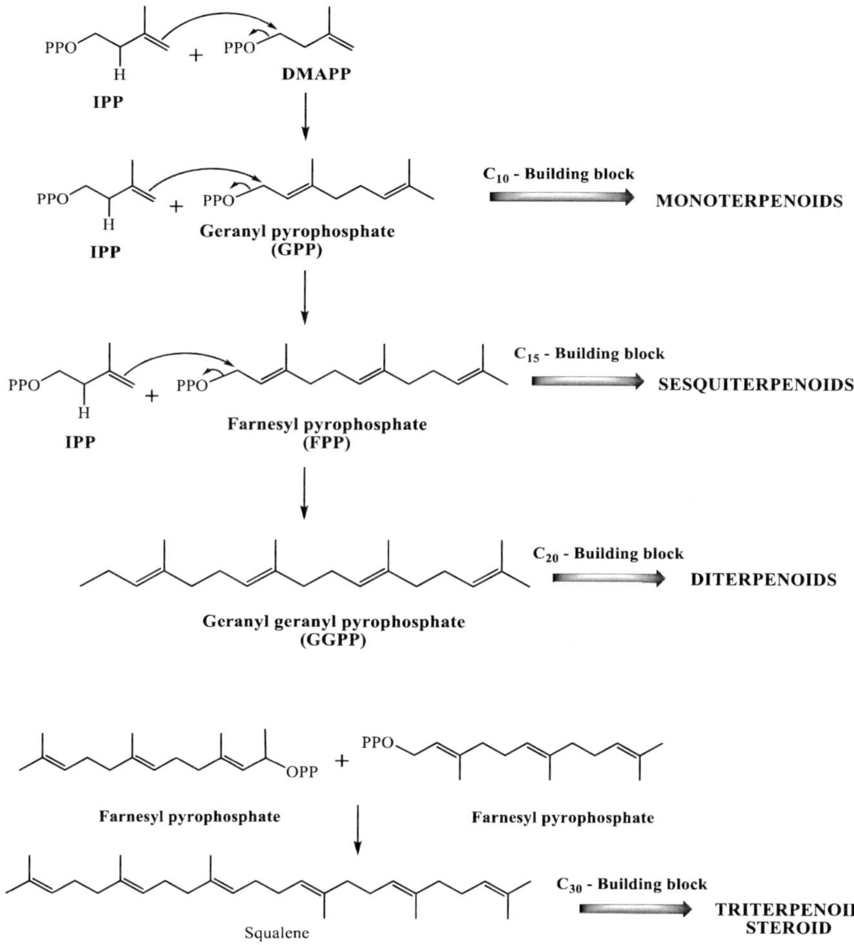

Figure 1. The mevalonic acid pathway (Rohdich et al., 2001 [43]).

A number of degraded/decomposed carotenoids fragments found in EOs are the ionones and the damascones (both have similar carbon skeleton). They are often degraded from the central part of the carotenoids. The site of oxidative degradation, in the case of the ionones, is three carbon atoms away from the carotenoid ring [52], while in damascones, oxygenation is found at the carbon chain next to the ring. α-ionone and β-ionone are both isomers, naturally occurring widely in variety of flowers, fruits, and leaves [53]. β-damascenone (occurs as low as 0.05% in the oil of the Damask rose) was the first to be isolated and characterised in its class such as safranal (70% component and a significant contributor to saffron EO), and cyclocitral [41].

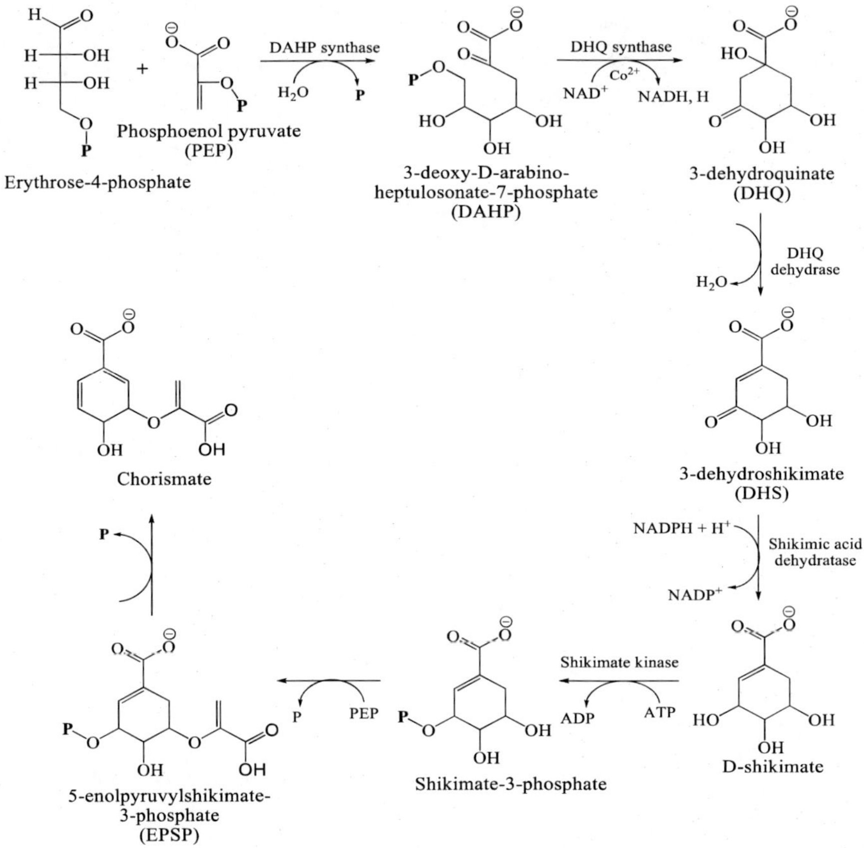

Figure 2. The Shikimate pathway [55].

Other important components of EOs, frequently present in smaller proportions but in significant quantities, are the phenylpropanoids (the aromatic and phenolic compounds) [5, 54]. They are plant secondary metabolites that have the benzene ring, with or without hydroxyl groups attached, as well as the free phenolic acid derivatives. Their biosynthetic origin is from the shikimate pathway (Figure 2). Examples are phenylalanine, cinnamic acid, ferulic acid, benzyl alcohol, benzaldehyde, vanillin (the key odour component of vanilla), eugenol (found in spices such as clove, cinnamon, allspice; in herbs like bay and basil; and in flower oils of rose, jasmine, and carnation), isoeugenol and methyleugenol (which makes 98% oil composition of some Melaleuca species) [55, 41].

Botanically identical plants (that is, plants of the same species) which differ significantly in chemical composition due to geographical or geological differences are referred to as chemotypes. They occur when there are variations in their biosynthetic pathways or environmental factors such as soil types, weather conditions, altitude, light intensity and temperature [37, 42]. Essential oil composition also changes between different plant parts or organs. This is referred to as phytochemical polymorphism [56]. These differences in the composition between parts such as the oil glands are more often due to the enormous number of individual cells present and the age of oil glands [57, 58, 59].

Further in this chapter, some EOs and their constituents that have been used in experimental studies in literatures, against various helminthes parasites and annelids, were highlighted. Plant EO extracts employed as anthelmintics, which were documented in our current research and publications, were also discussed. However, the plants of choice premised on their ethnobotanical survey in the treatment of one or more gastrointestinal troubles (GIT).

Anthelmintic Activity of Essential Oils Using Intestinal Parasites as Test Organism

Experimental studies on the use of plant essential oils (EOs) against various intestinal nematodes have been reported in literature. In folk medicine, *Croton zehntneri* and *Lippia sidoides* are used in the treatment of gastrointestinal disturbances in Brazil. According to Camurça-Vasconcelos *et al.*, [60], the anthelmintic activity of *C. zehntneri* and *L. sidoides* EOs, together with two major constituents from these oils, anethole and thymol, was carried out on the eggs and larvae of sheep gastrointestinal nematode *(Haemonchus contortus)*, and intestinal nematodes of mice. Two essential oil sample of *C. zehntneri* were obtained from plant parts collected at different periods of the year and were found to vary in the concentration of anethole. The oils exhibited significant activities against the intestinal nematodes of sheep and mice, at varying concentrations. At highest concentration of 1.25 μL/mL, both plant EOs showed statistical similarity in the egg hatch test while thymol and *L. sidoides* oils had similar results at 0.62 μL/mL. The EC_{50} value of *L. sidoides* was obtained at 0.40 μL/mL while the two EO samples of *C. zehntneri* had EC_{50} values at 0.55 μL/mL and 0.74 μL/mL respectively. It was further reported that the results obtained in their work are better than those achieved using other plants or extracts at higher concentrations.

The *in vitro* anthelmintic efficacy of *Eucalyptus staigeriana* EO was determined by the egg hatching test and the inhibition of larval development of *H. contortus* followed by an *in vivo* faecal egg count reduction assay according to Macedo et al., [61]. The *in vitro* and *in vivo* experiment presented a concentration and dose-dependent effect on the test organism with an EC_{50} of 0.324 mg/mL and 1.702 mg/mL for egg hatching and larval development tests respectively. The fecal egg count reduction after treatment varied from 61.40 to 76.57% for *E. staigeriana* EO and 85.59 to 67.34% for Ivermectin (control) at 8 and 15 days post-trcatment respectively. However, it was stated that the therapeutically required level of synthetic anthelmintics for its efficacy was not reached.

One of the species of plants with promising anthelmintic activities in a Brazilian study is *Cymbopogon citratus.* Macedo et al., [62] evaluated the efficacy of *C. citratus* EO and citral against *H. contortus* using *in vitro* egg hatch test, larval development test and an *in vivo* test utilising a *Meriones unguiculatus* (Gerbil) model – a model sometimes conducted to evaluate the anthelmintic activity of new drugs against *H. contortus in vivo* before studies in ruminants. The major constituents of the oil were geranial (57.30%) and neral (40.40%). The EO of the plant and citral (a natural combination of two isomeric aldehydes, neral and geranial) inhibited egg hatching at concentrations $\leq$ 0.62 mg/mL ($P < 0.05$) and their effective concentrations required to inhibit 50% of egg hatching (EC_{50}), were 0.14 and 0.13 mg/mL, respectively. From their findings, it was reported that *C. citratus* had better efficacy than for 300 mg/Kg and 1,000 mg/Kg concentrations of the essential oil and ethanolic extract of *Artemisia annua*, respectively, administered to gerbils for five days [63, 62].

Further in 2019, Macedo et al., [64] assessed the anthelmintic activity of *C. citratus* EO and *C. citratus* EO nanoemulsion on gastro-intestinal nematodes. Among the main constituents of the plant's EO are neral (*cis*-citral) (17.77%) and geranial (*trans*-citral) (18.98%). In the egg hatch test, the mean efficacy of *C. citratus* EO and its nanoemulsion indicated ovicidal activity at all tested concentrations in a dose-dependent manner, the effect similar to that of thiabendazole ($p > 0.05$) at higher concentration (1.25 mg/mL) and the EC_{50} values were 0.15 and 0.16 mg/mL, respectively. Determination of worm burden via the fecal egg count reduction test was conducted on sheep with *C. citratus* EO (500 mg/Kg) and its nanoemulsion (450 mg/kg) and fecal samples were collected before and after 7 and 14 days of treatment. Parasite species found were *H. contortus*, *Trichuris ovis, Oesophagostomum columbianum* and *Trichostrongylus colubriformis*. The total worm burden of groups treated with the test samples and the control group was similar ($p > 0.05$). Both tested samples; *C. citratus* EO and the nanoemulsified EO; were effective against *H. contortus* with reductions in adult worm burden at 66.40% and 83.10%, respectively of which the nanoemulsified sample was able to significantly reduce the parasite load of *H. contortus*. Moreover, similar results were reported when the anthelmintic efficacy of the free and nanoencapsulated EOs of *Eucalyptus citriodora* and *Eucalyptus staigeriana* was evaluated whereby inhibition of larvae hatching was enhanced by nanoencapsulation with 1% chitosan [64].

An *in vitro* anthelmintic assay was also evaluated on EOs of some plants against the developmental stages of trichostrongylids (*H. contortus* and *Trichostrogylus* spp.) from naturally infected sheep through the egg hatch assay (EHA), larval development assay (LDA), larval feeding inhibition assay (LFIA) and the larval exsheathment assay (LEA). The EOs of *Mentha piperita, Cymbopogon martinii* and *Cymbopogon schoenanthus* exhibited good activity. The EO of *C. schoenanthus* had the best activity against ovine trichostrongylids in all the *in vitro* tests employed, with an LC_{50} value of 0.045 mg/mL in the EHA, 0.063 mg/mL in the LDA, 0.009 mg/mL in the LFIA, and 24.66 mg/mL in the LEA [65]. Further in 2017, Katiki et al., [66] assessed the anthelmintic efficacy of the monoterpenoids carvacrol, carvone, cineole, linalool, limonene, thymol, and the phenylpropanoids cinnamaldehyde, anethole, vanillin, and eugenol for their individual anthelmintic efficacy and as a combined efficacy in mixtures of binary, ternary and quaternary combinations against *H. contortus* in order to identify which has/have the greatest individual anthelmintic efficacy and also the most powerful combinations. The lethal concentrations (mg/mL) of these common EOs constituents, producing 50% eggs mortality (LC_{50}), were calculated and ranked as follows: cinnamaldehyde (0.018), anethole (0.070), carvone (0.085), carvacrol (0.11), thymol (0.13), linalool (0.29), vanillin (0.57), eugenol (0.57), cineole (4.74), and limonene (207.5). For binary, ternary, and quaternary combinations, the synergism, additive effect, and antagonism were quantified and calculated. However, 16 different combinations were classified according to their combination index (CI) from which the combination of cinnamaldehyde:carvacrol (LC_{50}: 0.012 mg/mL) and anethole:carvone (LC_{50}: 0.013 mg/mL) produced the best anthelmintic effect (a synergistic activity) [66].

Investigation of anthelmintic effect of *Coriandrum sativum* Linn., *Ocimum gratissimum* Linn., *Ocimum lamifolium* Hochst. Ex Benth, *Ruta chalpensis* Linn., *Thymus schimperi* Ronniger and *Echinops kebericho* Mesfin EOs against *H. contortus* was documented by Hussien et al., [67] in an egg hatch assay. All the plants demonstrated promising inhibitory activities (observed in a dose dependent manner; $p < 0.05$) at all concentrations (from which efficacy was best for most plants at 1% concentration when compared with thiabendazole). *Ocimum gratissimum* EO ($IC_{50} = 0.0784\%$) and *R. chalpensis* leaf and fruit EOs ($IC_{50} = 0.0876\%$ and 0.0944%, respectively) were the most active of the oils.

Based on their ethno-pharmacological usage against worm infections in folk medicine, the EOs obtained from *Citrus aurantifolia* (Christm.) Swingle (Rutaceae) fruit peel, *Anthemis nobile* (syn. Chamaemelum nobilis (L.) All.) (Asteraceae) flowers and *Lavandula officinalis* (Chaix & Kitt.) (Lamiaceae) flowers were investigated for their egg hatch, larval development and adult worm motility inhibitory capabilities. The oils demonstrated significant *in vitro* anthelmintic activity, based on these three assays, in a dose-dependent manner. The egg hatching inhibitory effect of the oils was higher than 85-90% for the concentration range of 3.125 to 50 mg/mL with IC_{50} values of 0.316 g/mL, 0.694 mg/mL and 0.842 mg/mL for *L. officinalis*, *C. aurantifolia* and *A. nobile* respectively. The rate of larval development inhibition at a concentration of 0.187 mg/mL or higher by *C. aurantifolia* fruit peel oil was greater than 85%, thus implying the best inhibition and the lowest IC_{50} (0.044 mg/mL). *Anthemis nobile* oil achieved a larval development inhibition greater than 85% at a higher concentration of 0.375 mg/mL with IC_{50} of 0.117 mg/mL while the lowest inhibition was observed for *L. officinalis* flower oil showing larval development inhibition greater than 85% only for concentrations above 1.5 mg/mL with its IC_{50} value at 0.280 mg/mL [68].

According to a review by Mali and Mehta, [69], the major constituents of EO of *Occimum sanctum* Linn. (Lamiaceae), commonly known as Sacred Basil (*Tulsi*), were identified to be Eugenol (51%), β-caryophyllene (37%), alongside a number of monoterpenes and sesquiterpenes. In an *in vitro* anthelmintic assay against the nematode *Caenorhabditis elegans* using Levamisole as reference standard, the EO and Eugenol demonstrated potent activity, both exhibiting ED_{50} of 237.90 µg/mL and 62.10 µg/mL, respectively. It was further suggested that Eugenol could be reputed to enhance the anthelmintic activity. Also, a definite paralytic action on the nerve-muscular preparation of *Ascaris lumbricoids* was observed for the fruits EO of *Piper longum* Linn. (Piperaceae) when screened for its anthelmintic activity – an activity better than Piperazine citrate.

In another review article by Sunita et al., [70], the varying anthelmintic activity of several plant EOs against many test organism was highlighted, among which are as follows: profound strong and better anthelmintic activity of *Anacardium occidentale* (Anacardiaceae), *Buddlea asiatica* (Loganiaceae), *Callistemon viminalis* (Myrtaceae), *Chloroxylon swientenia* (Rutaceae), *Zanthoxylum limonella, Artemisia pallens* (Compositae), *Eupatorium triplinerve* (Compositae), *Artabotrys odoratissimus*

(Annonanceae), *Capillipedium foetidum* (Poaceae), *Cymbopogon martini* (Poaceae) and *Piper betle* EOs was reported against either of *Taenia solium* (tapeworms), hookworms and *Ascaris lumbricoides* parasites. The efficacy of some of these plants' EOs was also observed to either be comparable or even better than that of piperazine phosphate and hexylresorcinol. It was further reported that the oils of *Gardenia lucida* (Rubiaceae), *Cyperus rotendus* (Cyperaceae), *Inula racemosa* (Compositae), *Psitacia integrrima* (Anacardiaceae), *Litsea chinensis* (Lauraceae) and *Randia dumetorum* (Rubiaceae) seeds possess good anthelmintic activity against tapeworms and earthworms. Jeyathilakan et al., [71] in 2010, evaluated the *in vitro* efficacy of EOs of *Cymbopogan nardus* (citronella) and *Azadirachta indica* (neem) on *Fasciola gigantica* (Fluke). Similar to oxyclozanide, citronella oil showed flukicidal effect while neem oil exhibited less effect on flukes than citronella oil.

Anthelmintic Activity of Essential Oils Using Earthworm as Test Organism

The *in vitro* anthelmintic activities of various plant extracts and essential oils against earthworms has been documented in literature. This is due to their physiological and anatomical resemblance to human intestinal roundworm parasites. Worms such as the Indian adult earthworm, *Pheritima posthuma* and *Eudrilus eugeniae*, commonly referred to as the African night crawler [72, 73, 74, 75, 76, 77, 78, 79] have been employed. The activity of plant extracts/essential oils is determined by observing the time of paralysis and time of death of the worms, when compared to that of a control (usually drugs as standard). The following are reports from literature;

Oxygenated monoterpenoid dominated *Thymus bovei* essential oil (EO) exhibited significant potency against the adult Indian earthworm, *Pheretima posthuma*. *Trans*-geraniol (35.38%), α-citral (20.37%) and β-citral (14.76%) were the major constituents identified, comprising 70.51% of the oil. For the test oil sample and piperazine (control), the time of paralysis of the worm were 19.61 ± 0.88 and 24.25 ± 0.61 min, while the time of death were 47.32 ± 0.94 and 62.96 ± 0.29 min, respectively thus indicating a good anthelmintic activity compared to the reference standard [80].

The major constituents of allspice (*Pimenta dioica* (Linn.) Merill) leaf EO from Jamaica were reported to be eugenol, methyl eugenol, β-caryophyllene and Myrcene. However, the anthelmintic activity of eugenol rich *P. dioica* leaf EOs collected from plant samples between January to May (summer period) from South Canara, India, was evaluated against the Indian adult earthworms (*Pheretima posthuma*) in order to compare the variation in activity based on the months of collection. Significant activity in a concentration dependent trend was observed for all the EO samples but the oil from leaves collected in the month of April, showed best result ($p < 0.05$) with respect to time of paralysis as well as time of death at all concentrations when compared with Albendazole [75].

Against earthworms, tapeworms, hookworms and nodular worms, *Nigella sativa* Linn. (Ranunculaceae) showed fairly good activity against earthworms and tapeworms from which the active principles of the oil are thymoquinone, dimethyquinone-cymene and α-pinene. In a study, the EOs of both *Anacardium occidentale* Linn. and *Callistemon viminalis* (Soland.) Cheel were found to possess activity against earthworms, tapeworms and hookworms better than Piperazine phosphate and Hexyl resorcinol [69].

Anthelmintic Activity of Essential Oils from Our Studies

The essential oils (EOs) from four Fabaceae plants, namely; *Albizia adiantifolia* (Schumach) W.F. Wright, *Albizia zygia* (DC) J.F. Macbr., *Albizia odoratissima* (LF) Benth. and *Millettia thonningii* (Schum & Thonn) Baker were characterised and tested for their anthelminthic activities. The choice of these plants premised on their ethnobotanical survey in their usage in the treatment of one or more gastrointestinal troubles (GIT).

METHODS

Plant Sampling and Hydrodistillation

The leaves, stem bark and root bark of the four Fabaceae plants were collected from a secondary forest vegetation at Awotan area, Ibadan, South west Nigeria in July, 2013. Identification and authentication of each plant sample were carried out at the Forestry Research Institute of Nigeria (FRIN) Jericho, Ibadan, Nigeria where voucher specimens for *A. adiantifolia* (FHI 109922), *A. zygia* (FHI 109920), *A. odoratissima* (FHI 109729) and *M. thonningii* (FHI 109921) were registered and deposited at the herbarium section. Essential oils (EOs) present in the dried pulverised plant samples of the leaves (300 g), stem bark (350 g) and root bark (350 g) were extracted for 4 hours by hydro-distillation method in an all glass Clevenger apparatus designed in accordance with the British Pharmacopoeia specifications [81]. The EOs isolated in about 1.0 mL of hexane, displaced over water at the receiver arm of the Clevenger apparatus, were carefully collected over water into sample bottles (vials), dried over anhydrous sodium sulphate (Na_2SO_4) and stored inside the refrigerator at 4 °C prior to analysis.

Characterisation and Identification of the Essential Oil Constituents by Gas Chromatography-Mass Spectrometry (GC/GC-MS Analyses)

The gas chromatography analyses on all the EOs were carried out on HP-5890 gas chromatograph fitted with HP-Wax and HP-5 capillary columns (30 m x 0.25 mm, 0.25 mm film thickness). The GC oven temperature was programmed at 60 °C (held for 10 min), heated to 220 °C at 5 °C/min. The injector and detector temperatures were maintained at 250 °C. Helium was used as carrier gas at a flow rate of 2 mL/min. Gas Chromatography - Mass Spectrometry analysis was carried out on a Varian CP-3800 gas chromatograph interfaced to a Varian Saturn 2000 ion trap mass detector operated at 70 eV. Temperatures of the injector and transfer lines were 220 °C and 240 °C, respectively. The GC oven temperature was programmed from 60-240 °C at 3 °C/min. The carrier gas, Helium was used at a flow rate of 1 mL/min. Essential oil constituents were identified based on comparison of the retention times with those of the authentic samples, comparing their retention indices relative to the series of n-hydrocarbons, and by comparison of their mass spectra with those of reference compounds published by NIST, 2002. Calculating the integration of GC peak areas gave the relative concentrations of each constituent [82].

Evaluation of Anthelmintic Activity

In vitro anthelmintic activity for our study was carried out according to the method by Rao *et al.*, [75] with some modifications. The adult earthworms, *Eudrilus eugeniae*, were utilised while Albendazole (reference standard) and 10% v/v Tween-80 in distilled water served as the positive and negative controls, respectively. Each of the EOs and Albendazole were dissolved in 10 mL Tween-80 and diluted up to 30 mL to prepare five concentrations (1, 2, 3, 4 and 5% v/v). Time of paralysis and death were expressed as mean ± standard error of mean (SEM). Statistical analyses were carried out using GraphPad Prism, version 5.01 statistical software. At 95% confidence interval, activity ($p < 0.001$) was considered statistically significant.

Albizia adiantifolia (Schumach) W.F. Wright

Albizia adiantifolia (the West African Albizia or rough-bark flat-crown) is known as 'Ayinreta' or 'Igbabo' and 'Kawo' in the Southwestern and Northern parts of Nigeria respectively. Many parts of the plant have been used to treat various ailments, some of which include bronchitis, skin diseases, gonorrhea, malaria, diarrhea, abdominal pains, tapeworm infection, irregular menstruation, urinary and respiratory tracts infections and as well employed as a vermifuge, purgative and an antidote [83]. Hydro-distilled EOs of the leaves, stem bark and root bark of *A. adiantifolia* were evaluated for their *in vitro* anthelmintic activity using the adult earthworm

(*Eudrilus eugeniae*). Sesquiterpene hydrocarbons were the most dominant class of terpenoids in the leaves (39.50%), stem bark (67.30%) and root bark (42.60%), respectively. β-caryophyllene was the most abundant constituent characterised in the three EOs. The leaf EO exhibited highest activity than both the stem bark and root bark oils (time of paralysis and death with respect to the highest concentration was at 12.60 ± 1.21 and 60.20 ± 3.09 minutes, respectively). All the EOs showed significant activity ($p < 0.001$) compared to the standard drug (Albendazole) in a concentration dependent manner [83].

Albizia zygia (DC) J.F. Macbr.

Albizia zygia (West African Albizia) is locally known as 'Ayinre-weere' and 'Nyie avu' among the Yorubas and the Igbos in Nigeria, respectively [84, 85, 86]. It has been used as an aphrodisiac, an anti-parasite, an antidote, a purgative and as well in vermifuge purposes. It is also useful in the treatment of maladies such as malaria fever, diarrhea, bronchial diseases and female sterility [87].

The classes of compounds identified in the characterised EOs of *A. zygia* from our study [88] varied significantly in composition to those obtained by Oloyede and Ogunlade [89]. 1,8-cineole, β-caryophyllene and viridiflorol were the dominant constituents of the EOs but were only present in less significant quantities in the oils obtained by Oloyede and Ogunlade. Furthermore, the anthelmintic activity of *A. zygia* from our study [88] was evaluated based on time of paralysis and time of death (expressed as mean ± standard error of mean), utilising *Eudrilus eugeniae* worms. The time taken for both paralysis and death of worm to occur were compared with that of the control (Albendazole) at varying concentrations. The root bark oil, rich in 1,8-cineole (14.80%), showed the best activity followed by the leaves oil and then the stem bark oil. All the EOs demonstrated promising activities in a concentration dependent manner ($p < 0.001$) better than the control at all concentrations. The gastro protective effect [90] and potential anthelmintic activity [91] of plants rich in 1,8-cineole which of course was also obtained as one of the major constituents in *A. zygia* EOs further corroborates the ethno-medicinal uses of the plant as an anti-parasitic, a purgative and a vermifuge.

Albizia odoratissima (LF) Benth.

Albizia odoratissima (the fragrant *Albizia* or black siris), is a tropical small sized deciduous tree, domestically and commercially sort for products like fuel, timber, gum or resin [92]. Traditionally, it is used to treat leprosy, ulcers, cough [93], and found to possess analgesic, stimulant, diuretic and anthelmintic properties [94]. The plant had shown significant antimicrobial activities [95] and anti-diabetic potential [96, 97].

The hydro-distilled essential oils (EOs) from the leaves, stem bark and root bark of *A. odoratissima* (all colourless) yielded 0.240%, 0.228% and 0.260% (volume/dry weight) respectively. A total of 37, 27 and 33 constituents (Table 2) representing 96.50%, 96.00% and 97.10% of the total oil fractions were identified in the leaves, stem bark and root bark oils, respectively. The class of compounds identified in the complex EO mixtures consist of the monoterpene hydrocarbons (6.00%, 2.80% and 6.20%), oxygenated monoterpenes (36.90%, 29.60% and 15.10%), sesquiterpene hydrocarbons (12.60%, 6.80% and 39.90%), oxygenated sesquiterpenes (40.10%, 55.30% and 35.90%), all represented in the leaves, stem bark and root bark, respectively and non-terpene derivatives (1.50% and 1.50%) in the leaves and stem bark, respectively. Oxygenated sesquiterpenes were dominant in the leaves and stem bark oils while sesquiterpene hydrocarbons dominated the root bark oil. The non-terpene derivatives were present in low quantity.

Viridiflorol (31.60%), 1,8-cineole (29.20%) and α-terpineol (5.40%) were the major constituents in the leaves oil. The major constituents in the stem bark are viridiflorol (44.00%), 1,8-cineole (23.60%) and α-terpineol (5.60%) while the root bark oil constitutes majorly viridiflorol (18.50%), 1,8-cineole (13.60%) and β-caryophyllene (10.30%). Viridiflorol (the most abundant constituent) and 1,8-cineole dominated the three plant parts while α-terpineol was dominant in the leaves and stem bark oils. Other compounds found in significant quantities are caryophyllene oxide (4.70%), viridiflorene (4.20%) and β-selinene (4.20%), β-elemene (3.80%), limonene

(3.70%), α-humulene (3.40%) all present in the root bark and (2.80% in the leaves). The *Melaleuca* species are known for their medicinal EOs production and are very good source of 1,8-cineole often isolated alongside with viridiflorol in significant quantity. The EO composition of these species possesses some important biological activities such as insect repellent as well as in the relief of coughs and colds, headache and toothache, rheumatism and neuralgia, and applied in aromatherapy. The broad-spectrum antimicrobial activity of *M. alternifolia* EO (tea tree oil) was attributed to 1,8-cineole [98].

Table 2. Essential oil constituents of *Albizia odoratissima*

Constituents	L.R.I	L.R.I[A]	AOL	AOSB	AORB
2-heptanone[e]	891	889	0.6	-	-
α-pinene[a]	941	932	2.3	1.2	-
benzaldehyde[e]	962	952	0.5	-	-
β-pinene[a]	981	974	0.5	0.3	-
2-octanone[e]	993	988	0.2	-	-
p-cymene[a]	1028	1020	1.1	0.7	0.9
Limonene[a]	1032	1024	-	-	3.7
1,8-cineole[b]	**1034**	**1026**	**29.2**	**23.6**	**13.6**
(*Z*)-β-ocimene[a]	1042	1032	-	-	0.5
Dihydrotagetone[b]	1054	1046	0.2	-	-
Terpinolene[a]	1090	1086	-	-	1.1
p-cymenene[a]	1091	1089	2.1	0.6	-
neo-iso-pulegol [b]	1147	1144	0.3	-	-
4-terpineol [b]	1179	-	0.5	0.4	-
(*Z,E*)-undeca-1,3,5-triene[e]	1182	-	0.2	-	-
p-cymen-8-ol[b]	1185	1179	1.1	-	-
α-terpineol[b]	**1191**	**1186**	**5.4**	**5.6**	1.5
p-menth-4-en-3-one[b]	1251	-	0.2	-	-
α-copaene[c]	1377	1374	-	-	0.5
β-bourbonene[c]	1385	1387	-	-	0.6
β-elemene[c]	1392	1389	0.2	-	3.8
α-gurjunene[c]	1410	1409	0.3	-	-
β-caryophyllene[c]	1419	1417	3.2	1.9	**10.3**
β-copaene[c]	1430	1430	-	-	0.6
Aromadendrene[c]	1440	1439	0.9	0.4	-
α-humulene[c]	1455	1452	0.7	0.4	3.4
Alloaromadendrene[c]	1462	1458	1.1	0.6	-
γ-muurolene[c]	1478	1478	0.4	-	2.6

Constituents	L.R.I	L.R.I[A]	AOL	AOSB	AORB
Germacrene D[c]	1481	1484	-	-	2.2
β-selinene[c]	1487	1489	0.5	0.4	**4.2**
Valencene[c]	1493	1496	2.8	-	-
Viridiflorene[c]	1495	1496	-	2.0	**4.2**
α-muurolene[c]	1499	1500	-	-	0.7
α-bulnesene[c]	1507	1509	-	-	1.5
trans-γ-cadinene[c]	1514	1513	0.9	0.5	1.9
δ-cadinene[c]	1524	1522	1.0	0.6	2.5
Germacrene B[c]	1557	1559	-	-	0.9
(*E*)-nerolidol[d]	1564	1561	0.8	0.7	1.7
Ledol[d]	1566	1602	-	0.3	-
Spathulenol[d]	1577	1577	-	-	1.3
Caryophyllene oxide[d]	**1582**	1582	2.8	3.5	**4.7**
Viridiflorol[d]	**1591**	**1592**	**31.6**	**44.0**	**18.5**
Guaiol[d]	1596	1600	0.6	0.9	0.5
Humulene epoxide II[d]	1607	1608	0.3	0.3	0.7
β-oplopenone[d]	1608	1607	-	-	0.6
1-*epi*-cubenol[d]	1629	1627	0.5	0.7	1.0
γ-eudesmol[d]	1632	1630	0.4	0.6	1.1
T-cadinol[d]	1641	1638	0.9	1.4	2.5
2,6,10-trimethylpentadecane[e]	1642	-	-	1.5	-
β-eudesmol[d]	1650	1649	0.7	1.2	0.8
α-eudesmol[d]	1653	1652	1.0	1.7	-
Valerianol[d]	1656	1656	-	-	2.5
Acorenone[d]	1688	1692	0.5	-	-
[a]Monoterpene hydrocarbons			6.0	2.8	6.2
[b]Oxygenated monoterpenes			36.9	29.6	15.1
[c]Sesquiterpene hydrocarbons			12.0	6.8	39.9
[d]Oxygenated sesquiterpenes			40.1	55.3	35.9
[e]Non-terpene derivatives			1.5	1.5	0.0
Total identified			**96.5**	**96.0**	**97.1**

Major constituents are in bold form.

Key: L.R.I = Linear Retention Index on HP-5 column from this work.
L.R.I[A] = Linear Retention Index on DB-5 column from literature [82].
AOL = *Albizia odoratissima* leaves.
AOSB = *Albizia odoratissima* stem bark.
AORB = *Albizia odoratissima* root bark.

The anthelmintic activity of *A. odoratissima* EOs (Table 3) against *Eudrilus eugeniae* showed a reduction in time of paralysis and death as concentration increased. The leaf EO, with the highest composition of 1,8-cineole, showed the best activity such that at highest concentration, paralysis was observed at 8.40 mins and death at 38.00 mins. The activities exhibited by the stem bark and root bark oils are relatively similar. However, EOs in which 1,8-cineole was reported to be in abundance displayed anthelmintic activity. *Eucalyptus globules* Labill EO showed an efficacy of 87.30% against *H. contortus* in an egg-hatch inhibitory and larval developmental assay, from which 1,8-cineole (83.90% composition) was identified as the dominant constituent [99]. More to these, Oliveira et al., [91] reported the efficacy of 1,8-cineole rich *Piper aduncum* EO, with an egg-hatching inhibition of 95% against *H. contortus,* to be twice more effective than *E. globules* EO. *Albizia odoratissima* EOs were significantly more active, in terms of time of paralysis and death, than Albendazole in a dose-dependent manner ($p < 0.001$) while the time observed for paralysis and death of worm to take place in distilled water (negative control) was much greater than 300 minutes, after which the worms might have suffered from excess absorption of water by osmosis.

Table 3. Anthelmintic activity of *Albizia odoratissima* essential oils

Conc. (% v/v)	Time of Paralysis (Mean ± SEM) in minutes, n = 5			
	AOL	AOSB	AORB	ALBZ
1.00	23.80 ± 1.77	26.40 ± 1.50	28.60 ± 1.44	97.20 ± 1.39
2.00	20.20 ± 1.50	22.40 ± 1.89	22.60 ± 1.57	94.20 ± 1.77
3.00	14.08 ± 1.59	15.60 ± 0.98	15.00 ± 1.14	89.60 ± 1.29
4.00	10.00 ± 1.05	12.20 ± 1.07	11.60 ± 0.92	87.40 ± 1.08
5.00	8.40 ± 0.68	10.20 ± 0.73	10.00 ± 0.71	82.80 ± 1.28
Conc. (% v/v)	Time of Death (Mean ± SEM) in minutes, n = 5			
	AOL	AOSB	AORB	ALBZ
1.00	80.60 ± 2.29	84.40 ± 1.50	86.00 ± 1.87	154.60 ± 1.86
2.00	73.60 ± 1.97	75.40 ± 1.91	79.80 ± 1.98	149.20 ± 2.35
3.00	65.20 ± 2.62	67.00 ± 1.41	71.40 ± 2.09	140.60 ± 1.72
4.00	47.20 ± 1.77	50.80 ± 1.56	55.20 ± 1.60	135.00 ± 1.92
5.00	38.00 ± 1.26	41.60 ± 1.36	44.80 ± 1.56	130.20 ± 1.77

Key: AOL = Albizia odoratissima leaves.
AOSB = Albizia odoratissima stem bark.
AORB = Albizia odoratissima root bark.
ALBZ = Albendazole (Standard drug as positive control).
SEM = Standard error of mean.
n = number of worms in each petri-dish.

Millettia thonningii (Schum & Thonn) Baker

Millettia thonningii (Schum & Thonn) Baker, commonly referred to as 'Ito' and 'Turburku' by the Yorubas and the Hausas, respectively in Nigeria, is a deciduous tree often found on riverbanks. In traditional system of medicine, the plant is useful in worm expulsion, as a laxative/purgative, a blood purifier, in the treatment of diarrhea/dysentery, menstrual disorders and bronchitis. The leaf juice was also reported to be a poison to water snails [100, 101, 102, 103].

Millettia thonningii leaves, stem bark and root bark EOs were obtained in yields of 0.256%, 0.260% and 0.268% (v/w) respectively. Of the total oil fractions in the leaves, stem bark and root bark oils, a total of 21, 24 and 35 constituents representing 94.80%, 96.90% and 96.90%, respectively were identified (Table 4). The leaves, stem bark and root bark oils consist of monoterpene hydrocarbons (0.50%, 0.00%, and 0.20%, respectively), oxygenated monoterpenes (0.00%, 0.00% and 8.00%, respectively), sesquiterpene hydrocarbons (74.90%, 76.90% and 66.30%, respectively), oxygenated sesquiterpenes (6.80%, 18.90% and 21.90%, respectively),

Table 4. Essential oil constituents of *Millettia thonningii*

Constituents	L.R.I	L.R.I[A]	MTL	MTSB	MTRB
α-pinene[a]	941	932	-	-	0.2
1-octen-3-ol[f]	981	974	-	0.5	0.3
2-pentyl furan[f]	993	984	0.9	-	-
3-octanol[f]	994	988	-	0.6	-
Limonene[a]	1032	1024	0.5	-	-
1,8-cineole[b]	1034	1026	-	-	5.9
Naphthalene[f]	1181	1178	-	-	0.2
α-terpineol[b]	1191	1186	-	-	2.1
Cyclosativene[c]	1369	1369	-	-	0.2
α-copaene[c]	1377	1374	-	-	0.4
β-elemene[c]	1392	1389	1.0	0.7	0.8
Isocaryophyllene[c]	1405	-	1.2	-	0.2
(*E*)-β-damascone[e]	1412	1413	0.6	-	-
β-caryophyllene[c]	1419	1417	57.6	62.9	47.0
(*E*)-α-ionone[e]	1428	1428	1.8	-	-

Table 4. (Continued)

Constituents	L.R.I	L.R.I^{A}	MTL	MTSB	MTRB
α-humulene[c]	1455	1452	8.6	8.9	7.5
γ-muurolene[c]	1478	1478	0.9	0.5	0.9
ar-curcumene[c]	1483	1479	-	-	0.8
(*E*)-β-ionone[e]	1487	1487	1.3	0.6	1.5
β-selinene[c]	1487	1489	2.3	-	-
Viridiflorene[c]	1495	1496	1.0	0.7	0.7
α-zingiberene[c]	1496	1493	-	-	0.9
α-selinene[c]	1496	1498	2.0	0.5	2.4
α-bulnesene[c]	1507	1509	0.7	1.0	0.8
β-bisabolene[c]	1508	1505	-	0.2	-
trans-γ-cadinene[c]	1514	1513	-	-	0.4
δ-cadinene[c]	1524	1522	0.6	0.7	-
β-sesquiphellandrene[c]	1525	1521	-	-	0.6
Kessane[c]	1530	1529	-	0.2	-
Elemol[c]	1550	1548	-	-	1.2
(*E*)-nerolidol[d]	1564	1561	-	0.3	0.6
Caryophyllene oxide[d]	1582	1582	5.0	13.2	13.6
Viridiflorol[d]	1591	1592	-	-	1.1
Guaiol[d]	1596	1600	-	-	0.3
Humulene epoxide II[d]	1607	1608	0.6	1.7	1.5
1-*epi*-γ-eudesmol[d]	1622	1622	-	0.1	0.2
1-*epi*-cubenol[d]	1629	1627	-	0.3	0.4
γ-eudesmol[d]	1632	1630	-	-	0.2
Caryophylla-4(14),8(15)-dien-5-ol[d]	1636	1639	-	0.3	0.3
Cubenol[d]	1641	1645	-	0.3	0.4
2,6,10-trimethylpentadecane[f]	1642	-	1.8	-	-
β-eudesmol[d]	1650	1649	-	0.3	0.3
Selin-11-en-4α-ol [d]	1655	1658	-	0.6	0.8
Valerianol[d]	1656	1656	-	0.5	1.3
Aromadendrene oxide-(1)[d]	1673	-	-	1.3	0.9
1-tetradecanol[f]	1675	1671	0.8	-	-
Acorenone[d]	1688	1692	1.2	-	-
Pentadecanal[f]	1716	-	4.4	-	-
[a]Monoterpene hydrocarbons			0.5	0.0	0.2
[b]Oxygenated monoterpenes			0.0	0.0	8.0
[c]Sesquiterpene hydrocarbons			74.9	76.9	66.3
[d]Oxygenated sesquiterpenes			6.8	18.9	21.9
[e]Apocarotenoids			4.7	0.0	0.0
[f]Non-terpene derivatives			7.9	1.1	0.5
Total identified			94.8	96.9	96.9

Major constituents are in bold form.

Key: L.R.I = Linear Retention Index on HP-5 column from this work.

L.R.I^{A} = Linear Retention Index on DB-5 column from literature [82].

MTL = *Millettia thonningii* leaves.

MTSB = *Millettia thonningii* stem bark.

MTRB = *Millettia thonningii* root bark.

apocarotenoids (4.70%, 0.00% and 0.00%, respectively) and non-terpene derivatives (7.90%, 1.10% and 0.50%, respectively) with the dominance of the sesquiterpene hydrocarbons. The major constituents identified in the leaves and stem bark oils, respectively are β-caryophyllene (57.60% and 62.90%), α-humulene (8.60% and 8.90%) and caryophyllene oxide (5.00% and 13.20%) while β-caryophyllene (47.00%), caryophyllene oxide (13.60%), α-humulene (7.50%) and 1,8-cineole (5.90%) dominated the root bark oil. Common in the three oils are β-caryophyllene, α-humulene and caryophyllene oxide from which β-caryophyllene is the most abundant as expressed in the stem bark oil.

Table 5. Anthelmintic activity of *Millettia thonningii* essential oils

Conc. (% v/v)	Time of Paralysis (Mean±SEM) in minutes, n = 5			
	MTL	**MTSB**	**MTRB**	**ALBZ**
1.00	31.80 ± 2.67	28.80 ± 2.78	23.80 ± 2.52	97.20 ± 1.39
2.00	24.80 ± 2.35	23.60 ± 2.56	17.20 ± 1.93	94.20 ± 1.77
3.00	16.80 ± 2.08	15.20 ± 2.18	13.00 ± 1.70	89.60 ± 1.29
4.00	12.60 ± 1.69	10.20 ± 1.39	9.80 ± 1.24	87.40 ± 1.08
5.00	9.00 ± 1.05	8.40 ± 1.03	8.60 ± 0.93	82.80 ± 1.28
Conc. (% v/v)	**Time of Death (Mean ± SEM) in minutes, n = 5**			
	MTL	**MTSB**	**MTRB**	**ALBZ**
1.00	88.00 ± 3.78	79.00 ± 4.39	73.40 ± 3.36	154.60 ± 1.86
2.00	77.20 ± 3.54	69.60 ± 3.78	66.80 ± 3.37	149.20 ± 2.35
3.00	61.80 ± 3.81	59.00 ± 3.67	57.60 ± 3.88	140.60 ± 1.72
4.00	49.20 ± 3.77	48.40 ± 3.75	45.40 ± 3.33	135.00 ± 1.92
5.00	38.00 ± 3.56	36.20 ± 2.85	35.80 ± 2.78	130.20 ± 1.77

Key: MTL = Millettia thonningii leaves.
MTSB = Millettia thonningii stem bark.
MTRB = Millettia thonningii root bark.
ALBZ = Albendazole (Standard drug as positive control).
SEM = Standard error of mean.
n = number of worms in each petri-dish.

CONCLUSION

This chapter reported the anthelmintic efficacy of various essential oils in literature as well as the activity of some of the essential oil constituents for their individual anthelmintic efficacy and a combined efficacy against different test organisms. It also provided information on the constituents, and compositional patterns of essential oils of some Nigerian medicinal plants used to treat gastro-intestinal troubles ethno-medicinally. Variation in composition due to either ecological factor, geographical origin, genetic make-up, climatic condition or physical factors plays important role in the activity of the oils, such that the constituents present often dictates the rate of activity. The encouraging activity of these oils and the combined efficacy of mixture of constituents could be attributed to the synergistic and additive effect among the multiple bioactive compounds contained in the essential oils. Promising combined formulations for parasite control could be explored further for dominant constituent of oils studies from Nigerian source and deserve further investigations and justification *in vivo*.

REFERENCES

[1] World Health Organisation (WHO) (2012). Soil-transmitted helminthiases: eliminating soil-transmitted helminthiases as a public health problem in children. Geneva: In *progress report 2001-2010 and strategic plan 2011-2020.* WHO Library Cataloguing-In-Publication Data, 20 p. WHO/HTM/NTD/PCT/2012.4. (http://www.who.int/about/licensing/copyright_form/en/index.html).

[2] Hotez, P. J., Brindley, P. J., Bethany, J. M., King, C. H., Pearce, E. J. and Jacobson, J. (2008). Helminth infections: the great neglected tropical diseases. *J. Clin. Invest.*, 118(4): 1311-1321.

[3] Brooke, E. M., Meagan, A., Greg, B., Michael, B., Yamilette, M. C. A., James, D. E., Mallory, F., Cody, H., Edward, E. H., Olivia, H., George, J. K., Aspen, M. M., José T. M., Paul, P., Lucy, F. R. and Bernhard, J. (2014). *The Atlas of infectious diseases.* Oregon State University. Carto group. www.cartograhy.oregonstate. edu.

[4] Norris, J., Adelman, C., Spantchak, Y. and Marano, K. (2012). Social and economic impact review on Neglected Tropical Diseases.

Economic policy/briefing paper, Hudson Institute (Washinton DC) and Global Network for Neglected Tropical Diseases, 36 p.

[5] Carson, C. F. and Hammer, K. A. (2011). Chemistry and bioactivity of essential oils. In: Thormar, H. (Ed.), *Lipids and essential oils as antimicrobial agents*. Wiley, United Kingdom. Chapter 9: 203-238.

[6] Hamid, A. A., Aiyelaagbe, O. O. and Usman, L. A. (2011). Essential oils: Its medicinal and pharmacological uses. *International Journal of Current Research*, 33(2): 086-098.

[7] Abad, M. J., Bedoya, L. M., Apaza, L. and Bermejo, P. (2012). The *Artemisia* L. Genus: a review of bioactive essential oils. *Molecules*, 17: 2542-2566.

[8] Castro, G. A. (1996). Helminths: Structure, classification, growth, and development (Chapter 86). Baron, S. (Ed.), *Medical Microbiology,* 4th Edition. Galveston (TX): University of Texas Medical Branch, Galveston.

[9] Rosso, D., Miller, J. and Marek, T. (1996). *Class action: Improving school performance in the developing world through better health and nutrition.* The World Bank, directions in development.

[10] Omitola, O. O., Mogaji, H. O., Oluwole, A. S., Adeniran, A. A., Alabi, O. M. and Ekpo, U. F. (2016). Geohelminth infections and nutritional status of preschool aged children in a periurban settlement of Ogun State. *Scientifica*, Volume 2016, Article ID 7897351, 9 pp.

[11] Hotez, P. J., Ottesen, E., Fenwick, A. and Molyneux, D. (2006). The neglected tropical diseases: the ancient afflictions of stigma and poverty, and the prospects for their control elimination. In: Pollard, A.J. and Finn, A. (Eds.), *Hot Tropics Infection and Immunity in Children III*. New York: Springer, US.

[12] Kealey, A. and Smith, R. (2010). Neglected tropical diseases: infection, modeling and control. *Journal of Health Care for the Poor and Underserved*, 21: 53-69.

[13] Bethany, J., Brooker, S., Albonico, M., Geiger, S. M., Loukas, A., Diemert, D. and Hotez, P. J. (2006). Soil-transmitted helminth infections: ascariasis, trichuriasis, and hookworm. *Lancet*, 367: 1521-32.

[14] Hotez, P. J., de Silva, N., Brooker, S. and Bethany. J. (2003). Soil transmitted helminth infections: the nature causes and burden of the condition. *Working paper No. 3, disease control priorities project,* Bethesda, Maryland. Fogarty International Center, National Institutes of Health.

[15] Sanchez, A. L., Gabrie, J. A., Usuanlele, M-T., Rueda, M. M., Canales, M. and Gyorkos, T. W. (2013). Soil-transmitted helminth infections and nutritional status in school-age children from Fural communities in Honduras. *PLoS Neglected Tropical Diseases*, 7(8): e2378.

[16] Hall, A., Hewitt, G., Tuffrey, V. and de Silva, N. (2008). A review and meta-analysis of the impact of intestinal worms on child growth and nutrition. *Matern. Child Nutr.*, 4(1): 118-236.

[17] Ezeamama, A. E., Friedman, J. F., Olveda, R. M., Acosta, L. P., Kurtis, J. D., Mor, V. and Mcgarvey, S. T. (2005). Functional significance of low-intensity poly-parasite helminth infections in anaemia. *Journal of Infectious Disease*, 192: 2160-2170.

[18] Stephenson, L. S., Latham, M. C. and Ottesen, E. A. (2000). Malnutrition and parasitic helminth infections. *Parasitology*, 121 Suppl: S23-38.

[19] Mulu, A, Kassu, A., Legesse, M., Erko, B., Nigussie, D., Shimelis, T., Belyhun, Y., Moges, B., Ota, F. and Elias, D. (2014). Helminths and malaria co-infections are associated with elevated serum IgE. *Parasites & Vectors*, 7:240.

[20] Mulu, A., Maier, M. and Liebert, U. G. (2013). Deworming of intestinal helminths reduces HIV-1 subtype C viremia in chronically co-infected individuals. *International Journal of Infectious Diseases*, 17: e897-e901.

[21] van Riet, E., Hartgers, F. C. and Yazdanbakhsh, M. (2007). Chronic helminth infections induce immunomodulaion consequences and mechanism. *Immunobiology*, 212(6): 475-479.

[22] Brooker, S., Clements, A. C., Hotez, P. J., Hay, S. I., Tatem, A. J., Bundy, D. A. and Snow, R. W. (2006). The co-distribution of

Plasmodium falciparum and hookworm among African schoolchildren. *Malaria Journal*, 5: 99.

[23] Druilhe, P., Tall, A. and Sokhna, C. (2005). Worms can worsen malaria: towards a new means to roll back malaria? *Trends in Parasitology*, 21(8): 359-362.

[24] Mkhize, B. T., Mabaso, M., Mamba, T., Napier, C. E. and Mkhize-Kwitshana, Z. L. (2017). The interaction between HIV and intestinal helminth parasites co-infection with nutrition among adults in KwaZulu-Natal, South Africa. *BioMed Research International*, Volume 2017, Article ID 9059523, 12 p.

[25] Simon, G. G. (2016). Impacts of neglected tropical disease on incidence and progression of HIV/AIDS, tuberculosis, and malaria: scientific links. *International Journal of Infectious Diseases*, 42: 54-57.

[26] Alemayehu, M., Birhan, W., Belyhun, Y., Sahle, M. and Tessema, B. (2014). Prevalence of smear positive tuberculosis, intestinal parasites and their co-infection among tuberculosis suspects in Gondar University Hospital and Gondar Poly Clinic, North West Ethiopia. *J. Microb. Biochem. Technol.*, 6(4): 179-184.

[27] Dada-Adegbola, H. O., Oluwatoba, O. A. and Falade, C. O. (2013). Asymptomatic malaria and intestinal helminth co-infection among children in a rural community in Southwest Nigeria. *Malaria World Journal*, 4(18): 1-6.

[28] Tian, L-G., Chen, J-X., Wang, T-P., Cheng, G-J., Steinmann, P., Wang, F-F., Cai, Y-C., Yin, X-M., Guo, J., Zhou, L. and Zhou, X-N. (2012). Co-infection of HIV and intestinal parasites in rural area of China. *Parasites & Vectors*, 5: 36.

[29] Tchinda, V. H. M., Ponka, R., Ndzi, E. S., Madocgne, A. K., Amédée, M., Tchinda, M. G. and Moyou, R. S. (2012). Prevalence of malaria and soil-transmitted helminth infections and their association with under-nutrition in school children residing in Mfou health district in Cameroon. *Journal of Public Health and Epidemiology*, 4(9): 253-260.

[30] Molefe, N. I., Tsotetsi, A. M., Ashafa, A. O. T. and Thekisoe, O. M. M. (2013). *In vitro* anthelmintic activity of *Cotyledon orbiculata, Hermannia depressa* and *Nicotiana glauca* extracts against parasitic gastrointestinal nematodes of livestock. *Journal of Medicinal Plants Research*, 7(9): 536-542.

[31] Albonico, M., Bickle, Q., Ramsan, M., Montresor, A., Savioli, L. and Taylor, M. (2003). Efficacy of mebendazole and levamisole alone or in combination against intestinal nematode infections after repeated targeted mebendazole treatment in Zanzibar. *Bulletin of the World Health Organization*, 81: 343-352.

[32] Zerdo, Z., Yohanes, T. and Tariku, B. (2016). Soil-transmitted helminth re-infection and associated risk factors among school-age children in Chencha district, Southern Ethiopia: A cross-sectional study. *Journal of Parasitology Research*, Volume 2016, Article ID 4737891, 7 pages.

[33] Speich, B., Moser, W., Ali, S. M., Ame, S. M., Albonico, M., Hattendorf, J. and Keiser, J. (2016). Efficacy and re-infection with soil-transmitted helminths 18-weeks post-treatment with albendazole-ivermectin, albendazole-mebendazole, albendazole-oxantel pamoate and mebendazole. *Parasites & Vectors*, 9:123.

[34] Grant, W., Bisset, S., Prichard, R. K., Hotez, P., Bethony, J., Gilleard, J., Sternberg, P., Gasser, R., Mardis, E. R., Wilson, R. K. and Mitreva, M. (2010). Anthelmintic resistance in parasitic nematodes. *A consortium.* 6 p.

[35] Sutherland, I. A. and Leathwick, D. M. (2011). Anthelmintic resistance in nematode parasites of cattle: a global issue? *Trends Parasitol.*, 27: 176-181.

[36] Gilleard, J. S. and Beech, R. N. (2007). Population genetics of anthelmintic resistance in parasitic nematodes. *Parasitol.*, 134(8): 1133-47.

[37] Edwards-Jones, V. (2013). Alternative antimicrobial approaches to fighting multidrug-resistant infections. In: Rai, M. K. and Kon, K. V. (Eds.), *Fighting multidrug resistance with herbal extracts, essential*

oils and their components. Academic press (Elsevier), London. Chapter 1: 1-9.

[38] Miguel, M. G. (2010). Antioxidant and anti-inflammatory activities of essential oils: A short review. *Molecules*, 15: 9252-9287.

[39] Carson, C. F., Hammer, K. A. and Riley, T. V. (2006). *Melaleuca alternifolia* (tea tree) oil: A review of antimicrobial and other properties. *Clin. Microbiol. Rev.* 19: 50-62.

[40] Keszei, A., Brubaker, C. L. and Foley, W. J. (2008). A molecular perspective on terpene variation in Australian Myrtaceae. *Aust. J. Bot.*, 56: 197-213.

[41] Sell, C. (2010). Chemistry of essential oils. In: Başer, K.H.C. and Buchbauer, G. (Eds.), *Handbook of Essential Oils: Science, Technology, and Applications*. Taylor & Francis Group, 6000 Broken Sound Parkway NW, Suite 300, Chapter 5: 121-150.

[42] Sadgrove, N. and Jones, G. (2015). A contemporary introduction to essential oils: Chemistry, bioactivity and prospects for Australian Agriculture. *Agriculture*, 5: 48-102.

[43] Rohdich, F., Eisenreich, W., Wingsintaweekul, J., Hecht, S., Schuhr, C. A. and Bacher, A. (2001). Biosynthesis of terpenoids. 2C-Methyl-D-erythritol-2,4-cyclodiphosphate synthase (IspF) from *Plasmodium falciparium. European Journal of Biochemistry*, 268(11): 3190-3197.

[44] Qidwai, T., Jamal, F., Khan, M. Y. and Sharma, B. (2014). "Exploring drug targets in isoprenoid biosynthetic pathway for *Plasmodium falciparum*". *Biochemistry Research International*, 2014: 657189.

[45] Zhao, L., Chang, W-c., Xiao, Y., Liu, H-w. and Liu, P. (2013). Methylerythritol Phosphate Pathway of Isoprenoid Biosynthesis. *Annu. Rev. Biochem.*, 82:497-530.

[46] Bohlmann, J. and Keeling, C. I. (2008). Harnessing plant biomass for biofuels and biomaterials - Terpenoid biomaterials. *Plant J.*, 54: 656-669.

[47] Dubey, V. S., Bhalla, R. and Luthra, R. (2003). An overview of the non-mevalonate pathway for terpenoid biosynthesis in plants. *J. Biosci.*, 28: 637-646.

[48] Croteau, R., Kutchan, T. M. and Lewis, N. G. (2000). Natural products (secondary metabolites). In: Buchanan, B., Gruissem, W. and Jones, R. (Eds.), *Biochemistry and Molecular Biology of Plants*, American society of plant biologists, Rockville, MD, USA, p. 1250-1268.

[49] Devon, T. K. and Scott, A. I. (1972). Handbook of naturally occurring compounds, *Vol. 2, The Terpenes*. New York: Academic Press.

[50] Jäger, W. (2010). Metabolism of terpenoids in animal models and humans. In: Başer, K. H. C and Buchbauer, G. (Eds.), *Handbook of Essential Oils: Science, Technology, and Applications*. CRC Press, Taylor and Francis Group, London, UK. Chapter 8: 209-234.

[51] Başer, K. H. C. and Demirci, F. (2007). Chemistry of essential oils. In: Berger R.G. (Ed.), *Flavours and fragrances Chemistry, bioprocessing and sustainability*. Springer, Berlin, Germany, p. 43-86.

[52] Sell, C. S. (2003). A fragrant introduction to terpenoid Chemistry. Cambridge: Royal Society of Chemistry.

[53] Sell, C. S. (2007). Terpenoids. In: *The Kirk-Othmer Encyclopedia of Chemical Technology*, 5th edition, Wiley, New York.

[54] Friedrich, H. (1976). Phenylpropanoid constituents of essential oils. *Lloydia*, 39: 1-7.

[55] Petrussa, E., Braidot, E., Zancani, M. Peresson, C., Bertolini, A., Patui, S. and Vanello, A. (2013). Plant flavonoids - Biosynthesis, transport and involvment in stress response. *International Journal of Molecular Sciences*, 14: 14950-14973.

[56] Johnson, C. B., Kazantzis, A., Skoula, M., Mitteregger, U. and Novak, J. (2004). Seasonal, populational and ontogenic variation in the volatile oil content and composition of individuals of *Origanum vulgare* subsp. *hirtum*, assessed by GC headspace analysis and by SPME sampling of individual oil glands. *Phytochem. Anal.*, 15: 286-292.

[57] Schmiderer, C., Grassi, P., Novak, J., Weber, M. and Franz, C. (2008). Diversity of essential oil glands of clary sage (*Salvia sclarea* L., Lamiaceae). *Plant Biol.*, 10: 433-440.

[58] Novak, J., Bahoo, L., Mitteregger, U. and Franz, C. (2006). Composition of individual essential oil glands of savory (*Satureja hortensis* L., Lamiaceae) from Syria. *Flavour Fragr. J.*, 21: 731-734.

[59] Grassi, P., Novak, J., Steinlesberger, H. and Franz, C. (2004). A direct liquid, non-equilibrium solid-phase micro-extraction application for analysing chemical variation of single peltate trichomes on leaves of *Salvia officinalis. Phytochem. Anal.*, 15: 198-203.

[60] Camurça-Vasconcelos, A. L. F., Bevilaqua, C. M. L., Morais, S. M., Maciel, M. V., Costa, C. T. C., Macedo, I. T. F., Oliveira, L. M. B., Braga, R. R. Silva, R. A. and Vieira, L. S. (2007). Anthelmintic activity of *Croton zehntneri* and *Lippia sidoides* essential oils. *Veterinary Parasitology*, 148: 288-294.

[61] Macedo, I. T. F., Bevilaqua, C. M. L., de Oliveira, L. M. B., Camurça-Vasconcelos, A. L. F., Vieira, L. S., Oliveira, F. R., Queiroz-Junior, E. M., Tomé, A. R. and Nascimento, N. R. F. (2010). Anthelmintic effect of Eucalyptus staigeriana essential oil against goat gastrointestinal nematodes. *Veterinary Parasitology*, 173: 93-98.

[62] Macedo, I. T. F., de Oliveira, L. M. B., Ribeiro, W. L. C., dos Santos, J. M. L., Silva, K. C., Filho, J. V. A., Camurça-Vasconcelos, A. L. F. and Bevilaqua, C. M. L. (2015). Anthelmintic activity of *Cymbopogon citratus* against *Haemonchus contortus. Braz. J. Vet. Parasitol.*, 24(3): 268-275.

[63] Squires, J. M., Ferreira, J. F. S., Lindsay, D. S. and Zajac, A. M. (2011). Effects of artemisinin and *Artemisia* extracts on *Haemonchus contortus* in gerbils (*Meriones unguiculatus*). *Vet. Parasitol.*, 175(1-2): 103-108.

[64] Macedo, I. T. F., de Oliveira, L. M. B., André, W. P. P., Filho, J. V. A., dos Santos, J. M. L., Rondon, F. C. M., Ribeiro, W. L. C., Camurça-Vasconcelos, A. L. F., de Oliveira, E. F., de Paula, H. C. B. and Bevilaqua, C. M. L. (2019). Anthelmintic effect of *Cymbopogon citratus* essential oil and its nanoemulsion on sheep gastrointestinal nematodes. *Braz. J. Vet. Parasitol.*, 28(3): 522-527.

[65] Katiki, L. M., Chagas, A. C. S., Bizzo, H. R., Ferreirad, J. F. S. and Amarante, A. F. T. (2011). Anthelmintic activity of *Cymbopogon*

martinii, *Cymbopogon schoenanthus* and *Mentha piperita* essential oils evaluated in four different *in vitro* tests. *Veterinary Parasitology*, 183: 103-108.

[66] Katiki, L. M., Barbieri, A. M. E., Araujo, R. C., Veríssimo, C. J., Louvandini, H. and Ferreira, J. F. S. (2017). Synergistic interaction of ten essential oils against *Haemonchus contortus in vitro*. *Veterinary Parasitology*, 243: 47-51.

[67] Hussien, J., Urgessa, K., Regassa, F., Jemal, A., Abajebel, S. and Hussien, N. (2011). Anthelmintic effects of the essential oil extracts of selected medicinal plants again *Haemonchus contortus*. *International Journal of Agricultural Research*, 6: 290-298.

[68] Ferreira, L. E., Benincasa, B. I., Fachin, A. L., Contini, S. H. T., França, S. C., Chagas, A. C. S. and Beleboni, R. O. (2018). Essential oils of *Citrus aurantifolia*, *Anthemis nobile* and *Lavandula officinalis*: *in vitro* anthelmintic activities against *Haemonchus contortus*. *Parasites & Vectors*, 11:269.

[69] Mali, R. G. and Mehta, A. (2008). A review on anthelmintic plants. *Natural Product Radiance*, 7(5): 466-475.

[70] Sunita, K., Kumar, P., Khan, M. A., Husain, S. S. A. and Singh, D. K. (2017). Anthelminthic/larvicidal activity of some common medicinal plants. *European Journal of Biological Research*, 7(4): 324-336.

[71] Jeyathilakan, N., Murali, K., Anandaraj, A., Latha, B. R. and Basith. S. A. (2010). Anthelmintic activity of essential oils of *Cymbopogan nardus* and *Azadirachta indica* on *Fasciola gigantica. Tamilnadu. J. Veterinary & Animal Sciences*, 6: 204-209.

[72] Pueblos, K. R. S., Lagare, J. P. B., Tapales, P. V. P. P., and Quimque, M. T. J. (2015). *In vitro* anthelmintic activity evaluation of the aerial part of *Ruellia tuberose* Linn. against *Eudrilus eugeniae*. International Symposium on Applied Chemistry. *Procedia Chemistry*, 16: 570-577.

[73] Subash, K. R., Rao, N. J., Cheriyan, B. V., Bhaarati, G. M., and Kumar, K. S. (2012). Anthelmintic activity of *Eupatorium triplinerve* and *Alpiniagalanga* in *Pheritima posthuma* and *Ascardia galli*. *Journal of Clinical and Diagnostic Research*, 6(6): 947-950.

[74] Bachani, M. H. (2012). *In vitro* anthelmintic activity of some medicinal plants: A review. *International Journal of Pharmaceutical Sciences Research*, 3(9): 3064-3075.

[75] Rao, P. S., Sheth, N. R., and Jayaveera, K. N. (2012). Anthelmintic activity of essential oil of *Pimentadioica* (Linn.) Merill, Family: Myrtaceae, collected in summer from South Canara, India. *European Journal of Experimental Biology*, 2(6): 2271-2275.

[76] Tandon, V., Yadav, A. K., Roy, B. and Das, B. (2001). Phytochemicals as cure of worm infections in traditional medicine systems. *Emerging trends in Zoology*, 16: 351-378.

[77] Dash, G. K., Suresh, P., Sahu, S., Kar, D., Ganapaty, S. and Panda, S. (2002). Evaluation of *Evolvulus alsinoides* Linn. for anthelmintic and antimicrobial activities. *J. Nat. Remedies*, 2:182-185.

[78] Ajaiyeoba, E. O., Onocha, P. A. and Olarenwaju, O. T. (2001). *In vitro* anthelmintic properties of *Buchholzia coriaceae* and *Gynandropsis gynandra* extract. *Pharm Biol.*, 39: 217-220.

[79] Akhtar, M. S., Iqbal, Z., Khan, M. N. and Lateef, M. (2000). Anthelmintic activity of medicinal plants with particular reference to their use in animals in the Indo-Pakistan subcontinent. *Small Ruminant Research*, 38: 99-107.

[80] Jaradat, N., Adwan, L., K'aibni, S., Shraim, N. and Zaid, A. N. (2016). Chemical composition, anthelmintic, antibacterial and antioxidant effects of *Thymus bovei* essential oil. *BMC Complementary and Alternative Medicine*, 16:418. 7p.

[81] Medicines and Healthcare products Regulatory Agency, MHRA (1980). *British Pharmacopoeia*, Vol. II; H.M. Stationery Office, Pharmaceutical Press: London, UK.

[82] Adams R. (2007). Identification of essential oil components by Gas Chromatography/Mass spectrometry. 4th ed. Allured Publishing Corporation, Carol Stream IL, USA.

[83] Akande, A., Aboaba, S. and Flamini, G. (2018a). Constituents and anthelmintic activity evaluation of *Albizia adiantifolia* (Schumach) W.F. Wright essential oils from Nigeria. *International Journal of Chemistry*, 10(2): 10-15.

[84] Ugbogu, O. A., Osiyemi, O. A. and Odewo, T. K. (2012). Checklist of ethno-medicinal trees and shrubs in Federal college of forestry, Ibadan, Oyo State, Nigeria. *Journal of Forestry Research and Management*, 9: 106-124.

[85] Lawal, I. O., Uzokwe, N. E., Igboanugo, A. B. I., Adio, A. F., Awosan, E. A., Nwogwugwu, J. O., Faloye, B., Olatunji, B. P. and Adesoga, A. A. (2010). Ethno-medicinal information on collation and identification of some medicinal plants in Research Institutes of South-west Nigeria. *African Journal of Pharmacy and Pharmacology*, 4(1): 1-7.

[86] Orwa, C., Mutua, A., Kindt, R., Jamnadass, R. and Simons, A. (2009). *Albizia zygia* (DC.) J.F.Macbr.: *Agroforestree Database: A tree reference and selection guide*, version 4.0. (http://www.worldagroforestry.org/sites/treedbs/treedatabases.asp). 5 p.

[87] Apetorgbor, M. M. (2007). *Albizia zygia* (DC.) J.F.Macbr. [Internet] Record from PROTA4U. Louppe, D., Oteng-Amoako, A. A. and Brink, M. (Editors). PROTA (*Plant Resources of Tropical Africa/Ressources végétales de l'Afrique tropicale*), Wageningen, Netherlands. (http://www.prota4u.org/search.asp).

[88] Akande, A., Aboaba, S. and Flamini, G. (2018b). Variation in chemical constituents and anthelmintic activity of *Albizia zygia* (DC.) J.F.Macbr. Essential oils from Ibadan, Nigeria. *Journal of Science Research*, Vol. 17.

[89] Oloyede, G. K. and Ogunlade, A. O. (2015). Free radical scavenging activity and toxicity of linalool and thymol dominated essential oils of *Albizia Zygia* (DC) J.F. Macbr. leaves and stem-bark. *Research Journal of Medicine and Medical Sciences,* 10(2): 33-40.

[90] Rocha, C. G. F., Oliveira, A. R. dS., Araújo, A. V., Lafayette, S. S. L., Albuquerque, G. S., Silva-Neto, J. dC., Costa-Silva, J. H., Ferreira, F., da Costa, J. G. M. and Wanderley, A. G. (2015). Gastroprotective mechanisms of the monoterpene 1,8-Cineole (Eucalyptol). *PLoS ONE*, 10(8).

[91] Oliveira, G. L., Vieira, T. M., Nunes, V. F., Ruas, M. dO., Duarte, E. R., Moreira, D. dL., Kaplan, M. A. C. and Martins, E. R. (2014).

Chemical composition and efficacy in the egg-hatching inhibition of essential oil of *Piper aduncum* against *Haemonchus contortus* from sheep. *Rev. Bras. Farma.*, 24: 288-292.

[92] Orwa, C., Mutua, A., Kindt, R., Jamnadass, R. and Simons, A. (2009). *Albizia Odoratissima* (L.F) Benth. *Agroforest tree Database: A tree reference and selection guide,* version 4.0. (http://www.worldagroforestry.org/sites/treedbs/treedatabases.asp). 5 p.

[93] Rao, Y. K., Reddy, M. V. B., Rao, C. V., Gunasekar, D., Blond, A., Caux, C. and Bodo, B. (2002). Two new 5-deoxyflavones from *Albizia odoratissima*. *Chem. Pharm. Bull.*, 50(9): 1271-1272.

[94] Rajan, M., Kumar, V. K, Kumar, P. S., Venkatachalam, T. and Anbarasan, V. (2011). Pharmacognostical and phytochemical studies of the leaves of *Albizia Odoratissima* (L.F.) Benth. *International Journal of Pharmacognosy and Phytochemical Research*, 3(3): 47-55.

[95] Kumar, D., Kohli, S., Kumar, S., Gupta, J., Jain, P. and Pundir, R. K. (2011a). Screening of methanolic bark extract of *Albizia odoratissima* for antimicrobial activity. *Pharmacognosy Communications*, 1(2): 47-49.

[96] Kumar, D., Kumar, S., Kohli, S., Arya, R. and Gupta, J. (2011b). Antidiabetic activity of methanolic bark extract of *Albizia odoratissima* Benth. in alloxan induced diabetic albino mice. *Asian Pacific Journal of Tropical Medicine*, p. 900-903.

[97] Arumugam, G., Manjula, P. and Paari, N. (2013). A review: Anti diabetic medicinal plants used for diabetes mellitus. *Journal of Acute Disease*, p. 196-200.

[98] Barbosa, L. C. A., Silva, C. J., Teixeira, R. R., Meira, R. M. S. A. and Pinheiro, A. L. (2013). Chemistry and biological activities of essential oils from *Melaleuca* L. Species. *Agric. Conspec. Sci.*, 78(1): 11-23.

[99] Macedo, I. T. F., Bevilaqua, C. M. L., Oliveira, L. M. B., Camurça-Vasconcelos, A. L. F., Vieira, L. S., Oliveira, F. R., Queiroz-Junior, E. M., Portela, B. G., Barros, R. S. and Chagas, A. C. S. (2009). Ovicidal and larvicidal activity *in vitro* of *Eucalyptus globulus* EOs on *Haemonchus contortus*. *Rev. Bras. Parasitol. Vet.*, 18: 62-66.

[100] Harrison, J. J. E. K., Dankyi, E., Kingsford-Adaboh, R. and Ishida, H. (2011). In search of new leads: A closer look at the therapeutic potential of the constituents of *Millettia thonningii, Millettia pachycarpa* and their structural analogues. *Int. J. Pharm. Pharm. Sci.*, 3(2): 71-81.

[101] Koné, W. M., Vargas, M. and Keiser, J. (2012). Anthelmintic activity of medicinal plants used in Côte d'Ivoire for treating parasitic diseases. *Parasitol. Res.*, 110:2351-2362.

[102] Orwa, C., Mutua, A., Kindt, R., Jamnadass, R. and Simons, A. (2009). *Millettia thonningii.* Agroforestree Database: A tree reference and selection guide, version 4.0. (http://www.worldagroforestry.org/af/treedb). 5 p.

[103] Banzouzi, J. T., Prost, A., Rajemiarimiraho, M. and Ongoka, P. (2008). Traditional uses of the African *Millettia* species (Fabaceae). *International Journal of Botany*, 4: 406-420.

In: What to Know about Essential Oils
Editor: Malene M. Kjeldsen
ISBN: 978-1-53617-986-6

Chapter 5

MEDICINAL BENEFITS OF LEMON, LAVENDER AND PEPPERMINT ESSENTIAL OILS

***Danielle McGlynn*[*]*, Kayla Broscious, Alexandra Ruth and Ajay Bommareddy*[†]**
Department of Pharmaceutical Sciences, Nesbitt School of Pharmacy,
Wilkes University, Wilkes-Barre, Pennsylvania, US

ABSTRACT

The purpose of this chapter is to describe the medicinal benefits of lemon, lavender and peppermint essential oils. Essential oils are liquid extracts from aromatic plants that possess a variety of uses. In order to extract the liquid oil from plants, the most common extraction processes are steam distillation, cold press and enfleurage. Quality assurance testing should be performed on the oils before they are used by consumers to minimize risk and maximize benefit. To obtain the benefits for the body, essential oils can be used by topical application, inhalation and ingestion

[*] Corresponding Author's Email: danielle.mcglynn1@wilkes.edu.
[†] Corresponding Author's Email: ajay.bommareddy@wilkes.edu.

as well as other techniques. Many studies have been performed to find the statistical significance behind therapeutic claims about these oils. Lemon oil has been proven to help with morning sickness, bacterial infections, skin inflammation, pain and cognitive function. Lavender oil has proven use for alopecia, postpartum depression, hypertension, insomnia, and skin conditions. Peppermint oil has shown use for irritable bowel syndrome, motion sickness, nausea, pruritus, migraines, chest pain, dysphagia, and to treat bacterial and fungal infections. Lemon, lavender and peppermint oils can treat some of the same conditions, such as anxiety and depression. These oils have an abundance of uses that have been studied and proven to have statistically significant outcomes. Essential oil use has been proven to be an influential holistic approach to treatment of various disease states and symptoms. Further research should be performed to discover even more uses for these oils so that we can gain the most benefit from use.

Keywords: essential oils, lemon oil, lavender oil, peppermint oil, health benefits

ABBREVIATIONS

5-HT	Serotonin
ACC	Anterior Cingulate Cortex
AChE	Acetylcholine
ANCOVA	Analysis of Covariance
AqEO	Aqueous Working of Essential Oil
BDNF	Brain-derived neurotrophic factor
BPH	Benign prostatic hyperplasia
CgA	Chlorogenic acid
Clp-EO	Citrus Limetta Peels
CYP	Cytochrome P450
DA	Dopamine
DES	Distal esophageal spasm
DOI	2,5-Dimethoxy-4-iodoamphetamine
EGJOO	Esophagogastric junction outflow obstruction
FDA	Food and Drug Administration
GABA	Gamma-Aminobutyric Acid

GBSS-J	Gottfries, Brane, Steen scale
GC/MS	Gas chromatography and mass spectrometry
IBS	Irritable Bowel Syndrome
IL-1β	Interleukin 1 beta
IL-6	Interleukin-6
LPS	Lipopolysaccharide
MAO-A	Monoamine Oxidase A
MBC	Minimal Bactericidal Concentration
MDR	Multi-drug resistant
MIC	Minimum Inhibitory Concentration
MiEO	Micelle Solution of Essential Oil
NMDA	N-methyl-D-aspartic acid
PSQI	Pittsburgh sleep quality index
PUQE-24	Pregnancy-Unique Quantification of Emesis and Nausea
SERT	Serotonin Transporter
TBAR	Xanax
TDAS	Tuberculosis Drug Activity
TNF-α	Tumor necrosis factor alpha
TPA	12-O-tetradecanoylphorbol-13-acetate
TSB	Tryptic Soy Broth
VAS	Visual Analogue Scale

1. Introduction

Essential oils are liquid extracts from aromatic plants that possess a variety of uses including bactericidal, virucidal, fungicidal, antiparasitic and insecticidal properties, and are widely used in industries ranging from the food and agricultural industries to the cosmetic industry (Aziz et al., 2018). Aromatic plants have been used for thousands of years as herbal medicines. It is suggested that several cultures in the world have used aromatic plants at some point in history, and their use not confined to a specific area. Centuries of analyzing essential oils and isolating the therapeutic compounds present led to the beginning of modern medicine (Buckle, 2015).

All essential oils are primarily composed of carbon, hydrogen and oxygen, and their aroma is determined by the number of carbon atoms found on the aromatic ring (Sherwood, 2016). After extraction, essential oils contain a variety of non-volatile as well as volatile compounds, such as terpenes, terpenoids, phenol-derived aromatic components and aliphatic components (Bakkali et al., 2008). Essential oils can be separated into two main groups, terpenes and oxygenated compounds. Terpenes are unsaturated hydrocarbons, while "oxygenated compounds encompass a large subset, including ketones, aldehydes, alcohols, acids, phenols, coumarins, and esters. Based on the species of the plant, growing environment, the origin and the extraction method, the components of the oil may differ" (Sherwood, 2016).

Essential oils are used in different ways to obtain physiological benefits in the body. The oils can be applied and massaged into the skin, inhaled by steam inhalation, vaporized by a diffuser, or placed in the warm water of a bath. The most popular method of using these essential oils is aromatherapy, which is accomplished by using any of the inhalation processes mentioned. When the essential oils' essences or aromas are inhaled, the unique scent will trigger the olfactory receptors of the nose, which sends a signal to the olfactory bulb, relaying the message through the central nervous system to the limbic system. The limbic system is directly connected to parts of the brain that control heart rate, blood pressure, breathing, memory, stress levels, and hormone balance. Therefore, essential oils can have biological effects on any of these systems when used as aromatherapy. Each essential oil will have different physiological effects since each oil triggers the olfactory receptors in different ways.

To release the essential oils found inside of plants, various extraction methods are used such as steam distillation, cold press and enfleurage. Specific extraction methods are optimal for certain plant types. Steam distillation extraction begins with the plant material being placed inside of the still. Pressurized steam is forced through the plant material and the essential oil is freed from the oil glands in the plant tissue. The steam mixture of water and oil is turned to liquid as it passes through a cold water condenser. The oil separates automatically from the distillate water due to its lighter density, allowing for a simple decanting of the oil layer. Some volatile oils need to be gathered through a different extraction method, expression or cold press, because they cannot be distilled without being broken down beforehand. These extraction methods are best for citrus fruits since they have tough outer peels that need to be pulverized to release the oils. The fruits are either ground or punctured with sharp objects to release the oil from the glands of the epidermis. Pressure is then applied with a metal plate to expel all of the juices and oils, which are then filtered to separate the two (Rassem et al., 2016). Lastly, enfleurage extraction is best to obtain the oils from flower petals. A chassis, which is a large glass plate, is covered with solid animal fat or vegetable oil and flower petals are placed on top. The vegetable oil works on the mechanism of dissolving the essential oils and capturing the aromas. New flower petals are introduced to the chassis until the fat is fully saturated, becoming a pomade. The pomade is then dissolved with alcohol to leave just the essential oils behind. Many times this process is needed because the amount of volatile oil present in flower petals is so small that the other methods would not yield enough essential oil (Soe'eib et al., 2016).

Quality assurance testing of essential oils is imperative to minimize risk for the consumer, ensuring they will not be harmed from impurities, and will gain the most benefit from the oils. However, the FDA does not regulate essential oil production or testing. It is at the discretion of the production company to test the oils, and the consumer to research whether the company carries out proper testing. Before testing the oils, marker components are set as standards. If the essential oil falls outside of just one marker, the oil does not meet therapeutic grade standards and the product should not be sold. Ways that companies should scientifically test the quality of oils are by GC/MS, and refractive index. GC/MS is a technique that determines the presence and quantity of chemical constituents. This method can detect whether two or more oils have been mixed together, if any phytochemicals have been removed, or if an oil has been diluted, which are all factors that would negatively affect the consumer. The refractive index is a measure of how fast light travels through the material. This can be used to confirm the identity of the sample and determine the purity of the oil by comparing it to a standard (Hanson, 2003). For companies that do choose to test, GC/MS and refractive index analysis are performed on every batch of essential oils to confirm quality ("Top"). Consumers can further confirm the quality of the oils by performing their own tests such as organoleptic analysis. Organoleptic testing is a learned skill where the five senses are used to identify adulterants or extenders ("Essential"). Adulterants and chemically synthesized versions of the oils are added to essential oils because they are inexpensive. Consumers can learn this skill from a licensed aromatherapist who will help to confirm that they are purchasing grade oils. It is necessary to examine the quality of essential oils to gain evidence behind the bioavailability and metabolism in the body to prove the mechanism of action in treating diseases and conditions.

The bioavailability of essential oils has not been heavily tested in humans and limited data exists. Many previously conducted studies were performed in mouse models and cannot be relied upon for evidence-based information or decision making. Most essential oils are rapidly absorbed after dermal, oral, or pulmonary administration and cross the blood-brain barrier to interact with receptors in the central nervous system, affecting biological functions. The majority of components of essential oils are metabolized and eliminated by phase one enzyme metabolism in the kidneys, or exhaled from the lungs as carbon dioxide. The fast metabolism and short half-life of essential oil compounds has led researchers to believe that there is minimum risk of toxicity (Djilani et al., 2006). More studies will need to be implemented in human subjects to form evidence behind the proposed notions of the bioavailability of essential oils.

The three essential oils that are spotlighted throughout this chapter are lemon, lavender and peppermint oils. The versatility of these oils is immense and can be used as a therapeutic benefit to many ailments. There have been numerous studies discovering the pathways and receptors that these oils act on and have proven relief to various symptoms. In this chapter, each oil is introduced and research studies are presented to substantiate the therapeutic claims.

2. Lemon Oil

Although lemon essential oil has been used for centuries, we are just now gathering medical evidence to support claims stating that lemon oil is able to reduce anxiety and depression, ease morning sickness, improve skin health, relieve pain, soothe a sore throat, improve cognitive function, treat acne, heal wounds and act as an antifungal. Several pathological diseases such as diabetes, cardiovascular diseases, inflammation, hepatobiliary dysfunction and neurodegenerative disorders have been treated using citrus lemon (Falls et al., 2018). Many of its properties may be due to the major compounds present in the oil: limonene (37.5%), β-pinene (17.9%) and α-pinene (19.2%) (Man et al., 2019).

2.1. Anxiety and Depression

In a 2006 study on the anti-stress effects of lemon oil vapor via modulating the 5-HT and DA activities in mice, conducted by Komiya, Takeuchi, and Harada, mice were made to complete three tasks: an elevated plus-maze task, a forced swimming task, and an open field task. This was done in order to support the claim that lemon oil can reduce anxiety and depression. A regulatory mechanism of the lemon oil was explored by observing pretreatments with agonists or antagonists of benzodiazepine, 5-HT, DA and adrenaline receptors by elevated plus-maze task and forced swimming task. When pretreated with a benzodiazepine receptor antagonist, frumazenil, or a nonselective DA receptor agonist, apomorphine, the lemon oil anti-stress effect was greatly reduced. However, the anti-stress effect of lemon oil was not altered when agonists or antagonists of the 5-HT and alpha-2 adrenergic receptors were administered. The findings suggest that the anti-depressant effects of lemon oil are tied to the serotonergic pathway, especially the 1A receptor due to the fact that buspirone, 2,5-Dimethoxy-4-iodoamphetamine, and mianserine blocked the antidepressant effect, but WAY-100635, a piperazine drug thought to work as a 5-HT1A antagonist, did not (Komiya et al., 2006).

A randomized controlled clinical trial was done to determine the impact of lemon essential oil on patients' anxiety after orthopedic surgery. Eighty-two patients were divided into intervention and control groups, making sure the samples were homogeneous for age, gender, education and marital status, after being referred to the hospital for a distal radius fracture. The patients in the intervention group were treated by inhaling three drops of lemon oil placed on a cloth for 30 minutes. Anxiety levels were measured prior to surgery, 8 hours, and 16 hours after surgery, using the visual analog scale (VAS). When the intervention and control groups were compared prior to surgery there was no significant difference. After intervention with lemon essential oil, anxiety was significantly reduced 8 hours and 16 hours post surgery compared to anxiety in the control group. This supports the statement that lemon essential oil can help relieve anxiety post-surgery in patients with fractures (Kamrani et al., 2016).

2.2. Morning Sickness

Pregnant women commonly complain of nausea and vomiting, with as many as 50-80% having experienced some degree of morning sickness. Many women are interested in the use of herbal products due to their apprehension of medications causing adverse effects. In a double-blinded, randomized, controlled clinical trail including 100 pregnant women, there was a statistically significant difference between the mean scores of nausea and vomiting on the second and fourth days between the intervention group and the control group. The women in the study were referred to the health-medical centers of Birjand city, Iran, having mild to moderate nausea, with a score of 3-12 on the PUQE-24 questionnaire and were six to sixteen weeks pregnant. They were randomly divided into control and intervention groups through a four- and six-random block sampling method and treated for four days, measuring nausea, vomiting, and retch intensity. The placebo was made using carrot coloring in combination with almond oil, to imitate the intervention of ten cc of lemon oil, produced via solvent distillation. After analyzing the data through descriptive tests such as Chi-square, t-test and

ANCOVA statistical test, it was found that the mean nausea and vomiting scores were only statistically significant on days two and four, not days one and three. Therefore, this study provided evidence for the support of lemon oil use in easing morning sickness (Kia et al., 2014).

2.3. Antibacterial

Due to the variety of essential oil products, depending on the manufacturing process and microbial diversity, many publications on antibacterial properties have yielded irregular results, leaving space for more research. A study completed in 2019 explored the effects of commonly used essential oils on pathogenic bacteria. The essential oils frankincense (resin from *Boswellia sacra*), myrtle (*Myrtus communis*), thyme (*Thymus vulgaris*), lemon (*Citrus limon*), oregano (*Origanum vulgare*) and lavender (*Lavandula angustifolia*), were tested against six gram-negative and gram-positive bacteria. Methicillin sensitive *Staphylococcus aureus*, methicillin resistant *Staphylococcus aureus*, *Enterococcus faecalis*, *Escherichia coli*, *Klebsiella pneumoniae*, *Pseudomonas aeruginosa* were maintained in TSB medium with glycerin, at −70°C. Two broth microdilution methods were completed, the one method creating a micelle solution of essential oil and the other an aqueous working solution of essential oil. The minimum inhibitory concentrations were found using concentrations of 50%, 25%, 12.5%, 6.25%, 3.13%, 1.56%, 0.78%, 0.39%, 0.20%, 0.10%, 0.05% and 0.025% v/v in final volume in 96-well plates, one for AqEO and another for MiEO. The studied bacterial strains were checked for purity after being revitalized on Columbia blood agar 48 hours prior to the study. 100 μL of 10 μL inoculum: 9990 μL 2x Mueller-Hinton broth were transferred to 100 μL of AqEO/MiEO creating a bacterial inoculum of 2 × 104 CFU/well. Each plate contained a negative and positive control. Over 18 hours the plates were incubated at 35°C and normal atmospheric conditions. The last well where bacterial growth was not visible for each essential oil was interpreted as the MIC. 3 μl of the last three wells for each essential oil displaying no bacterial growth were spot-inoculated on blood-agar plates. After incubation at 35°C, minimum bactericidal concentration was noted where no bacterial colonies were developed. All of the values found were normalized against the MIC/MBC of pure ethanol, indicating whether the activity of the essential oil was lower or higher than the alcohol. The oils with the highest activity were oregano, thyme, lemon and lavender, with the greatest activity being achieved by the micelle suspensions. Aqueous solutions were not sufficient against all strains of bacteria compared to ethanol. The bacteria most sensitive to the essential oils were the Gram-positive cocci, with the *Enterobacteriaceae* family following. The bacteria with the highest resistance to majority of the essential oils, besides oregano and lemon oil, was *Pseudomonas aeruginosa.* Although the largest statistical differences between MiEO and AqEO occurred with oregano oil, lemon oil also possessed statistical differences between the two, demanding lower concentrations of micellar suspensions. The results concluded that essential oils containing a high amount of terpenes and terpenoids in a colloid form, including oregano, thyme, and lemon oil, are effective against various bacterial species (Man et al., 2019).

2.4. Skin Inflammation

After hydro-distillation was completed to extract the essential oil from Citrus limetta peels, the profile of the essential oil constituents were assessed via gas chromatography. Its anti-inflammatory effects were evaluated through the use of in vitro and in vivo models. It was found that the major components of the Clp-EO were monoterpene, hydrocarbon, and limonene. Pro-inflammatory cytokines, such as TNF-α, IL-6, IL-1β, in LPS- induced inflammation and reactive oxygen species in H2O2-induced oxidative stress were inhibited upon pretreatment with Clp-EO to macrophages. When the in vitro portion of the study was observed, topical administration of Clp-EO was found to lessen ear thickness, ear weight, lipid peroxidation, pro-inflammatory cytokines and improve ear tissue damage, induced by TPA, supporting the statement that Clp-EO can aid in treating inflammation (Maurya et al., 2018).

2.5. Pain

More research is needed to determine how lemon oil alters pain experienced by humans. However, it is believed that the anti-stress and antidepressant effects described above may aid our bodies to deciphering pain without overreacting. A 2014 study on mice was done to view how their brains responded to painful stimuli with and without lemon oil, leading to the evidence that lemon oil altered the way the mice responded to pain. By observing the anterior cingulate cortex and the descending pain inhibitory system of mice, as well as their behaviors when formalin was injected into their hind paw, inducing pain, it was noted that pain behavior decreased, the number of c-fos expression was significantly increased in the ACC, periaqueductal grey, nucleu raphe magnus and locus ceruleus, and decreased in the spinal dorsal horn with the use of lemon oil. Overall, the results implied that dopamine-related activation of ACC and the descending pain inhibitory system allowed for the inhibition of pain through lemon oil (Ikeda et al., 2014).

2.6. Cognitive Function

A 2008 study found aromatherapy to be an effective non-pharmacological therapy for dementia and may better cognitive function, especially in Alzheimer's patients. The study was completed with 28 elderly people, 17 of whom also had Alzheimer's disease. Aromatherapy, consisting of rosemary and lemon oils in the morning, and lavender and orange in the evening, was performed for 28 days, following a control period of 28 days and preceding a 28 day wash out period. Before the control period, after the control period, after aromatherapy, and after the washout period, the Japanese version of Gottfries, Brane, Steen scale, Functional Assessment Staging of Alzheimer's disease, a revised version of Hasegawa's Dementia, and the Touch Panel-type Dementia Assessment Scale, designed to rate cognitive dysfunction, were used to evaluate the effects of aromatherapy. Overall, the GBSS-J and the TDAS scores showed that patients' cognitive function improved, especially Alzheimer's patients, who demonstrated much higher TDAS scores (Jimbo et al., 2009).

Often times, learning environments only incorporate auditory and visual stimuli, excluding any olfactory stimuli that may also support students learning. Although this study did not observe the mechanism by which olfactory stimuli aids in learning and retaining information or whether the type of essential oil had an impact, it was shown that lemon aroma as an olfactory stimulus improved student's learning and achievement. Fifty-eight fourth grade students were separated into control and experimental groups. Both groups did not differ significantly on the 20-item test prior to the start of the study. However, after four weeks of learning English, the experimental group significantly outscored the control group, even one month after treatment was terminated. This study does not prove that the increase in scores was due to lemon essential oil, or olfactory stimuli, but there is an obvious correlation between lemon oil aromatherapy and memory and cognition (Akpinar, 2005).

A recent study investigated the effects of lemon oil on the memory of Swiss young Albino mice, both unstressed and stressed. Various groups of unstressed and stressed mice were given lemon oil and donepezil for three weeks, evaluating their nootropic movement with elevated plus maze and Hebbs Williams maze. In order to assess disease and drug effects, levels of acetylcholinesterase, plasma corticosterone, reduced glutathione, lipid peroxidation, superoxide dismutase and catalase, as well as histopathology were evaluated. The use of lemon oil was able to enhance movement of stress induced mice, significantly lower acetylcholinesterase and elevate catalase, superoxide dismutase and reduced glutathione, alter and reverse scopolamine induced amnesia, and aid in managing corticosterone levels. This study presumed that the memory enhancement was in part due to the reduction of AChE and TBAR (Falls et al., 2018).

Lemon oil is an extremely useful oil whether it is being applied topically or inhaled via aromatherapy. It has been found to be advantageous in various circumstances from post surgery anxiety to improved concentration and retention when learning. Although there were many studies performed in support of the clinical use of lemon oil, there are endless possibilities for new studies further enhancing our understanding of how lemon oil is able to aid in the treatment of numerous disease states.

3. Lavender Oil

Lavender essential oil is one of the most versatile oils with many therapeutic benefits. The main constituents found within lavender oil that are credited with these therapeutic benefits are linalool and linalyl-acetate (Garzoli et al., 2019). It can be used for personal use or in clinical settings such as surgical suites or inpatient facilities to treat ailments that patients are experiencing. The calming effect that lavender produces when introduced with the skin has been a proven remedy for conditions such as alopecia and various inflammatory skin conditions. Inhalation of lavender oil has also been proven as a remedy for conditions such as anxiety, depression, postpartum depression, hypertension, insomnia and other sleep disorders. The published studies that prove these claims are elaborated in this chapter.

3.1. Alopecia

Lavender produces a calming effect and hair growth increase to the scalp of patients who have been diagnosed with alopecia. Lavender oil was applied to the backs of C57BL/6 mice once a day, five times a week for four weeks. The results showed an increased number of hair follicles, deepened hair follicle depth, and thickened dermal layer which indicated that lavender could be used as a hair growth promoting agent. However, more studies need to be performed on humans to find extensive evidence regarding alopecia treatment (Lee et al., 2016).

3.2. Antidepressant

The mechanism of action of lavender oil in producing antidepressant effects was studied by looking at well established targets in the central nervous system including MAO-A, SERT, GABA and NMDA receptors as well as *in vitro* models of neurotoxicity. The results of this study showed that lavender oil, specifically linalool found within lavender oil, interacts with the NMDA and SERT receptors by acting as an antagonist and producing antidepressant effects (López et al., 2017).

The effects of lavender oil in boosting mood and decreasing depressive symptoms was studied via Sprague Dawley rats that were treated with chronic administration of high dose corticosterone to induce a depressive-like state. The rats were assigned to one of four groups which were control, corticosterone group with high dose of corticosterone, lavender essential oil group with daily exposure to lavender essential oil by inhalation, and lavender essential oil with corticosterone. Treatment was performed for fourteen days with behavioral testing along with serum samples were taken to measure brain-derived neurotrophic factor (BDNF, a factor in major depressive disorder), corticosterone and oxytocin levels (Phillips, 2017). Results of the behavior testing showed that the lavender essential oil group had significantly decreased depressive-like behavior after treatment compared to the other groups. It was also found that two to three days after the treatment with corticosterone, the levels of BDNF significantly increased in the lavender essential oil and lavender essential oil with corticosterone groups. This study proved that in rat models, lavender acted as an antidepressant when treating a depressive-like state induced by corticosterone. More studies need to be performed before conclusions can be drawn on the efficacy of lavender oil to treat depression in human subjects (Sánchez-Vidaña, 2019).

3.3. Anxiety

In a recent 2018 study, the phytochemical linalool, which is a main component of lavender essential oil, was found to cause the anxiolytic and calming therapeutic benefits when lavender was used as aromatherapy. The anxiolytic effects of linalool were studied with the light/dark box test and elevated plus maze on mice, of which half had the ability to smell and half did not. The mice that had the ability to smell were exposed to linalool odor and had anxiolytic outcomes without motor impairment. The mice that did not have the ability to smell did not have any beneficial outcomes from the linalool odor. This finding proved that the anxiolytic response to linalool is due to action on olfactory receptors. The mice that had the ability to smell were treated with flumazenil (a GABA antagonist) and found the anxiolytic effect being antagonized by this treatment. This further proved that the anxiolytic effect of linalool odor is due to (GABA)ergic transmission by the benzodiazepine-responsive GABA receptors. The effects of linalool are similar to that of benzodiazepines but without the motor impairment side effects. This study has shown the scientific background on the immense therapeutic benefits from linalool in treating and minimizing anxiety. By recognizing this mechanism of action, more studies on the anxiolytic properties of linalool within lavender essential oil can be made with more specific applications (Harada et al., 2018).

A mixed-methods study in 2019 determined that the use of overnight lavender aromatherapy skin patches eliminated or significantly reduced measurable anxiety symptoms for inpatient hematology-oncology patients (Shady et al., 2019). This study proved that overnight lavender aromatherapy skin patches are a beneficial option to improve quality of care in an inpatient setting.

In another study, individuals awaiting dental procedures were stimulated with the odor of lavender and anxiety levels, mood, alertness and calmness were assessed. Statistical analysis proved that compared to the control group, the odor of lavender reduced anxiety and improved mood in these individuals. This study further confirmed the notion that lavender oil can be used to ease anxiety and improve emotional state (Lehrner et al., 2005).

A 2019 randomized clinical trial studied the effects of lavender essential oil inhalation on perioperative oral surgery patients undergoing wisdom tooth removal under local anesthesia. Patients who expressed anxiety through the Dental Anxiety Questionnaire were enrolled in the study. The factors that were assessed were anxiety, mood, and vital signs including blood pressure, respiratory rate, heart rate, and saturation which were noted pre, intra and post-operatively. Statistical analysis proved that compared to the control group, the group that received the lavender oil inhalation had significant positive changes in blood pressures post-operatively, indicating reduced anxiety levels (Karan, 2019).

Anxiety and vital signs of BPH patients prior to undergoing BPH surgery (open prostatectomy surgery and transurethral resection of the prostate) were analyzed. The experimental group showed a statistically significant reduction in symptoms of anxiety and the posttest mean vital signs showed a decrease in respiration and an increase in oxygen saturation compared to the control group. The inhalation of lavender oil not only relieved anxiety symptoms but also improved the vital signs of patients (Genc et al., 2019).

A 2019 randomized control trial studied patients who were awaiting breast surgery. Before the surgery began, patients were given both a Personal Information Form and the State Anxiety Inventory to collect information on how they were feeling. Patients were split into a control and an experimental group prior to surgery. The experimental group was given lavender oil inhalation before the surgery began. It was determined that the experimental group State Anxiety Inventory post-test scores decreased significantly compared to the pre-test scores. This study proved that lavender oil can be used prior to surgery to reduce anxiety levels in patients (Beyliklioğlu et al., 2019).

A 2019 systematic review and meta-analysis of randomized controlled trials investigated whether published studies about the anxiolytic efficacy of lavender were considered strong evidence. Twenty two published randomized controlled trials that studied the anxiolytic effects of lavender oil in patients with and without clinical anxiety were chosen. The variables that were studied included self-rated anxiety, vital signs, and salivary cortisol and CgA levels. Through the meta-analysis, it was found that lavender aromatherapy had significant outcomes in reducing anxiety, systolic blood pressure, heart rate, salivary cortisol and CgA levels. Lavender essential oil reduces anxiety symptoms in patients who are or are not diagnosed with clinical anxiety and can also improve vital signs that are linked to anxiety. This meta-analysis proved that published trials involving anxiolytic efficacy of lavender aromatherapy are strong evidence for the use of lavender oil to reduce anxiety due to its calming properties (Kang et al., 2019).

3.4. Hypertension

Due to the anxiolytic and calming effects that lavender can have on the body, it has been proven that lavender oil can be used to decrease systolic blood pressure and supplementally treat hypertension. In a single-blind trial, a group of patients who had open-heart surgery were chosen. The blood pressure and heart rate of the patients were measured ten minutes after extubation, then a cotton swab saturated with lavender oil was placed in the patients' oxygen mask and inhaled for ten minutes. Thirty minutes after the lavender oil treatment, the patients' blood pressure and heart rate was measured again. There was a significant decrease in systolic blood pressure, diastolic blood pressure and heart rate compared to the levels recorded prior to the inhalation therapy. This study proved that lavender essential oil can be used to lower blood pressure and heart rate (Salamati et al., 2017).

In a study, participants who were hypertensive were randomly sorted into the experimental or control group. The experimental group received a blend of oils including lavender, lemon and ylang ylang and inhaled the oil blend for two minutes, twice a day, for the duration of three weeks. The systolic blood pressure and heart rate variability of the experimental group significantly decreased compared to the control group. Although this study determined there was a statistically significant decrease in systolic blood pressure, more research needs to be performed solely on lavender essential oil to determine if lavender has a direct effect compared to the oil blend used in this experiment (Cha et al., 2010).

A blend of essential oils composed of lavender, ylang ylang, marjoram, and neroli, lavender being the highest amount in the blend, was used as aromatherapy in a group of hypertensive and prehypertensive patients. The subjects in the experimental group were given a necklace, which contained the essential oil blend, to wear during the day and an aroma stone to set by the bedside with two drops of the oil blend so that there was 24-hour aromatherapy. The placebo group was given an artificial fragrance and the control group was not given any treatment. Subjects' blood pressure was taken using a 24-hour ambulatory blood pressure and salivary cortisol level was observed. The daytime systolic and diastolic blood pressure measurements and salivary cortisol concentrations were significantly decreased compared to both the placebo and control groups (Kim et al., 2012). Again, although this study proved that there was a statistically significant decrease in blood pressure, more studies involving only lavender essential oil for the use of hypertension treatment needs to be performed to gain greater scientific evidence.

3.5. Insomnia and Sleep Disorders

As we age, serum melatonin levels tend to decrease which can cause insomnia or other sleep disorders. The effect of lavender aromatherapy on serum melatonin levels in older adults was studied. Serum melatonin levels were measured before and after eight lavender aromatherapy sessions for four weeks. After the use of lavender aromatherapy, mean serum melatonin levels were found to significantly increase. This study proved that lavender aromatherapy can be used to increase serum melatonin levels in older adults, and therefore treat insomnia or other sleep disorders (Velasco-Rodríguez et al., 2019).

A study involving thirty elderly patients who live in nursing homes began with the patients' answering questions about sleep quality and being ranked on the PSQI scale. Then, lavender oil was dropped on patients' pillows and inhaled before sleep for one week. It was found that the patients experienced improved sleep quality which was proven with significantly lower PSQI scores at the end of the week of aromatherapy (Faydalı et al., 2018).

3.6. Postpartum Depression

A sample of pregnant women were selected who were all being cared for at the same facility and split into three groups: intervention with lavender oil, control with other oils and control with no oils. Depression level was determined using the Edinburgh questionnaire before the intervention, at thirty-five to thirty-seven weeks of pregnancy, two weeks after delivery and six weeks after delivery. The intervention with lavender oil group placed seven drops of lavender oil on a cloth, held it up to their mouths and inhaled deeply ten times before bed and then placed the cloth next to their pillow so that it was beside them throughout the duration of the night. The intervention group mean depression score significantly decreased compared to the two control groups. This study proved that lavender essential oil can be used as a preventative measure or to decrease feelings and symptoms of depression in pregnant patients who are at risk for postpartum depression (Moshirenia et al., 2018). The mechanism of action of lavender essential oil as an antidepressant was discussed above under the antidepressant section.

In a clinical trial, women who had just given birth at the hospital were split into either an aromatherapy group or a non-aromatherapy group right after delivery. The intervention group inhaled three drops of lavender essential oil every eight hours for four weeks. The women were assessed using the 21-item Depression, Anxiety, and Stress Scale and the Edinburgh questionnaire after two weeks, one month, and three months after delivery. The results of the study showed that the women in the intervention group had depression, anxiety and stress scores significantly lower than the women in the control group at two weeks, one month and three months after delivery. This study further confirmed that lavender essential oil can be used to reduce symptoms of postpartum depression such as depression, anxiety, and stress (Kianpour et al., 2016).

3.7. Skin Conditions

In determining the uses for skin conditions, it was found that applying lavender oil topically can treat blemishes and ease inflammation by scavenging free radicals (Orchard et al., 2017). Lavender oil has been proven to ease inflammation in other areas of the body as well. During this discovery, the effects of lavender essential oil, linalyl acetate and linalool on the expression of TNF-α induced cell adhesion molecules in bEnd.3 cells were evaluated. The bEnd.3 cells were treated with lavender oil, linalyl acetate or linalool and subjected to TNF-α. Lavender essential oil and linalyl acetate suppressed TNF-α-induced E-selectin, P-selectin, vascular cell adhesion molecule-1 and intercellular adhesion molecule-1. These results indicated that lavender essential oil and linalyl acetate suppress NF-κB activation and may be used as an alternative anti-inflammatory agent (Aoe et al., 2017).

The versatility of lavender oil is due to the calming properties of linalyl acetate and linalool, the two main constituents of lavender oil. Whether lavender oil is applied topically or inhaled, it can be very beneficial to a persons' overall health. Lavender oil has many therapeutic benefits and can help to dampen or even eliminate conditions such as anxiety, depression, postpartum depression, hypertension, alopecia, insomnia, or skin conditions. Although many studies have been performed and supported by scientific evidence, there are still many opportunities to study lavender oil and discover even more benefits of its use.

4. Peppermint Oil

Peppermint is known as one of the most versatile oils in the world, sharing the title with lavender oil. Peppermint's main phytochemical that has its biological effects is menthol. Menthol has cooling properties which are especially helpful in relieving muscle pain and soothing a sore throat. Menthol contains cyclic monoterpenes which allows it to block calcium channels and have antispasmodic effects on skeletal and smooth muscles

(Alam et al., 2013). Peppermint oil has been proven to help with conditions such as irritable bowel syndrome, nausea & motion sickness, pruritus, and restlessness, which includes relieving migraines, insomnia, anxiety, and stress. Although peppermint oil can help with these conditions, those that take medications that are metabolized by CYP 3A4 enzyme cannot use peppermint oil because a 2002 study found that peppermint oil (and the phytochemicals found in peppermint oil such as menthol, menthyl acetate, and ascorbyl palmitate) is a reversible inhibitor of this enzyme (Dresser et al., 2002). Therefore, peppermint oil will interact with medications that are metabolized by CYP 3A4. In the following paragraphs, it is explained how peppermint oil helps with the listed conditions above, along with studies proving peppermint oil's ability.

4.1. IBS

Peppermint oil (*Mentha piperita*) is most commonly used in the treatment of digestive ailments, which include IBS, Crohn's disease, diarrhea, gas, bloating, and heartburn. IBS affects 7 to 16% of the US population and is characterized by diarrhea, constipation, or both (Ford et al., 2017). When peppermint oil is used to help alleviate these conditions, menthol's cooling properties soothes the stomach and eases the pain because menthol can block calcium channels, which causes inhibition of the smooth muscle contractions in the intestines that are experienced with IBS or other gastrointestinal conditions. In order to relieve the symptoms of these conditions, the diluted oil is topically massaged onto the stomach to facilitate the absorption of the oil into the body. A systematic review and meta-analysis was done in 2014 on peppermint oil for the treatment of IBS. Nine studies were evaluated in which 726 patients were identified. The patients ingested the peppermint oil in the form of enteric coated capsules, rather than using the application of the oil to the stomach. Peppermint oil was found to be significantly superior to the placebo group for global improvement of IBS symptoms and improvement of abdominal pain.

Therefore, peppermint oil is a safe and effective short-term treatment for IBS (Khanna et al., 2014).

A double-blind randomized placebo-controlled study which assessed the efficacy of peppermint oil in diarrhea predominant IBS. This study focused on peppermint oil's ability in relieving symptoms and improvement in quality of life. There were 74 patients that participated in the study, and were randomly assigned to the placebo or treatment group, but only 65 patients completed the study in its entirety. The treatment group used peppermint oil three times a day for 6 weeks while the control group received a placebo in replacement of the peppermint oil. The symptoms of the patients were assessed in three week intervals, as well as assessed two weeks after the study concluded. The data were analyzed using a paired and unpaired t-test. It was concluded that in a six week period, abdominal pain improved in the treatment group compared to the placebo group, which shows a statistically significant improvement. Unfortunately, two weeks after the study concluded, pain levels increased. Therefore, Peppermint oil is effective in relieving abdominal pain in diarrhea predominant IBS transiently (Alam et al., 2013).

4.2. Nausea and Motion Sickness

Peppermint is commonly used for treating nausea and motion sickness and is safe to use in pregnancy related nausea. Peppermint oil acts as an anesthetic on the walls of the stomach, which eases vomiting and nausea. Symptoms of nausea are typically relieved upon inhalation of peppermint oil. A study conducted in 2016 analyzed inhaled peppermint oil for post-op nausea patients undergoing cardiac surgery and concluded that peppermint oil inhalation is a viable first-line treatment. Antiemetics are commonly given to post-op patients, but these agents have many adverse reactions such as dysrhythmias and drowsiness, so peppermint oil could serve as an effective alternative. One hundred twenty-three patients participated in this study, inhaling the peppermint oil through a nasal inhaler. The average rating for nausea before inhalation was a 3.29 on a scale of 0-5, with 5 being the greatest feeling of nausea. Two minutes after inhalation, the average nausea rating decreased to 1.44. The study concluded that peppermint oil is a viable treatment option for nausea in postoperative cardiac surgery patients (Briggs et al., 2016).

4.3. Pruritus

Pruritus, also known as itchiness, is a common skin complaint. Peppermint oil has been shown to relieve symptoms of itchiness and soothe the skin. A study conducted in 2016 evaluated the effectiveness of topical peppermint oil on symptomatic treatment of chronic pruritus. In the study, fifty patients, previously diagnosed with chronic pruritus due to hepatic, renal, or diabetic cause, were divided into two groups. Group 1 was instructed to hydrate the skin and then apply the peppermint oil to the skin, while group 2 was instructed to use petrolatum instead of peppermint oil. The applications were performed twice daily for two weeks. The severity of pruritus was assessed before and after the study using the 5-D itch scale. It was found that there was a significant improvement in symptoms of pruritus with group 1 but no significant improvement in symptoms with group 2. The total scores from both groups were compared and it was found that improvement of pruritus favored the use of peppermint oil over petrolatum. (Elsaie et al., 2016). In conclusion, peppermint oil can serve as an effective alternative to other pharmacological agents that are used for chronic pruritus as it is easy to use, safe, and can be less irritating and tolerated than other products.

4.4. Migraines

Peppermint oil is not only effective in treating migraines but also in relieving muscle pain. Symptoms associated with headaches are typically relieved when peppermint oil is massaged into the neck, temples, and/or forehead, or when a few drops of the oil are placed on a cool wet towel and used as a compress on the forehead. A double- blind clinical trial published in 2019 compared the effects of intranasal lidocaine 4% to peppermint essential oil drop 1.5% on migraine attacks. A sample of 120 adult patients with a diagnosis of migraine based on the International Headache Society criteria, were treated with lidocaine, peppermint oil, or placebo. All patients recorded their symptoms 30 minutes after administration. The patients continued on these treatments for two months. At the conclusion of the study, it was found that there was a significant difference among groups in headache intensity after treatment compared to placebo. In the placebo group, fewer patients responded to the treatment, whereas 41.5% of patients in the lidocaine group and 42.1% of patients in the peppermint oil group responded to the treatment. Therefore, nasal application of peppermint oil caused reduction in the intensity and frequency of headaches, and relieved the majority of patients' pain similar to that of lidocaine (Hasanpour-Dehkordi et al., 2019).

Another study explored peppermint oil's active ingredient, menthol and its effectiveness on treating migraines. Specifically, the study researched the cutaneous application of menthol 10% as an abortive treatment of migraine without aura (light). This study was a randomized, double-blind, placebo-controlled, crossover study. Patients were separated into two groups in which one group received 10% menthol (treatment group) and the other group received 0.5% menthol (placebo) in which the solutions were applied to the forehead and temporal area. Pain was measured using a questionnaire with the following endpoints of pain free, pain relief, sustained pain free, and sustained pain relief. The intention-to-treat population consisted of 35 patients with 118 migraine attacks, and was found to be statistically significant compared to the placebo group for 2 hours pain free, 2 hours pain relief, sustained pain free and sustained pain relief end-points. It was also found that the menthol solution was more effective in alleviating nausea, vomiting, phonophobia, or photophobia (Borhani Haghighi et al., 2010). Therefore, peppermint oil and its active constituent, menthol can serve as an effective, safe, and tolerable therapeutic option in treatment of migraines.

4.5. Antibacterial/Antifungal

Bacterial resistance has been on the rise and poses a threat to clinical settings in treating severe infectious diseases. A study performed in 2019, explored the effects of peppermint oil on various multi-drug resitant (MDR) gram-negative bacteria such as carbapenem-resistant *Enterobacteriaceae, Pseudomonas aeruginosa* or *Acinetobacter baumannii*, and extended-spectrum cephalosporin-resistant *Enterobacteriaceae* (Muntean et al., 2019). The essential oil was extracted by steam distillation and tested on six reference bacterial strains and on the MDR strains that were collected from patients. The antibacterial activity was evaluated by agar disc diffusion method and microdilution method. The peppermint oil demonstrated bactericidal effects on both the reference strains as well as the MDR strains obtained from hospitalized patients. The MIC was lower (20 mg/mL) for *Staphylococcus aureus, Escherichia coli* and *Proteus mirabilis* and higher (40 mg/mL) for *Klebsiella pneumoniae, Pseudomonas aeruginosa* and *Acinetobacter baumannii* strains. The MBC was equal to the MIC, with the exception of *Pseudomonas aeruginosa*, where MBC was double to the MIC. Peppermint oil can be a possible therapeutic option in the future in the treatment of infections caused by MDR bacteria such as *Staphylococcus aureus, Escherichia coli, Klebsiella pneumoniae*, *Proteus mirabilis, Pseudomonas aeruginosa* and *Acinetobacter baumannii* (Muntean et al., 2019).

Peppermint oil (*Mentha piperita*) is very versatile and can be widely used, inexpensively, for treating the conditions of irritable bowel syndrome, motion sickness, nausea, pruritus, migraines, and bacterial and fungal infections. Menthol, the main active ingredient of peppermint oil has been shown to have vasodilatory and antispasmodic effects. Although peppermint oil is still being learned about and not widely known as a medical substitute, it will become more and more known in the near future as an effective alternative medicine for these conditions.

Conclusion

Essential oil use has been proven to be an influential holistic approach to treatment of various disease states and symptoms. Various phytochemicals present in the essential oils when used in their highest purity may produce beneficial effects to the body. Lemon, lavender and peppermint essential oils are uniquely diverse. Lemon oil has been proven to help with morning sickness, bacterial infections, skin inflammation, pain and cognitive function. Evidence has shown that lavender oil can be used for alopecia, postpartum depression, hypertension, insomnia, and skin conditions. Peppermint oil has proven use for irritable bowel syndrome, motion sickness, nausea, pruritus, migraines, chest pain, dysphagia, and to treat bacterial and fungal infections. In the same sense, lemon, lavender and peppermint oils can treat some of the same conditions such as anxiety and depression. These oils have an abundance of uses that have been studied and proven to have statistically significant outcomes. Further research should be performed to discover even more applications of these oils for their maximum benefit to humans.

References

Akpinar, Burhan. (2005). "The Effects of Olfactory Stimuli on Scholastic Performance." *The Irish Journal of Education*, 86–90.

Alam, MS, et al., (2002). "Efficacy of Peppermint Oil in Diarrhea Predominant IBS - a Double Blind Randomized Placebo - Controlled Study." *Mymensingh Medical Journal*, 2(2).

Aoe, Michinori, et al., (2017). "Lavender Essential Oil and Its Main Constituents Inhibit the Expression of TNF-α-Induced Cell Adhesion Molecules in Endothelial Cells." *Pub Med*, U.S. National Library of Medicine.

Aziz, Zarith Asyikin Abdul, et al., (2018). "Essential Oils: Extraction Techniques, Pharmaceutical and Therapeutic Potential - A Review." *Current Drug Metabolism*, 19(13): 1100–1110.

Bakkali, F., et al., (2008). "Biological Effects of Essential Oils – A Review." *Food and Chemical Toxicology*, 46(2): 446–475.

Beylikli̇oğlu, Ayşe, and Sevban Arslan. (2019). "Effect of Lavender Oil on the Anxiety of Patients Before Breast Surgery." *Journal of PeriAnesthesia Nursing*, 34(3): 587–593.

Briggs, Patricia. (2016). "Inhaled Peppermint Oil for Postop Nausea in Patients Undergoing Cardiac Surgery." *Nursing*, 46(7): 61–67.

Buckle, Jane. (2015). *Clinical Aromatherapy: Essential Oils in Healthcare*. 3rd ed, Elsevier.

Cha, Jung-Hee, et al., (2010). "Effects of Aromatherapy on Changes in the Autonomic Nervous System, Aortic Pulse Wave Velocity and Aortic Augmentation Index in Patients with Essential Hypertension." *Journal of Korean Academy of Nursing*, 40(5): 705.

Djilani, Abdelouaheb, and Amadou Dicko. (2012). "The Therapeutic Benefits of Essential Oils." Nutrition, Well-Being and Health.

Dresser, George K. (2002). "Evaluation of Peppermint Oil and Ascorbyl Palmitate as Inhibitors of Cytochrome P4503A4 Activity in Vitro and in Vivo*." *Clinical Pharmacology & Therapeutics*, 72(3): 247–255.

Elsaie, Lotfy. (2016). "Effectiveness of Topical Peppermint Oil on Symptomatic Treatment of Chronic Pruritus." *Clinical, Cosmetic and Investigational Dermatology*, 9: 333–338.

Faydalı, Saide, and Funda Çetinkaya. (2018). "The Effect of Aromatherapy on Sleep Quality of Elderly People Residing in a Nursing Home." *Holistic Nursing Practice*, 32(1): 8–16.

Ford, Alexander C., et al., (2017). "Irritable Bowel Syndrome." *New England Journal of Medicine*, 376(26): 2566–2578.

Garzoli, Stefania, et al., (2019). "Liquid and Vapour Phase of Lavandin (Lavandula × Intermedia) Essential Oil: Chemical Composition and Antimicrobial Activity." *US National Library of Medicine National Institutes of Health*, 24(15): 2701.

Genc, Hasan, and Serdar Saritas. (2019). "The Effects of Lavender Oil on the Anxiety and Vital Signs of Benign Prostatic Hyperplasia Patients in Preoperative Period." *Explore*.

Haghighi, A. Borhani. (2010). "Cutaneous Application of Menthol 10% Solution as an Abortive Treatment of Migraine without Aura: a Randomised, Double-Blind, Placebo-Controlled, Crossed-over Study." *International Journal of Clinical Practice*, 64(4): 451–456.

Hanson, John. (2003). Refractometry." *Refractometry: Introduction*. www2.ups.edu/faculty/hanson/labtechniques/refractometry/intro.htm.

Harada, Hiroki, et al., (2018). "Linalool Odor-Induced Anxiolytic Effects in Mice." *Frontiers in Behavioral Neuroscience*, vol. 12.

Hasanpour-Dehkordi, Ali. (2019). "Comparing the Effect of Intranasal Lidocaine 4% with Peppermint Essential Oil Drop 1.5% on Migraine Attacks: A Double-Blind Clinical Trial." *International Journal of Preventive Medicine*, 10(1): 121.

Ikeda, Hiroshi, et al., (2014). "Contribution of Anterior Cingulate Cortex and Descending Pain Inhibitory System to Analgesic Effect of Lemon Odor in Mice." *Molecular Pain*, vol. 10.

Jimbo, Daiki, et al., (2009). "Effect of Aromatherapy on Patients with Alzheimer's Disease." *Psychogeriatrics*, 9(4): 173–179.

Kamrani, Farhad, et al., (2016). "Effect of Aromatherapy With Lemon Essential Oil on Anxiety after Orthopedic Surgery." Iranian Journal of Rehabilitation Research in Nursing, 2(4): 26–31.

Kamrani, Farhad, et al., (2016). "Effect of Aromatherapy With Lemon Essential Oil on Anxiety after Orthopedic Surgery." *Iranian Journal of Rehabilitation Research in Nursing*, 2(4): 26–31.

Kang, Hyun-Ju, et al., (2019). "How Strong Is the Evidence for the Anxiolytic Efficacy of Lavender?: Systematic Review and Meta-Analysis of Randomized Controlled Trials." *Asian Nursing Research*, vol. 13(5): 295–305.

Karan, Nazife Begüm. (2019). "Influence of Lavender Oil Inhalation on Vital Signs and Anxiety: A Randomized Clinical Trial." *Physiology & Behavior*, vol. 211: 112676.

Khalaf, Mohamed H. G. (2019) "Impact of Peppermint Therapy on Dysphagia and Non-Cardiac Chest Pain: A Pilot Study." *Digestive Diseases and Sciences*, vol. 64(8): 2214–2218.

Khanna, Reena, (2014) "Peppermint Oil for the Treatment of Irritable Bowel Syndrome." *Journal of Clinical Gastroenterology*, 48(6): 505–512.

Kia, Parisa Yavari, et al., (2014). "The Effect of Lemon Inhalation Aromatherapy on Nausea and Vomiting of Pregnancy: A Double-Blinded, Randomized, Controlled Clinical Trial." *Iranian Red Crescent Medical Journal*, 16(3).

Kianpour, Maryam, et al., (2016). "Effect of Lavender Scent Inhalation on Prevention of Stress, Anxiety and Depression in the Postpartum Period." *Iranian Journal of Nursing and Midwifery Research*, 21(2): 197.

Kim, In-Hee, et al., (2012). "Essential Oil Inhalation on Blood Pressure and Salivary Cortisol Levels in Prehypertensive and Hypertensive Subjects." *Evidence-Based Complementary and Alternative Medicine*, pp. 1–9.

Komiya, Migiwa, et al., (2006). "Lemon Oil Vapor Causes an Anti-Stress Effect via Modulating the 5-HT and DA Activities in Mice." *Behavioural Brain Research*, 172(2): 240–249.

Lee, Boo Hyeong, et al., (2016). "Hair Growth-Promoting Effects of Lavender Oil in C57BL/6 Mice." *Toxicological Research*, 32(2): 103–108.

Lehrner, J., et al., (2005). "Ambient Odors of Orange and Lavender Reduce Anxiety and Improve Mood in a Dental Office." *Physiology & Behavior*, 86(1-2): 92–95.

López, Víctor, et al., (2017). "Exploring Pharmacological Mechanisms of Lavender (Lavandula Angustifolia) Essential Oil on Central Nervous System Targets." *Frontiers in Pharmacology*, vol. 8.

Man, Adrian, et al., (2019). "Antimicrobial Activity of Six Essential Oils Against a Group of Human Pathogens: A Comparative Study." *Pathogens*, 8(1).

Maurya, Anil Kumar, et al., (2018). "The Essential Oil from Citrus Limetta Risso Peels Alleviates Skin Inflammation: In-Vitro and in-Vivo Study." *Journal of Ethnopharmacology*, 212: 86–94.

Moshirenia, Fateme, et al., (2018). "The Effects of Inhalation Aromatherapy with Rose and Lavender at Week 38 and Postpartum Period on Postpartum Depression in High-Risk Women Referred to Selected Health Centers of Yazd, Iran in 2015." *Iranian Journal of Nursing and Midwifery Research*, 23(5): 395.

Muntean, Delia, (2019) "Evaluation of Essential Oil Obtained from Mentha×Piperita L. against Multidrug-Resistant Strains." *Infection and Drug Resistance*, 12: 2905–2914.

Orchard, Ané, Vuuren, Sandy V. (2017) "Commercial Essential Oils as Potential Antimicrobials to Treat Skin Diseases." *Evidence-Based Complementary and Alternative Medicine*, 2017: 1–92.

Phillips, Cristy. (2017). "Brain-Derived Neurotrophic Factor, Depression, and Physical Activity: Making the Neuroplastic Connection." *Neural Plasticity*, 2017: 1–17.

Rassem, Hesham, et al., (2016). "Techniques Available for the Extraction of Essential Oils from Plants: A Review." *Australian Journal of Basic and Applied Sciences*. 117–127.

Salamati, Armaiti, et al., (2017). "Effect of Inhalation of Lavender Essential Oil on Vital Signs in Open Heart Surgery ICU." *Iranian Journal of Pharmaceutical Research*, 16: 404–409.

Sánchez-Vidaña, Dalinda Isabel, et al., (2019). "Lavender Essential Oil Ameliorates Depression-like Behavior and Increases Neurogenesis and Dendritic Complexity in Rats." *Neuroscience Letters*, 701: 180–192.

Shady, Kathryn, et al., (2019). "Lavender Aromatherapy: Examining the Effects of Lavender Oil Patches on Patients in the Hematology-Oncology Setting." *Clinical Journal of Oncology Nursing*, 23(5): 502–508.

Sherwood, Bella. (2016). *Aromatherapy: A Clinical Guide to Essential Oils for Holistic Healing*. Create Space.

Soe'eib, Siswati, et al., (2016). "Enfleurage Essential Oil from Jasmine and Rose Using Cold Fat Absorbent." *Journal Kmiah Widya Teknik*, 15(1): 58–61.

Velasco-Rodríguez, R., et al., (2019). "The Effect of Aromatherapy with Lavender (Lavandula Angustifolia) on Serum Melatonin Levels." *Complementary Therapies in Medicine*, vol. 47.

BIOGRAPHICAL SKETCH

Ajay Bommareddy, PhD
Nesbitt School of Pharmacy, Wilkes-Barre, PA, US

Education: BPharm; PhD

Business Address: 84 W South St, Wilkes-Barre, PA, US

Research and Professional Experience: I primarily work in the area of natural products and cancer prevention employing various cancer models both *In vitro* and *In vivo* and have more than 16 years of experience in cancer research. Thus far, I have published 30 articles in reputed cancer research journals, presented research findings at different conferences with more than 35 conference proceedings, and published abstracts. At my current position, my primary responisiblilites include teaching students in the professional PharmD program and engage interested students in research endeavors.

Professional Appointments:

05/01/15-present	Department of Pharmaceutical Sciences, Associate Nesbitt College of Pharmacy, Wilkes University Professor Wilkes Barre, PA (With Tenure)
08/17/09-04/30/15	Department of Pharmaceutical Sciences, Assistant Nesbitt College of Pharmacy, Wilkes University Professor Wilkes Barre, PA
07/01/07-08/16/09	Department of Pharmacology & Chemical Research Biology, University of Pittsburgh School of Medicine, Associate, University of Pittsburgh Cancer Institute, Pittsburgh, PA.

Honors:

- 2018, Awarded "Overall Teacher of the Year" award, Nesbitt School of Pharmacy, Wilkes University, Wilkes-Barre, PA.
- 2017, Awarded "Outstanding advisor" award, Teacher Recognition and Effectiveness Committee, Wilkes University, Wilkes-Barre, PA.
- 2009, University of Pittsburgh Cancer Institute Director's award for scientific excellence: First place in Translational & Clinical research section, poster presentation at 21st Annual University of Pittsburgh Cancer institute, Pittsburgh, PA.
- 2005, Rho Chi honor society, South Dakota State University, Brookings, SD.

Publications from the Last 3 Years:

Bommareddy A, Knapp K, Nemeth A, Steigerwalt J, Landis T, Vanwert AL, Gorijavolu HP, Dwivedi . Alpha-Santalol, a Component of Sandalwood Oil Inhibits Migration of Breast Cancer Cells by Targeting the β-catenin Pathway. *Anticancer Research*. 2018, 38 (8) 4475-4480.

Bommareddy A, Brozena S, Steigerwalt J, Landis T, Hughes S, Mabry E, Knopp A, VanWert AL, Dwivedi C. *Medicinal properties of alpha-santalol, a constituent of sandalwood oil, Nat Prod Res.* 2017 Nov 13:1-17.

In: What to Know about Essential Oils
Editor: Malene M. Kjeldsen
ISBN: 978-1-53617-986-6

Chapter 6

Relevance of Essential Oils in Food Preservation, the Extension of Shelf Life and Post-Harvest Research, Therapeutic Effects, Wound Healing, Aromatherapy, Mosquito Repellent and Bee Behavior: A Review

Olufunke O. Fajinmi and Johannes Van Staden*
Research Centre for Plant Growth and Development,
School of Life Sciences, University of KwaZulu-Natal,
Pietermaritzburg, South Africa

Abstract

Essential oils are secreted in the glands of plants as volatile oils and are responsible for the scents emitted from different plant parts. When plant parts are used as spices, the essential oil present in them enhances the

---

* Corresponding Author's Email: rcpgd@ukzn.ac.za.

palatability of the cooked food. Irrespective of the high price of most essential oils, it remains an important item needed for human daily living as it is used in the production of soaps, creams, lotions, perfumes, roll-ons and deodorizers. It improves mood, enhances self-esteem, ignites romance and helps to relieve stress. In addition, essential oils have a variety of applications such as preservation of food and drinks, control of insects and pests, air freshener, and the treatment of diseases and infections. The therapeutic value of essential oils cannot be over emphasized. They have been used to cure diseases for several centuries. In this article, the medicinal use of essential oils from ancient times to the present are highlighted. Irrespective of their history, caution must be taken when using essential oils as they are easily absorbed by the skin and then find their way into the blood stream. Thus, indiscriminate use of essential oils may lead to serious health hazards. This article therefore highlights various usage, its mosquito repellent activities, and reaction of bees to essential oil (EO) volatiles, toxicity, side effects and applications of EO.

Introduction

Essential oil (EO) has been utilized since ancient times. The Egyptians utilized aromatic oils as early as 4500 BC as an ingredient in the production of cosmetics and ointments [1]. The use of EOs was first recorded in the Chinese and Indian traditional medicine systems between 3000 and 2000 BC [1]. The documented history of China and India traditional medicine systems record more than 700 substances which included cinnamon, ginger, myrrh, and sandalwood as being effective for healing [2]. Greek history documented the use of various EOs for the first time between 500 and 400 BC. The recorded EOs included saffron, marjoram, cumin, peppermint and thyme [3].

Use of Essential Oil in Food Preservation and Extension of Food Shelf Life

In the present era of civilization, much interest has been paid to the use of EO in the food packaging industry to extend shelf-life as a result of their antimicrobial and antioxidant activities. Oregano and sage EOs protect minced meat samples from autoxidation [4]. Thyme is a common species, highly utilized in the Spanish meat industry [5] as a result of its antimicrobial and antioxidant activities. Oregano EO protects extra virgin olive oil from oxidation during storage and extends the shelf life of sea bream [6].

Essential oils are composed of a variety of highly bioactive compounds which are volatile in nature and therefore makes EO unstable and liable to degradation. As a result of this instability of EOs in food matrices, different methods of protection which can prevent the degradation of EOs when used to prolong food shelf-life have been developed [5]. Encapsulation has emerged as an effective alternative to improve EO stability [5]. The encapsulation of EOs using different materials and methods has been widely studied [7] and EOs have been encapsulated in polymeric particles, liposomes, and solid lipid nanoparticles, which enhances its stability and efficacy [5]. Recent developments in nanotechnology have made the development of novel carrier agents for the delivery and control release of EOs in food systems with improved chemical, oxidative, and thermal stability, possible [8]. EOs have also been utilized as additives in bio-degradable films and coatings for food packaging [9, 10] as it enhances the films and coatings with antioxidant and/or antimicrobial properties, depending both on their composition and the interactions with the polymer matrix [5]. The antioxidant activity of EO depends not only on the specific antioxidant activity of the oil compounds but also on the film's oxygen permeability [5]. Their incorporation into edible films can promote the antimicrobial capacity of EOs [5]. The effectiveness of the edible film against microbial growth is highly dependent on the oil's nature and the types of microorganism [5]. EOs have proven to be effective in the inhibition of various microorganisms responsible for diseases and infections in humans.

Essential Oils Role in the Inhibition of Human Disease-Causing Microorganisms

The germ tube formation which is generally regarded as an important tool of pathogenicity of *C. albicans* [11, 12, 13] was highly inhibited by clove oil and eugenol [14]. The essential oil from *Citrus sinensis* epicarp is composed of 84.2% limonene and capable of inhibiting the growth of *Aspergillus niger* and in the process leads to irreversible deleterious morphological alterations [15]. Essential oil extract of Lemon Cui (*Citrus microcarpa)* skin has an inhibitory effect on *Trichophyton rubrum* growth [16]. Application of thyme essential oil on sheepskin leather for lining finished with synthetic film completely inhibited the development of *Trichophyton interdigitale*, with no increase in growth for 28 days [17]. Several investigations have shown the superior activity of *Ocimum gratissimum* L. EO over benzyl peroxide-based products in the reduction of lesions (papules and pustules) [18].

Wound Healing Properties of Essential Oils

Recently, the therapeutic effect of several plant EOs especially for the treatment of wounds has received great attention as the EOs have demonstrated a number of wound-healing effects which are rare to find with pharmaceuticals [19]. Lavender EO improves the formation of scar tissues and is therefore commonly used to treat wounds, cuts, burns, and sunburns [3]. The oil can also be applied to protect the wounds from developing infections [20]. Tea tree oil increased monocytic differentiation *in vitro* and reduce inflammation, thus assisting in the healing of chronic wounds [2]. Tea tree oil has demonstrated effective *in vitro* activity on several strains of methicillin-resistant *Staphylococcus aureus* (MRSA) isolated from wounds [21] and therefore justifies its use as a treatment for wounds. The development of ointment from EOs could offer an effective treatment of first degree burns as EOs have antiinflamatory, antioxidant, wound healing and disinfectant properties. The potency of many EOs is linked to their volatile components.

ESSENTIAL OIL PROPERTIES, ITS COMPONENTS AND ITS SIGNIFICANCE IN AROMATHERAPY

At room temperature, the atmospheric pressure is naturally high, thus making EOs to be mostly found in a partial vapor state [22]. EOs are highly soluble in volatile compounds such as alcohol, ether, and fixed oils but lipophilic i.e., insoluble in water [22]. EOs extracted from cinnamon, sassafras, vetiver, and other natural sources are liquid in nature and colourless at room temperature [23]. As a result of this, they are widely utilized in cosmetic formulations and the aromatherapy industry [22]. The presence of volatile compounds such as ketones, aldehydes, and aromatic compounds in the EOs play key roles in aromatherapy as inhalation of these compounds is highly effective in the reduction of mental and physical stresses [22]. In the late 20th century, EO-based aromatherapy gained much popularity as a result of its importance, and widespread use [22]. Inhalation and external application of some EO volatiles are used for therapeutic purposes which include mental and physical balance, which is the basis of aromatherapy [22]. Essential oils are highly utilized for various therapeutic purposes such as massage aromatherapy, psycho-aromatherapy and olfactory-aromatherapy [22]. Inhalation of the volatiles of certain EO is believed to play a crucial role in relieving stress as it rejuvenates and regenerates the body. Inhalation of essential oil volatiles, especially floral scents is believed to ignite romance and elevate mood and increase sex drive. Essential oil diffuser and aromatic floral bouquets are often used in rooms of some five-star hotels in order to offer a serene, romantic atmosphere for customers to enjoy. These floral scents also play crucial roles in the control of insects and flies.

Essential Oil Insecticidal Property against Mosquito, Scientific Reports and Shortcomings of Essential Oil Volatiles

Globally, mosquitoes are a menace as they are responsible for malaria which is the cause of high mortality rate especially among children. The insecticidal activity of different EOs of various plants have been reported in scientific literature. Diseases transmitted by mosquitoes include malaria, filariasis, yellow fever, Japanese encephalitis and dengue fever [24]. The valuable properties of EOs and aromatic plants as insect repellent properties of plant essential oils against mosquitoes and insects were well known before the invention of synthetic chemicals (insecticide sprays) to repel mosquitoes and control their populations. For centuries, several methods that could be used to control mosquitoes have been developed [24]. Pharmaceutical companies across the globe have been developing synthetic drugs, antibiotics and insect repellents to combat fever resulting from mosquito bites and control the population of mosquitoes especially in Africa where the climatic condition favors the growth and multiplication of these dreadful insects. However, their products have one shortcoming or the other and in many cases are not affordable for, and accessible to, the majority of the populace. Generally, EOs are known to be environmentally friendly, easily biodegradable and minimally toxic to mammals and have displayed repellent [25, 26], toxicant [27, 28, 29], growth and/or reproduction inhibition and oviposition deterrent, [30, 31] activities against different mosquito species. Hence, use of aromatic plants and EOs still remain the most accessible, affordable, effective and viable method of controlling mosquitoes growth and dealing with inflammation and discomfort associated with mosquito bites among some urban dwellers and the majority of the rural dwellers.

Traditionally, essential oils from different plants, especially plants of the genus *Cymbopogon* have been used as insect repellents in Africa. In Nigeria, and other West African countries, members of these families, especially lemon grass is utilized either by burning dry plant material on a tray or by hanging the twigs at the door, on the window or under the beds to repel mosquitoes and or inhibit an increase in their population. Dry peels of Citrus species such as orange and or lemon are also burnt on trays to repel mosquitoes. The EOs of lemon-grass (*Cymbopogon excavatus*), citronella (*Cymbopogon nardus*), eucalyptus (*Eucalyptus maculata*), cedar (Juniper virginiana), geranium (*Pelargonium reniforme*), peppermint (*Mentha piperita*) are the most studied in scientific literature and have been reported to have potent insecticidal activity against different species of mosquitoes. The monoterpenoids and sesquiterpenes are responsible for the repellent activity of several EOs [32].

Some of the EO volatiles and or compounds responsible for insecticidal activity against species of mosquitoes have been incorporated into commercial sprays. Citronella EO is obtained from the aerial parts (leaves and stems) of different species of Cymbopogon popularly referred to as lemon grass. Citronella is one of the most popular natural repellents on the market, with concentrations ranging from 5-10% which is lower than that of most commercial repellents, but a higher concentration could lead to skin sensitivity [33]. Skin sensitivity to a high concentration of topically administered EO is a common occurrence especially among children. The components of EOs responsible for these allergic reactions/ sensitivities are yet unknown. However, the volatile components of the EO have been reported to be responsible for their various bioactivities. In some cases, the activity of these compounds is more effective, or it has longer duration than commercially used synthetic chemicals [34, 35].

Geraniol is a plant-derived alcohol and is considered completely safe for use and thus listed on the US Food and Drug Administration (US FDA) Generally Regarded as Safe (GRAS) list [36]. It has been reported to be effective in repelling mosquitoes [37, 38] and other insects such as houseflies, stable flies [39] and ticks [40]. In a study carried out in Israel, 5% geraniol candles were reported to be about twice as effective as those with 5% linalool and were about 5 times as effective as 5% citronella candles in protecting a person from being bitten by mosquitoes when used indoors [41]. Revay et al., 2012 [36] investigated the extent of protection offered by a timed-released, water-based emulsion of 0.3% geraniol mist dispensed by a pressurized spray can in an area known for high mosquito biting pressure in Israel. Dispensed aerosolized geraniol reduced biting pressure (landing, probing and biting mosquitoes) of *Culex pipiens* and *Aedes albopictus* [36]. Geraniol-based products are available commercially in several countries and in several forms [36]. Similarly, Mosi-Guard, a commercial mosquito repellent contains 50% Eucalyptus oil [36].

However, despite their efficacy, affordability and minimal toxicity, EOs still do not have a widespread application due to some limitations such as their high volatility, composition variability and strong smell [43]. Most EOs are highly volatile and this characteristic is responsible for their poor longevity as mosquito repellents [33]. However, this shortcoming can be addressed by using fixatives or effective formulation to improve their longevity [33]. For example, EOs of turmeric and hairy basil combined with 5% vanillin repelled three species of mosquitoes under cage conditions for 6-8 hours depending on the species [44]. The EOs of *Artemisia verlotiorum* Lamotte (Asteraceae), *Lavandula dentata* L. (Lamiaceae), and *Ruta chalepensis* L. (Rutaceae) had substantial skin repellent activity against *Aedes albopictus* [43]. The EOs deterred *Ae. albopictus* oviposition in the field and exerted a strong larvicidal activity [43].

Relationship between Essential Oil Volatiles and Behavioral Patterns of Bees

The vapour phase of essential oils plays a variety of biological roles in plants [45] as it attracts pollinating insects [46, 47, 48]. The bees are one of the key players in pollination on the field. They are also solely responsible for honey production which is a globally utilised product. However, the relationship between EO scents/volatiles and the bees is not well explored. The role of scents in bee farming is not well documented. Researchers from the University of Queensland carried out research to test the effect of floral scents on calming an aggressive beehive. They discovered that the effect of alarm pheromones, the odour released by aggressive bees to communicate with other bees that there is a threat and they should join them during bees attack can be reduced by a floral scent which indicates the presence of food nearby. According to the researchers, the floral scent does not act to mask the odours of the pheromone but acts to tame the bees as floral scent to bees means food is somewhere around them. The authors proved that specific floral scents such as linalool, 2-phenylethanol and lavender have the capacity to block recruitment for attack by the pheromone. On the other hand, banana makes bees very aggressive as a result of isoamyl acetate which is a compound responsible for banana scent/aroma. Several reports from blogs show that bees get aggressive after perceiving the smell of banana and visiting a beehive after eating banana makes you a target. The EO volatiles makes up the scent plants emit on the field and they play crucial roles in plant survival.

Essential Oil and Its Crucial Role for Plant Survival in the Field

The EO vapour phase/scents play a crucial role in natural defence mechanisms against a variety of pathogens and predators, which includes microbes, insects and herbivores [46, 47, 48]. Volatile compounds of essential oil are low molecular weight, lipophilic molecules that have a tendency to volatise at relatively low temperatures [46, 49]. Volatile EOs are made up of a complex mixture of compounds that are mostly composed of monoterpenes and sesquiterpenes [50]. The volatile components of EOs are usually categorized into various chemical classes such as aldehydes, ketones, alcohols, amines, amides, phenols and mainly, terpenes [22]. Among these components, alcohols, aldehydes, and ketones are responsible for the aromatic effects of fruits and other parts of certain plants [22]. The major compounds of EO include alcohols, aldehydes, esters, ketones, phenols, oxides, coumarins and phenylpropenes [51]. The antioxidant potential of many EOs results from the inherent ability of some of their components, particularly the phenols, to stop or delay aerobic oxidation of organic matter [52]. However, there are phenol-free EOs with antioxidant potentials linked to some terpenoids and other volatile constituents (e.g., sulphur containing components) [18].

Application of Essential Oils Postharvest, an Emerging Area of Global Interest

The postharvest sector faces the challenge of how to prevent the growth of microorganisms/pathogens that could initiate the process of decay/rot and growth of toxins in fruits, vegetables and cereals. There has been a growing interest globally in the efficient ability of some EOs to extend shelf-life of agricultural produce and thus reduce postharvest loss. Several studies have reported the effective inhibition of EOs of food pathogen even at a very low concentration. Clove EO extracted from *Syzygium aromaticum* (L.) Merr. & Perry has a bioactive substance as a result of its active component the monoterpene, eugenol which acts against *Botrytis cinerea*, *Monilinia fructigena*, *Penicillium expansum* Link, and *Phlyctema vagabunda* Desm. in apples [53]. Globally, there is a growing interest in the use of EOs in the postharvest industries as effective natural substitutes for synthetic antimicrobial drugs. Oregano EO and its main constituent carvacrol effectively inhibited mycelium growth of *Neofabraea alba* in apples [54]. Other studies also highlighted the presence of significant fungicidal effects of some plant EOs such as thyme and vervain which surpass chemical preparations in postharvest treatments against *Monilinia laxa*, *M. fructigena*, and *M. fructicola* on peach fruit [55, 56]. Essential oils of fennel (*Foeniculum sativum* Mill.), marjoram, oregano, and sage displayed a fungicidal effect against *Botrytis cinerea* and, *Penicillium expansum* in apples [57]. Elshafie et al. (2015) [56] demonstrated that the EOs obtained from *T. vulgaris* and *V. officinalis* can be effective for the control of brown rot infection on peach fruit caused by *Monilinia laxa*, *M. fructicola*, and *M. fructigena*. Santoro et al. [58] reported the effect of thyme EO and savory EOs in the control of postharvest diseases and quality of peaches and nectarines, while Banani et al. [59] reported its efficacy on apples. Post-harvest synthetic fungicide treatments affect the quality of stored grain [61].

Thus, natural essential oils have great benefits over synthetic agents due to their biodegradable nature and low toxicity [62]. Papaya sachets incorporated with cinnamon, oregano and lemon grass EOs showed a significant reduction in the growth of mesophilic aerobic bacteria, yeasts and moulds, with the cinnamon sachet demonstrating the best reduction of microorganisms at the end of the storage time [63]. Physicochemical parameters of papaya, such as weight loss, colour, firmness, total soluble solids/titratable acidity ratio and pH were not significantly altered by the presence of cinnamon, oregano and lemon grass EO sachets, thus not affecting the natural ripening process of the papaya [63]. Sánchez-González et al. (2011) [64] found that incorporation of bergamot essential oil significantly reduced mould, yeast, and mesophilic counts on table grapes. Essential oils from different plants have been utilized as a preventive measure against fungal growth and mycotoxin accumulation in cereals [65, 66]. Especially oils from aromatic and spice plants have been used as a result of their safety and their common use in the food industry [62]. It is believed that the benefits of the use of essential oil volatiles surpass the direct application of the oils as a whole [47]. This includes reduced toxicity (compared to direct contact) and ease of application [49]. Essential oil could therefore minimize losses involved during shipment of fruit produce to other countries as it will inhibit microorganisms responsible for deterioration and spoilage and lead to extended shelf life of the produce thus offering export produce which is palatable and presentable. The antimicrobial activities of EOs against microorganisms responsible for human diseases and infections have been reported in scientific literature.

Effect of Essential Oil and Its Volatiles in the Treatment of Human Conditions and Anti-Inflammatory Activities

Inhalation of essential oil volatiles may have a great significance in the treatment and/or prevention of lung infections [46]. Inhalation of EO volatiles alleviated the symptoms of various medical conditions which include bronchitis and sinusitis, and some oil volatiles relieve the symptoms of asthma [67-69]. Vapour activity of volatiles of 72 essential oils against *Trichophyton mentagrophytes* demonstrated that essential oils with phenol as major constituent demonstrated the most potent vapour activity [70]. According to available literature, EOs have been used since the Middle Ages by Arabs as a result of their antiseptic, bactericidal, virucidal, and fungicidal properties [71]. They are utilized for embalming and preservation of foods and they exhibit antimicrobial, analgesic, sedative, anti-inflammatory, spasmolytic, and local anaesthetic properties [72]. The effective use of EOs in clinical procedures has been given great attention [73-75]. Lavender EO is well documented to be effective as an immune booster and for the treatment of inflammatory conditions such as abrasions, muscular pain, burns; and stress, headaches and skin problems [76, 77]. Lemon EO could act to accelerate the production of white blood cells, boost the immune system, and aid digestion [76]. The major constituents of lemon EO have displayed antiseptic, astringent, and detoxifying properties against blemishes related with oily skin [78]. The EOs in frankincense and geranium are released as a result of high temperature when their leaves are burnt and act as antiseptic agents to purify and scent the atmosphere in homes.

Essential Oil Toxicity and Interactions with Clinical Medications

Irrespective of the various uses and numerous applications and advantages of EO, indiscriminate use and abuse of essential oil is a serious issue as it can cause health hazards. Essential oil poisoning is on the rise globally, especially among children and toxicity of EOs could lead to health-related problems. For example, a 17-month old male who ingest less than 10 ml Melaleuca oil (Australian tea tree oil) developed ataxia and drowsiness [79]. When applied to the skin, EOs are easily absorbed by the skin and can find their way into the blood stream. An overdose could be fatal, and EOs must therefore be used with great caution. Some studies have also suggested its interference with the absorption and/or metabolism and efficacy of clinical medication. Evaluation of garlic oil for its potential effect on CYP enzymes in clinical trials suggest that garlic oil may selectively inhibit CYP2E1, but not other CYP isoforms (such as CYP1A2, CYP3A4 or CYP2D6) [80-84]. Some clinical data suggest that peppermint oil might increase the levels of drugs metabolized by CYP3A4 such as felodipine [85]. It is important to consult a medical practitioner before using essential oil for the treatment of health complaints. The quality of essential oil is another factor that needs to be taken into consideration as some essential oils could have a high microbial load resulting from its production process or environment. There are different methods of extraction of essential oils Common methods include cold-press extraction, solvent extraction, CO_2 extraction, maceration, enfleurage, steam distillation and water distillation. Steam distillation and water distillation could leave traces of water in the essential oil which is often removed using sodium sulphate. The absence of water even in minute traces, will prevent the growth of any microorganism in the oil as microorganisms need a hydrated substrate to grow and multiply. The use of high quality EOs in the right dosages could be beneficial to humans.

In conclusion, essential oil remains an indispensable gift of nature. Its potential could be maximized in the areas of post-harvest and clinical trials. Further in-depth research needs to be carried out to verify their efficacies and mode of action on host specific activities. These research activities could open new and exciting channels into the discovery and formulation of potential cures for life threatening diseases, especially those related to the respiratory tract.

ACKNOWLEDGMENT

Dr O. O Fajinmi is grateful to the University of KwaZulu-Natal for a Post-doctoral fellowship.

REFERENCES

[1] Baser, K; Husnu Can, *Gerhard Buchbauer. Handbook of essential oils: science, technology, and applications*. CRC press, 2015.

[2] Elshafie, Hazem S., Ippolito Camele. "An overview of the biological effects of some mediterranean essential oils on human health." *BioMed Research International*, 2017, (2017).

[3] Pauli, Alexander and Heinz Schilcher. "12 In Vitro Antimicrobial Activities of Essential Oils Monographed in the European Pharmacopoeia 6th Edition." *Essential*, (2010): 353.

[4] Amorati, Riccardo, Mario C. Foti and Luca Valgimigli. "Antioxidant activity of essential oils." *Journal of Agricultural and Food Chemistry*, 61, no. 46, (2013): 10835-10847.

[5] Fernández-López, Juana, and Manuel Viuda-Martos. *Introduction to the special issue: application of essential oils in food systems*. (2018): 56

[6] Goulas, Antonios E., and Michael G. Kontominas. "Combined effect of light salting, modified atmosphere packaging and oregano essential oil on the shelf-life of sea bream (Sparus aurata): Biochemical and sensory attributes." *Food Chemistry*, 100, no. 1 (2007): 287-296

[7] El Asbahani, A., K. Miladi, W. Badri, M. Sala, EH Aït Addi, Hervé Casabianca, Abdelhamid El Mousadik et al. "Essential oils: from extraction to encapsulation." *International Journal of Pharmaceutics*, 483, no. 1-2 (2015): 220-243.

[8] Prakash, Bhanu, Anupam Kujur, Amrita Yadav, Akshay Kumar, Prem Pratap Singh, and N. K. Dubey. "Nanoencapsulation: An efficient technology to boost the antimicrobial potential of plant essential oils in food system." *Food Control*, 89 (2018): 1-11.

[9] Atarés, Lorena and Amparo Chiralt. "Essential oils as additives in biodegradable films and coatings for active food packaging." *Trends in Food Science and Technology*, 48, (2016): 51-62.

[10] Ribeiro-Santos, Regiane, Mariana Andrade, Nathália Ramos de Melo, Ana Sanches-Silva. "Use of essential oils in active food packaging:

Recent advances and future trends." *Trends in Food Science and Technology*, 61, (2017):132-140.

[11] Calderone, Richard A., and William A. Fonzi. "Virulence factors of Candida albicans." *Trends in Microbiology*, 9, no. 7 (2001): 327-335.

[12] Hammer, K. A., Carson, C. F., and Riley T. V. "Melaleuca alternifolia (tea tree) oil inhibits germ tube formation by Candida albicans." *Medical Mycology*, 38, no. 5 (2000): 354-362.

[13] Pinto, Eugénia, Isabel Cristina Ribeiro, Nuria Joana Ferreira, Catia Eliana Fortes, Patrícia Alexandra Fonseca, Maria Helena Figueiral. "Correlation between enzyme production, germ tube formation and susceptibility to fluconazole in Candida species isolated from patients with denture-related stomatitis and control individuals." *Journal of Oral Pathology and Medicine*, 37, no. 10, (2008): 587-592.

[14] Pinto, Eugenia, Luís Vale-Silva, Carlos Cavaleiro, Lígia Salgueiro. "Antifungal activity of the clove essential oil from Syzygium aromaticum on Candida, Aspergillus and dermatophyte species." *Journal of Medical Microbiology*, 58, no. 11, (2009): 1454-1462.

[15] Sharma, Neeta, Abhishek Tripathi. "Effects of Citrus sinensis (L.) Osbeck epicarp essential oil on growth and morphogenesis of Aspergillus niger (L.) Van Tieghem." *Microbiological Research*, 163, no. 3, (2008): 337-344.

[16] Pinontoan, Sabrina, Nurmila Sunati, Befani Febriana, Elne Vieke Rambi. *Antifungal Activity of Essential Oil Extract of Lemon Cui (Citrus microcarpa) Skin against Trichophyton rubrum Growth*, (2019).

[17] Chirilă, Corina, Viorica Deselnicu, Mariana Daniela Berechet. "Footwear Protection against Fungi Using Thyme Essential Oil." *Leather and Footwear Journal*, 17, no. 3, (2017): 173.

[18] Pauli, Alexander, Heinz Schilcher. "Specific selection of essential oil compounds for treatment of children's infection diseases." *Pharmaceuticals*, 1, no. 1, (2004): 1.

[19] Stea, Susanna, Alina Beraudi, Dalila De Pasquale. "Essential oils for complementary treatment of surgical patients: state of the art."

Evidence-Based Complementary and Alternative Medicine, 2014, (2014).

[20] Pauli, Alexander. *Identification strategy of mechanism-based lipophilic antimicrobials*, 2007.

[21] Halcón, Linda, Kelly Milkus. "Staphylococcus aureus and wounds: a review of tea tree oil as a promising antimicrobial." *American Journal of Infection Control*, 32, no. 7, (2004): 402-408.

[22] Bhavaniramya, Sundaresan, Selvaraju Vishnupriya, Mohammad Saleh Al-Aboody, Rajendran Vijayakumar, Dharmar Baskaran. "Role of essential oils in food safety: Antimicrobial and antioxidant applications." *Grain and Oil Science and Technology*, (2019).

[23] Dhifi, Wissal, Sana Bellili, Sabrine Jazi, Nada Bahloul, Wissem Mnif. "Essential oils' chemical characterization and investigation of some biological activities: a critical review." *Medicines*, 3, no. 4, (2016): 25.

[24] Kalita, Bhupen, Somi Bora, Anil Kumar Sharma. "Plant essential oils as mosquito repellent-a review." *IJRDPL*, 3, (2013):143-150.

[25] Koliopoulos, George, Danae Pitarokili, Elias Kioulos, Antonios Michaelakis, Olga Tzakou. "Chemical composition and larvicidal evaluation of Mentha, Salvia, and Melissa essential oils against the West Nile virus mosquito Culex pipiens." *Parasitology Research*, 107, no. 2, (2010): 327-335.

[26] Gleiser, Raquel M., Maria A. Bonino, and Julio A. Zygadlo. "Repellence of essential oils of aromatic plants growing in Argentina against Aedes aegypti (Diptera: Culicidae)." *Parasitology Research*, 108, no. 1 (2011): 69-78.

[27] Kamsuk, K., W. Choochote, U. Chaithong, A. Jitpakdi, P. Tippawangkosol, D. Riyong, and B. Pitasawat. "Effectiveness of Zanthoxylum piperitum-derived essential oil as an alternative repellent under laboratory and field applications." *Parasitology Research*, 100, no. 2 (2007): 339.

[28] Mathew, Nisha, M. G. Anitha, T. S. L. Bala, S. M. Sivakumar, R. Narmadha, and M. Kalyanasundaram. "Larvicidal activity of Saraca indica, Nyctanthes arbor-tristis, and Clitoria ternatea extracts against

three mosquito vector species." *Parasitology Research*, 104, no. 5 (2009): 1017-1025.

[29] Conti, Barbara, Angelo Canale, Alessandra Bertoli, Francesca Gozzini, Luisa Pistelli. "Essential oil composition and larvicidal activity of six Mediterranean aromatic plants against the mosquito Aedes albopictus (Diptera: Culicidae)." *Parasitology Research*, 107, no. 6, (2010): 1455-1461.

[30] Rajkumar, S., and Jebanesan, A. "Repellency of volatile oils from Moschosma polystachyum and Solanum xanthocarpum against filarial vector Culex quinquefasciatus Say." *Tropical Biomedicine*, 22, no. 2, (2005): 139-142.

[31] Pushpanathan, T., A. Jebanesan, and M. Govindarajan. "Larvicidal, ovicidal and repellent activities of Cymbopogan citratus Stapf (Graminae) essential oil against the filarial mosquito Culex quinquefasciatus (Say)(Diptera: Culicidae)." *Tropical Biomedicine*, 23, no. 2 (2006): 208-212.

[32] Nerio, Luz Stella, Jesus Olivero-Verbel, Elena Stashenko. "Repellent activity of essential oils: a review." *Bioresource Technology*, 101, no. 1, (2010): 372-378.

[33] Maia, Marta Ferreira, and Sarah J. Moore. "Plant-based insect repellents: a review of their efficacy, development and testing." *Malaria Journal* 10, no. 1 (2011): S11.

[34] Moore, Sarah J., Annick Lenglet, Nigel Hill. "Field evaluation of three plant-based insect repellents against malaria vectors in Vaca Diez Province, the Bolivian Amazon." *Journal of the American Mosquito Control Association*, 18, no. 2, (2002): 107-110.

[35] Omolo, Maurice O., Denis Okinyo, Isaiah O. Ndiege, Wilber Lwande, and Ahmed Hassanali. "Repellency of essential oils of some Kenyan plants against Anopheles gambiae." *Phytochemistry*, 65, no. 20 (2004): 2797-2802.

[36] Revay, Edita E., Amy Junnila, Daniel L. Kline, Rui-De Xue, Ulrich R. Bernier, Vasiliy D. Kravchenko, Zoya A. Yefremova, Günter C. Müller. "Reduction of mosquito biting pressure by timed-release 0.3% aerosolized geraniol." *Acta Tropica*, 124, no. 1, (2012): 102-105.

[37] Barnard, Donald R., and Rui-De Xue. "Laboratory evaluation of mosquito repellents against Aedes albopictus, Culex nigripalpus, and Ochlerotatus triseriatus (Diptera: Culicidae)." *Journal of Medical Entomology*, 41, no. 4 (2004): 726-730.

[38] Kaufman, Phillip E., Rajinder S. Mann, and Jerry F. Butler. "Evaluation of semiochemical toxicity to Aedes aegypti, Ae. albopictus and Anopheles quadrimaculatus (Diptera: Culicidae)." *Pest Management Science*, 66, no. 5 (2010): 497-504.

[39] Mann, Rajinder S., Phillip E. Kaufman, Jerry F. Butler. "Evaluation of semiochemical toxicity to houseflies and stable flies (Diptera: Muscidae)." *Pest Management Science*, 66, no. 8, (2010): 816-824.

[40] Weldon, Paul J., John F. Carroll, Matthew Kramer, Robert H. Bedoukian, Russell E. Coleman, Ulrich R. Bernier. "Anointing chemicals and hematophagous arthropods: responses by ticks and mosquitoes to citrus (Rutaceae) peel exudates and monoterpene components." *Journal of Chemical Ecology*, 37, no. 4, (2011): 348-359.

[41] Müller, Günter C., Amy Junnila, Vasiliy D. Kravchenko, Edita E. Revay, Jerry Butler, Yosef Schlein. "Indoor protection against mosquito and sand fly bites: a comparison between citronella, linalool, and geraniol candles." *Journal of the American Mosquito Control Association*, 24, no. 1, (2008): 150-153.

[42] Khater, Hanem Fathy, Abdelfattah M. Selim, Galal A. Abouelella, Nour A. Abouelella, Kadarkarai Murugan, Nelissa P. Vaz, Marimuthu Govindarajan. "Commercial mosquito repellents and their safety concerns." In *Malaria*. IntechOpen, 2019.

[43] Bedini, S., G. Flamini, R. Ascrizzi, F. Venturi, G. Ferroni, A. Bader, J. Girardi, and B. Conti. "Essential oils sensory quality and their bioactivity against the mosquito Aedes albopictus." *Scientific Reports*, 8, no. 1 (2018): 1-10.

[44] Tawatsin, Apiwat, Steve D. Wratten, R. Roderic Scott, Usavadee Thavara, Yenchit Techadamrongsin. "Repellency of volatile oils from plants against three mosquito vectors." *Journal of Vector Ecology*, 26, (2001): 76-82.

[45] Cavanagh, Heather MA. "Antifungal activity of the volatile phase of essential oils: a brief review." *Natural Product Communications*, 2, no. 12, (2007): 1934578X0700201222.

[46] Utama, I. Made S., Ron BH Wills, Shimshon Ben-yehoshua, and Clem Kuek. "In vitro efficacy of plant volatiles for inhibiting the growth of fruit and vegetable decay microorganisms." *Journal of Agricultural and Food Chemistry*, 50, no. 22 (2002): 6371-6377.

[47] Creelman, Robert A., John E. Mullet. "Biosynthesis and action of jasmonates in plants." *Annual Review of Plant Biology*, 48, no. 1, (1997): 355-381.

[48] Hines, Pamela J. *The invisible bouquet.*, (2006): 803-803.

[49] Pichersky, Eran, Joseph P. Noel, Natalia Dudareva. "Biosynthesis of plant volatiles: nature's diversity and ingenuity." *Science*, 311, no. 5762, (2006): 808-811.

[50] Dorman, HJD; Stanley G. Deans. "Antimicrobial agents from plants: antibacterial activity of plant volatile oils." *Journal of Applied Microbiology*, 88, no. 2, (2000): 308-316.

[51] Dorman, HJD; Deans, SG. Antimicrobial agents from plants: antibacterial activity of plant volatile oils. *Journal of Applied Microbiology*, 88, (2000): 308–316.

[52] Valgimigli, L. "Essential oils: an overview on origins, chemistry, properties and uses." *Essential oils as natural food additives*. Nova Science Publishers, (2012): 24.

[53] Amiri, Achour, Robert Dugas, Anne L. Pichot, Gilbert Bompeix. "In vitro and in vitro activity of eugenol oil (Eugenia caryophylata) against four important postharvest apple pathogens." *International Journal of Food Microbiology*, 126, no. 1-2, (2008): 13-19.

[54] Tabanca, Nurhayat, Betul Demirci, Sara L. Crockett, Kemal Hüsnü Can Başer, David E. Wedge. "Chemical composition and antifungal activity of Arnica longifolia, Aster hesperius, and Chrysothamnus nauseosus essential oils." *Journal of Agricultural and Food Chemistry*, 55, no. 21, (2007): 8430-8435.

[55] Mancini, Emilia, Ippolito Camele, Hazem S. Elshafie, Laura De Martino, Carlo Pellegrino, Daniela Grulova, Vincenzo De Feo.

"Chemical composition and biological activity of the essential oil of Origanum vulgare ssp. hirtum from different areas in the Southern Apennines (Italy)." *Chemistry and biodiversity*, 11, no. 4, (2014): 639-651.

[56] Elshafie, Hazem S., Emilia Mancini, Ippolito Camele, Laura De Martino, Vincenzo De Feo. "In vivo antifungal activity of two essential oils from Mediterranean plants against postharvest brown rot disease of peach fruit." *Industrial Crops and Products*, 66, (2015): 11-15.

[57] Lopez-Reyes, Jorge Giovanny, Davide Spadaro, Maria Lodovica Gullino, Angelo Garibaldi. "Efficacy of plant essential oils on postharvest control of rot caused by fungi on four cultivars of apples in vivo." *Flavour and Fragrance Journal*, 25, no. 3, (2010): 171-177.

[58] Santoro, Karin, Marco Maghenzani, Valentina Chiabrando, Pietro Bosio, Maria Lodovica Gullino, Davide Spadaro, Giovanna Giacalone. "Thyme and savory essential oil vapor treatments control brown rot and improve the storage quality of peaches and nectarines, but could favor gray mold." *Foods*, 7, no. 1, (2018): 7.

[59] Banani, Houda, Leone Olivieri, Karin Santoro, Angelo Garibaldi, Maria Lodovica Gullino, Davide Spadaro. "Thyme and savory essential oil efficacy and induction of resistance against Botrytis cinerea through priming of defense responses in apple." *Foods*, 7, no. 2, (2018): 11.

[60] Osman, K. A., and H. T. Abdulrahman. "Risk assessment of pesticide to human and the environment." *Saudi Journal of Biological Sciences*, 10 (2003): 81-106.

[61] Anžlovar, Sabina, Matevž Likar, Jasna Dolenc Koce. "Antifungal potential of thyme essential oil as a preservative for storage of wheat seeds." *Acta Botanica Croatica*, 76, no. 1, (2017): 64-71.

[62] Espitia, Paula Judith Perez, Nilda de Fátima Ferreira Soares, Laura Costa Moreira Botti, Nathália Ramos de Melo, Olinto Liparini Pereira, Washington Azevêdo da Silva. "Assessment of the efficiency of essential oils in the preservation of postharvest papaya in an

antimicrobial packaging system." *Brazilian Journal of Food Technology*, 15, no. 4, (2012): 333-342.

[63] Sánchez-González, Laura, Clara Pastor, María Vargas, Amparo Chiralt, Chelo González-Martínez, Maite Cháfer. "Effect of hydroxypropylmethylcellulose and chitosan coatings with and without bergamot essential oil on quality and safety of cold-stored grapes." *Postharvest Biology and Technology*, 60, no. 1, (2011): 57-63.

[64] Batish, Daizy R., Harminder P. Singh, Nidhi Setia, Shalinder Kaur, Ravinder K. Kohli. "Chemical composition and phytotoxicity of volatile essential oil from intact and fallen leaves of Eucalyptus citriodora." *Zeitschrift für Naturforschung C*, 61, no. 7-8, (2006): 465-471.

[65] Sumalan, Renata-Maria, Ersilia Alexa, Mariana-Atena Poiana. "Assessment of inhibitory potential of essential oils on natural mycoflora and Fusarium mycotoxins production in wheat." *Chemistry Central Journal*, 7, no. 1, (2013): 32.

[66] Burrow, A., Eccles, R., Jones, AS. "The effects of camphor, eucalyptus and menthol vapour on nasal resistance to airflow and nasal sensation." *Acta oto-laryngologica*, 96, no. 1-2, (1983): 157-161.

[67] Shubina, L. P., S. A. Siurin, and V. M. Savchenko. "Inhalations of essential oils in the combined treatment of patients with chronic bronchitis." *Medical Practice*, 5 (1990): 66-67.

[68] Frohlich, E. "Lavender oil; review of clinical, pharmacological and bacteriological studies. Contribution to clarification of the mechanism of action." *Wiener Medizinische Wochenschrift*, 118, (1968): 345-350.

[69] Inouye, Shigeharu, Katsuhisa Uchida, Shigeru Abe. "Vapor activity of 72 essential oils against a Trichophyton mentagrophytes." *Journal of Infection and Chemotherapy*, 12, no. 4, (2006): 210-216.

[70] Luna, Emanuela Coutinho, Isadora Silva Luna, Luciana Scotti, Alex France M. Monteiro, Marcus Tullius Scotti, Ricardo Olímpio de Moura, Rodrigo Santos Aquino de Araújo et al. "Active essential oils and their components in use against neglected diseases and

arboviruses." *Oxidative Medicine and Cellular Longevity*, 2019, (2019).

[71] Bakkali, Fadil, Simone Averbeck, Dietrich Averbeck, Mouhamed Idaomar. "Biological effects of essential oils–a review." *Food and Chemical Toxicology*, 46, no. 2, (2008): 446-475.

[72] Ou, Ming-Chiu, Tsung-Fu Hsu, Andrew C. Lai, Yu-Ting Lin, Chia-Ching Lin. "Pain relief assessment by aromatic essential oil massage on outpatients with primary dysmenorrhea: A randomized, double-blind clinical trial." *Journal of Obstetrics and Gynaecology Research*, 38, no. 5, (2012): 817-822.

[73] Safajou, Farzaneh, Mahnaz Shahnazi, and Hossein Nazemiyeh. "The effect of lemon inhalation aromatherapy on nausea and vomiting of pregnancy: a double-blinded, randomized, controlled clinical trial." *Iranian Red Crescent Medical Journal*, 16, no. 3 (2014).

[74] Watanabe, Eri, Kenny Kuchta, Mari Kimura, Hans Wilhelm Rauwald, Tsutomu Kamei, Jiro Imanishi. "Effects of bergamot (Citrus bergamia (Risso) Wright & Arn.) essential oil aromatherapy on mood states, parasympathetic nervous system activity, and salivary cortisol levels in 41 healthy females." *Complementary Medicine Research*, 22, no. 1, (2015): 43-49.

[75] Tisserand, R., and T. Balacs. "The skin." *Essential Oil Safety: A Guide for Health Care Professionals* (1995): 77-89.

[76] Kim, Sioh, Hyun-Jae Kim, Jin-Seok Yeo, Sung-Jung Hong, Ji-Min Lee, Younghoon Jeon. "The effect of lavender oil on stress, bispectral index values, and needle insertion pain in volunteers." *The Journal of Alternative and Complementary Medicine*, 17, no. 9, (2011): 823-826.

[77] Tisserand, Robert, Rodney Young. *Essential oil Safety-E-Book: A guide for health care professionals*. Elsevier Health Sciences, 2013.

[78] Del, MA Beccaro. "Melaleuca oil poisoning in a 17-month-old." *Veterinary and Human Toxicology*, 37, no. 6, (1995): 557-558.

[79] Markowitz, John S; Lindsay DeVane, C; Kenneth D. Chavin, Robin M. Taylor, Ying Ruan, Jennifer L. Donovan. "Effects of garlic (Allium sativum L.) supplementation on cytochrome P450 2D6 and

3A4 activity in healthy volunteers." *Clinical Pharmacology and Therapeutics*, 74, no. 2, (2003): 170-177.

[80] Gurley, Bill J., Stephanie F. Gardner, Martha A. Hubbard, D. Keith Williams, W. Brooks Gentry, Yanyan Cui, and Catharina YW Ang. "Clinical assessment of effects of botanical supplementation on cytochrome P450 phenotypes in the elderly." *Drugs and Aging*, 22, no. 6, (2005): 525-539.

[81] Gurley, Bill J., Stephanie F. Gardner, Martha A. Hubbard, D. Keith Williams, W. Brooks Gentry, Yanyan Cui, Catharina YW Ang. "Cytochrome P450 phenotypic ratios for predicting herb-drug interactions in humans." *Clinical Pharmacology and Therapeutics*, 72, no. 3, (2002)., 276-287.

[82] Jabbari, Abbas, Hassan Argani, Amir Ghorbanihaghjo, Reza Mahdavi. "Comparison between swallowing and chewing of garlic on levels of serum lipids, cyclosporine, creatinine and lipid peroxidation in renal transplant recipients." *Lipids in Health and Disease*, 4, no. 1, (2005): 11.

[83] Cox, Michael C; Jennifer Low, James Lee, Janice Walshe, Neelima Denduluri, Arlene Berman, Matthew G. Permenter; et al. "Influence of garlic (Allium sativum) on the pharmacokinetics of docetaxel." *Clinical Cancer Research*, 12, no. 15, (2006)., 4636-4640.

[84] Dresser, George K., Vincent Wacher, Susan Wong, Harrison T. Wong, David G. Bailey. "Evaluation of peppermint oil and ascorbyl palmitate as inhibitors of cytochrome P4503A4 activity in vitro and in vivo." *Clinical Pharmacology and Therapeutics*, 72, no. 3, (2002)., 247-255.

In: What to Know about Essential Oils
Editor: Malene M. Kjeldsen
ISBN: 978-1-53617-986-6

Chapter 7

JASMINUM GRANDIFLORUM ESSENTIAL OIL: CHEMICAL CONSTITUENTS, MULTIPLE BIOLOGICAL ACTIVITIES WITH HEALTH PROMOTING EFFECTS

***Hajer Riguene*[1], *Ghayth Rigane*[1,2,*] *and Ridha Ben Salem*[1]**

[1]Organic Chemistry Laboratory, Sciences of Sfax Faculty, Chemistry Department, University of Sfax, Tunisia

[2]Faculty of Sciences and Technology of Sidi Bouzid, Department of Physics and Chemistry, Sidi Bouzid, University of Kairouan, Sidi Bouzid, Tunisia

ABSTRACT

Jasminum grandiflorum essential oil has received a great interest worldwide for its multiple biological activities due to its chemical constituents. Indeed, the application of *jasminum grandiflorum* essential

---

* Corresponding Author's Email: gaith.rigane@yahoo.fr.

oil in cosmetic and personal hygiene products is gradually increasing. Also, it has been widely used in the traditional medicine for centuries, in the treatment of respiratory diseases, common cold, influenza, and sinus congestion. This review addressed chemical composition and ethno-pharmacological aspects of *jasminum grandiflorum* plants, as also its *in vitro* and *in vivo* pharmacological activities, and current insights with regards to clinical efficacy and safety.

Keywords: *Jasminum grandiflorum,* essential oil, pharmacological activities, health promoting effects

INTRODUCTION

Jasmine is an important group of flowering plants. It is a *genus* of shrubs and vines in the olive family *Oleaceae* (Table 1) which possess about 2000 *species*. Jasmine varieties originated from India, but are also well-known in the Mediterranean countries of Europe, Asia, and Africa, the Comoro Islands, India and China (Jirovetz et al. 2007) (Figure 1). *Jasminum grandiflorum* Linn is small shrub, among different jasmine *species.Jasminum grandiflorum* is one of most important and remunerative crop for loose flower production and oil extraction purpose. It is known as a night blooming flowering plant with peak fragrance in the night (Pragadheesh et al. 2017). The jasmine crop has been cultivated in the open fields since ancient times for its peculiar and delicate fragrance and also for its aromatic and medicinal value (Mohanasundari et al. 2018). The traditional use of this plant suggests spasmolytic, antiinflammatory, antimicrobial, antioxidant, antiulcer, cytoprotective, chemo preventive, wound healing and antiacne activities (Sachan et al. 2009). Jasmineessential oil has a sweet and floral aroma. It is regarded as unique, as it blends well with other floral extracts and which is highly valued throughout the world for its high grade perfumes, which is used in soap and cosmetic industries and in flavoring mouth wash liquids. It is extensively used for oil extraction and also for the preparation of jasmine concrete.

Table 1. Taxonomical Classification

Kingdom	**Plantae**
Subkingdom	Tracheobionta – Vascular plants
Super division	Spermatophyta – Seed plants
Division	Magnoliophyta – Flowering plants
Class	Magnoliopsida – Dicotyledons
Sub class	Asteridae
Order	Scrophulariales
Family	Oleaceae – Olive family
Genus	Jasminum – Jasmine
Species	Grandiflorum Linn.

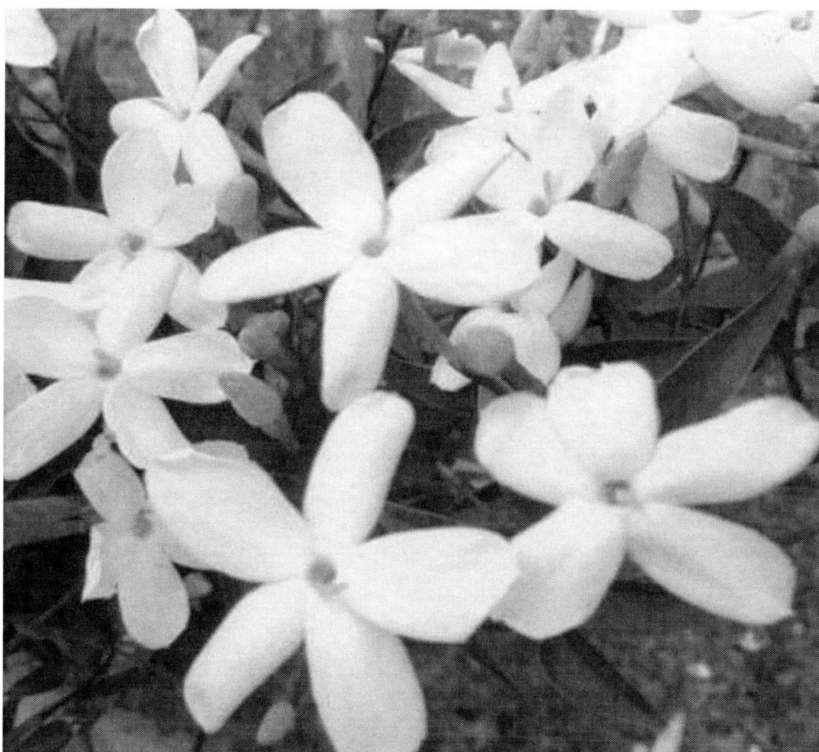

Figure 1. *Jasminum grandiflorum* L. plant.

Essential oil of*jasminum grandiflorum* can be useful as an antidepressant, as a calming agent to soothe stress, pain and anxiety, and as an aphrodisiac (Arun et al. 2016). The present review will highlight the analytical techniques used to study the chemical composition as well as the ethno-pharmacological aspects of *jasminum grandiflorum* essential oils of plants by different authors.

BOTANICAL CHARACTERISTICS

Jasminum grandiflorum, with an intensely floral, warm, rich and highly diffusive odor. It is a large scrambling suberect twining ever green shrub, which grows up to 10 to 15m high (Figure 1). The leaves are shining dark green with 5-7 leaf lets. This is twining shrub with pendulous branches. They can be simple, trifoliate, or pinnate. Flowers are very fragrant, 3.0 – 3.8cm across. Its color is white with a purplish tinge underneath. They are borne in cymose clusters with a minimum of three flowers, though they can also be solitary on the ends of branchlets. Each flower has about four to nine petals, two locules, and one to four ovules. (Mohanasundari et al. 2018; Arun et al. 2016) (Figure 2).

JASMINE ESSENTIAL OIL EXTRACTION

Different extraction techniques, such as hydrodistillation, maceration, CO_2 extraction, etc., are widely used for obtaining essential oils from *jasminum grandiflorum*.

The oils were extracted by maceration. Five gram flower buds were taken along with citric acid. It was grinded with mortar and pestle. Grinding was carried out for about ½ hour. The pulp mixture was transferred in a beaker. Juice was collected after filtration. Then it was subjected with ether for oil separation. Finally, it was stabilized by adding sodium sulphate salts and dried ether by gentle heat (40°C).

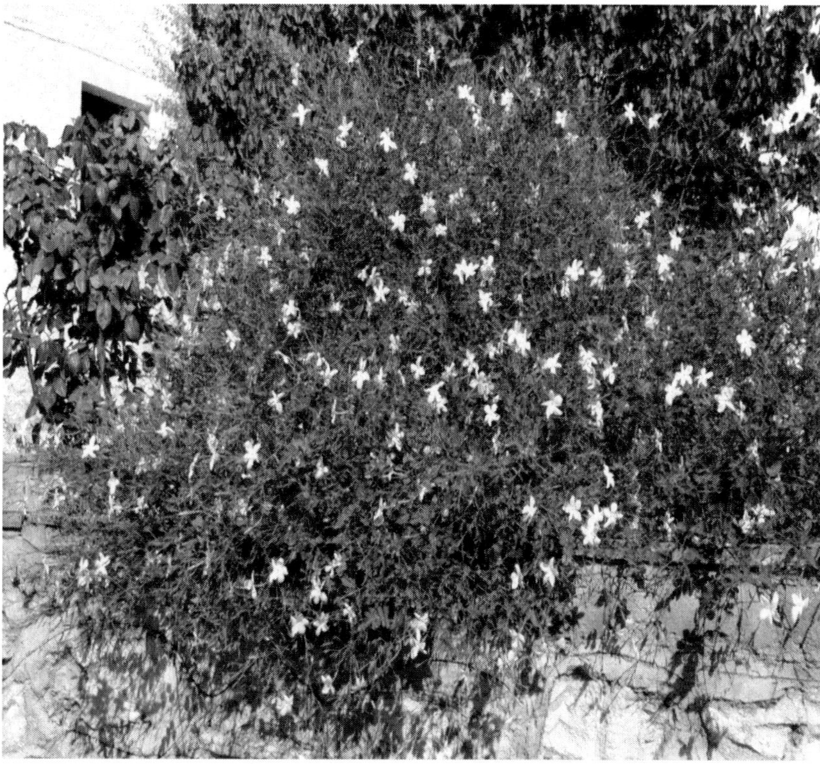

Figure 2. Flower of *jasminum grandiflorum* L. plant.

Prakash et al. (2012) have studied the advantages of CO_2 extraction of *jasminum grandiflorum.* Liquid CO_2 extraction appeared to be a simple process for obtaining a fine jasmine fragrance that was free from solvent residues and with low amounts of non-volatile components. The extract is enriched in volatiles making the product more acceptable for high value perfume compositions. Our process needs relatively simple equipment, requiring no compressors or high-pressure pumps for transfer of liquid CO_2, and thus the operating cost has been minimized. The extract was enriched with terpenoids and benzenoids, which might be suitable for use in aromatherapy and fine perfumer. They have studied the extraction of jasmine flowers with 22°C and 62 bar (Prakash et al. 2012). However, Wei et al. (2015) have studied the extraction of *jasminum grandiflorum* using hydrodistillation for 3h. The essential oil obtained was stored in a sealed glass tube with a screw cap in a refrigerator at 4°C until analyzed.

ESSENTIAL OIL ANALYSIS TECHNIQUES

The essential oils were analyzed using high performance liquid chromatography (HPLC), gas chromatography (GC) and gas chromatography–mass spectrometry (GC–MS). GC–MShas been proven to be a powerful and suitable tool for the determination of various types of essential oil because of its high separation efficiency and sensitive detection and identied a number of has never been reported before. But, gas chromatography–mass spectrometry (GC–MS) and FTIR spectra, combined with chemometrics, have been used to identify the different volatile oil components of raw medicinal materials from different species and different habitats (Table 2).

THE CHEMICAL COMPOSITION OF JASMINE ESSENTIAL OILS

Essential oils are liquid that are generally distilled from various parts of plant that have strong aromatic components such as from the leaves, stems, flowers and roots.

The chemical composition of *jasminumgrandiflorum* has been reported in Table 3. Extraction of flowers with liquid CO_2 yielded a product that contained the lowest amounts of fatty components (2.5%) and hydrocarbons (0.8%), with an improved percentage of oxygenated monoterpenes and polar compounds (C<11) (17.2%), and benzenoids (42.4%). The major compounds in the liquid CO2 extract were (Z)-3-hexenyl acetate (5.5%), linalool (9.6%), benzyl acetate (12.0%), methyl anthranilate (3.1%), (E,E)-α-farnesene (20.0%) and (Z)-3-hexenyl benzoate (24.8%).

Table 2. Essential oil analysis techniques of *jasminum grandiflorum* L.

Essential oil analysis techniques of *jasminum grandiflorum*	**Conditions**	**Major component**	**References**
GC-MS, GC/FID	The columns were 30m x 0.32mm bonded FSOT-RSL200 fused silica, with a film thickness of 0.25µm (Biorad, Germany) and 30m x 0.32mm bonded Stabilwax, with a film thickness of 0.50µm.The temperature program was: 40°C/5min to280°C/5min, with a heating rate of 6°C/min	Benzyl acetate (23.7%), Benzyl benzoate (20.7%), Phytol (10.9%), Linalool (8.2%), Isophytol (5.5%),	Jirovetz et al. 2007
GC-MS	100°C initial temperature, increased to 270°C at 4°C/min, final temperature 270°C and held for 7.5min.	Phytol (25.77%), 3,7,11trimethyldodeca-1,6,10-trien-3-ol (12.54%) Isophytol (12.42%). Hexadecanoic acid (9.16%) Perhydrofarnesyl Acetone (4.85%)	Wei et al. 2015
GC-FID, GC/MS	A 30m x 0.25mm WCOT column, coated with 0.25µm 5% diphenyl dimethyl siloxane (DB-5) Helium was used as the carrier gas at a flow rate of 1.2mL/min at a column pressure of 42 KPa. Component separation was achieved following a linear temperature program of 60°-210°C (2°C/min), and 210°C (50 min). MS parameters: ionization voltage (EI) 70 eV, peak width 2 s, mass range 40-400 amu and detector voltage 1.5 volts	Linalool (7.1%), Benzyl acetate (18.3%), (E,E)-α-farnesene (26.2%), (Z)-3-hexenyl acetate (12.2%) α-cadinol (7.2%).	Prakash et al. 2012

Table 3. Screening of important essential oil isolated from *Jasminum Grandiflorum* L.

No.	Chemical name	Identification Method	References
1	Benzylacetate	GC, GC-MS, GC-FID	Jirovetza et al. 2007; Wei et al. 2015; Prakash et al. 2012.
2	*trans*-Nerolidol	GC-MS, GC-FID	Jirovetza et al. 2007; Prakash et al. 2012; Wei et al. 2015.
3	Cedrol	GC-MS	Wei et al. 2015.
4	Methyl myristate	GC-MS	Wei et al. 2015.
5	7-Tetradecene	GC-MS	Wei et al. 2015.
6	Benzyl benzoate	GC, GC-MS	Jirovetza et al. 2007; Wei et al. 2015; Tyagi et al. 2017.
7	Neophytadiene	GC-MS	Wei et al. 2015.
8	PerhydrofarnesylAcetone	GC-MS	Wei et al. 2015.
9	Phytol acetate	GC-MS	Wei et al. 2015.
10	Nonadecane	GC-MS	Wei et al. 2015.
11	Geranyl linalool	GC, GC-MS	Jirovetza et al. 2007; Wei et al. 2015.
12	Linalool	GC-MS; GC-FID	Prakash et al. 2012; Jirovetza et al. 2007.
13	Methyl palmitate	GC-MS	Wei et al. 2015;
14	Isophytol	GC-MS	Wei et al. 2015; Jirovetza et al. 2007.
15	Hexadecanoic acid	GC-MS	Wei et al. 2015.
16	Methyl phytanate	GC-MS	Wei et al. 2015.
17	α -Methyl linolenate	GC-MS	Wei et al. 2015; Jirovetza et al. 2007.
18	Heneicosane	GC-MS	Wei et al. 2015.
19	Phytol	GC, GC-MS	Jirovetza et al. 2007; Wei et al. 2015.
20	Octadecanoic acid methyl ester	GC-MS	Wei et al. 2015.
21	9,12,15-Octadecatrienoic acid	GC-MS	Wei et al. 2015.
22	Docosane	GC-MS	Wei et al. 2015.
23	Tricosane	GC-MS	Wei et al. 2015.
24	Tetracosane	GC-MS	Wei et al. 2015.
25	Pentacosane	GC-MS	Wei et al. 2015.
26	Hexacosane	GC-MS	Wei et al. 2015.
27	Heptacosane	GC-MS	Wei et al. 2015.
28	Octacosane	GC-MS	Wei et al. 2015.

No.	Chemical name	Identification Method	References
29	Squalene	GC-MS	Wei et al. 2015.
30	Nonacosane	GC-MS	Wei et al. 2015.
31	*cis*-Jasmone	GC-MS; GC-FID	Jirovetza et al. 2007; Prakash et al. 2012.
32	*trans*-Jasmone	GC-MS	Jirovetza et al. 2007.
33	Methyl anthranilate	GC-MS	Jirovetza et al. 2007; Tyagi et al. 2017.
34	(E,E)-α-farnesene	GC-MS; GC-FID	Jirovetza et al. 2007; Prakash et al. 2012.
35	(Z)-3-hexenyl acetate	GC-MS; GC-FID	Jirovetza et al. 2007; Prakash et al. 2012.
36	α-cadinol	GC-MS; GC-FID	Prakash et al. 2012.
37	T-Cadinol	GC-MS; GC-FID	Prakash et al. 2012.
38	δ-Cadinene	GC-MS; GC-FID	Prakash et al. 2012.

The liquid CO_2 extract contained improved amounts of some minor compounds like methyl salicylate (0.3%), indole (0.3%), (Z)-jasmone (0.2%), (Z)-methyl jasmonoate (0.2%) and (Z)-methyl epi-jasmonoate (0.3%), which contribute towards the fragrance characteristics of the floral extract (Prakash et al. 2012).

In addition, *jasminum grandiflorum* absolute from India has been reported by Jirovetz et al. (2007). The chemical composition of a sample of *jasminum grandiflorum* L. was analyzed by GC and GC/MS. The major compounds identified were benzyl acetate (23.7%), benzyl benzoate (20.7%), phytol (10.9%), linalool (8.2%), isophytol (5.5%), geranyl linalool (3.0%), methyl linoleate (2.8%) and eugenol (2.5%). But the results of Wei (2015) using GC/MS technique show that phytol was the major volatile component of *jasminum grandiflorum*. The major volatile components of the flower were phytol(25.77%), 3,7,11 trimethyldodeca -1,6,10-trien-3-ol (12.54%) and 3,7,11,15 - tetramethyl -1-Hexadecen-3-ol (12.42%) (Figure 3).

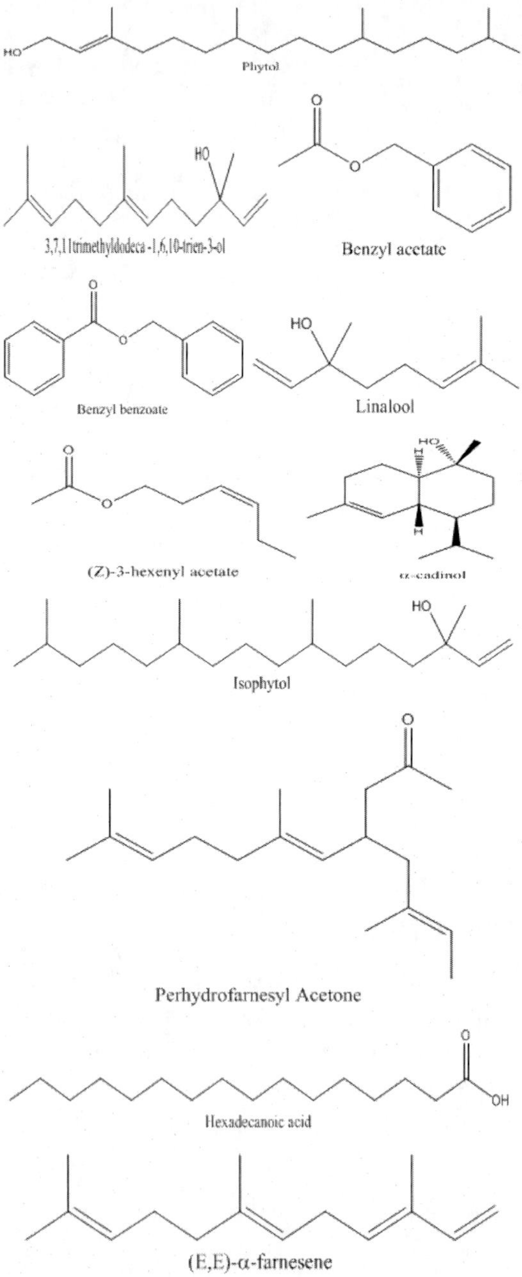

Figure 3. Chemical structure of some major constituents of *Jasminum Grandifluriom* L.

THE BIOLOGICAL ACTIVITIES OF JASMINE OIL

The data show that phytol is the major essential component of *jasminum grandiflorum*, and this component may have some of the pharmacological effects of *jasminum grandiflorum* plant itself and acute administration of phytol exerts an anxiolytic-like effect on mice by producing sedative and anxiolytic activities. In open field test, phytol (25, 50 and 75mg/kg) increased the number of crossings and rearings. In pentobarbital sleeping time test, phytol 75mg/kg decreased for latency of sleeping and phytol (25, 50 and 75mg/kg) increased the sleep time when compared to negative control (Costa et al. 2014).

The antimicrobial activities of the *jasminum grandiflorum* sample and of some of its main and minor compounds were tested against Gram-positive and Gram-negative bacteria, as well as against the yeast Candida albicans, using agar dilution and agar diffusion methods.

The jasmine absolute showed medium to high activity (reference compounds: eugenol and three synthetic antibiotics) against the Gram-positive bacterium *Enterococcus faecalis*, against the Gram-negative bacteria *Escherichia coli*, *Pseudomonasaeruginosa*, *Klebsiellapneumoniae* and *Salmonellasp.*, as well as against the yeast *Candidaalbicans* (Jirovetz et al. 2007).

Epilepsy is a common chronic neurological disorder that affects 1–2% of the world population. Phytol exhibits anticonvulsant activity by modulating of neurotransmitter systems. It was reported that phytol (25, 50 and 75mg/kg, i.p.) increased latency to first seizure and decreased percentage of these seizures.

Moreover, phytol also protected the animals against status epilepticus induced by pilocarpine, and decreased the mortality rate. Mice treated with pilocarpine (n = 24) presented 100% of mortality during the first hour of observation. In turn, phytol-pretreated animals within 30 min before the administration of pilocarpine (400mg/kg) remained alive during thefirst hour of observation (Costa et al. 2012).

The peroxisome proliferator-activated receptor (PPAR) is one of the indispensable transcription factors for regulating lipid metabolism in various tissues. Phytol is functional as a PPARa ligand and that it stimulates the expression of PPARa-target genes in intact cells. Because PPARa activation enhances circulating lipid clearance, phytol may be important in managing abnormalities in lipid (Goto et al. 2005).

Phytol exhibits a good antioxidant activity because of the allylic nature of the alcohol group. It is able to scavenge reactive oxygen and/or nitrogen species (ROS/RNS) produced by cellular stress and metabolism (Guo et al. 2014).

Some of the bioactivities of phytol which could be related to its redox properties are its reported in vitro anticancer effects, anti-teratogenic activity, tumor-promotor and anti-tumor activity. Furthermore, trans-phytol inhibits the biosynthesis of estrogen in human ovarian granulose cells by aromatase (CYP19) (Guo et al. 2014).

Anti-acne activity of essential oil of *jasminum grandiflorum* was evaluated towards Propionibacterium acnes and in vitro toxicology against three human cancer cell lines. Results demonstrated that the essential oil was found to effective against Propionibacterium acnes and showed significantly stronger cytotoxicity of essential oil on human prostate carcinoma cell (PC-3) than on human lung carcinoma (A549) and human breast cancer (MCF-7) cell lines.

Use of essential oils as mosquito larvicide has been suggested by different studies. Jasmine oil shows best results for larvicidal activity against Aedes aegypti larvae as 42.85 ppm and 78.18ppm while it shows higher LC50 and LC90 of 73.52 ppm, 399.05 ppm against *Anopheles stephensi larvae* (Tyagi et al. 2017).

Jasminum grandiflorum was checked for its antibacterial activity against selected human pathogens viz., *Escherichia coli*, *Bacillus* sp., *Streptococcus* sp., *Salmonella* sp., *Pseudomonas* sp., *Serratiamarcescens*, *Klebsiellapneumonia* and *Staphylococcusaureus*. It was found that the samples showed antimicrobial activity against some of the pathogens (Shekhar et al. 2015).

Jasmine oil could be used as blended massage oil or diluted in the bath for almost everything like addiction, post natal depression, relaxation, muscle pain, coughs, tension, stress and nervousness. It is also used as a base cream or lotion for dry or greasy and sensitive skin, as well as for scratch marks and scars.

Conclusion

The results of this study showed that there was a great variation in the constituent of the essential oil from *jasminum grandiflorum*, with the major component being phytol. It is clear that jasmine essential oils posses a wide variety of bioactivities (antidepressant, antimicrobial, anticonvulsant, antioxidant, anti-cancer and anti-acne activities, *etc.*). The commercial uses of essential oil (blended massage oil, diluted in the bath, parfum, *etc.*) are simple, less expensive and eco-friendly.

References

Arun Mittal, Sardana Satish and Pandey Anima. 2015. "Phytopharmacological Profile of *Jasminum Grandiflorum* Linn. (Oleaceae)." *Chinese Journal of Integrative Medicine,* 22(4):311-20. Accessed April, 2016. doi: 10.1007/s11655-015-2051-3.

Costa Jessica, Pereira, Guilherme, Antonio L. de Oliveiraa, Antonia Amanda de Almeidaa, Md. Torequl, Islama, Damiao Pergentino de Sousacand Rivelilson Mendes de Freitasa. 2014. "Anticonvulsant effect of phytol in a pilocarpine model in mice". *Brain Research,* 1547:34 - 42. AccessedDecember 10, 2013. doi:10.1016/j.brainres.2013.12.003.

Costa Jéssica Pereira, Paulo Michel Pinheiro Ferreira, Damião P. De Sousa, Joaquin Jordan and Rivelilson Mendes De Freitas. 2012. "Anxiolytic-like effects of phytol: Possible involvement of GABAergic transmission". *Neuroscience Letters,* 523:115-118. Accessed June 20, 2012. doi.org/10.1016/j.neulet.2012.06.055.

Goto Tsuyoshi, Nobuyuki Takahashi, Sota Kato, Kahori Egawa, Shogo Ebisu, Tatsuya Moriyama, Tohru Fushiki, Teruo Kawada. 2005. "Phytol directly activates peroxisome proliferator-activated receptor a (PPARa) and regulates gene expression involved in lipid metabolism in PPARa-expressing HepG2 hepatocytes". *Biochemical and Biophysical Research Communications,* 337:440 - 445. Accessed September 21, 2005. doi:10.1016/j.bbrc.2005.09.077.

Guo Jiajia, Yun Yuan, Danfeng Lu, Baowen Du, Liang Xiong, Jiangong Shi, Lijuan Yang, Wanli Liu, Xiaohong Yuan, Guolin Zhang and Fei Wang. 2014. "Two natural products, trans-phytol and (22E)-ergosta-6,9,22-triene-3β,5α,8α-triol, inhibit the biosynthesis of estrogen in human ovarian granulosa cells by aromatase (CYP19)". *Toxicology and Applied Pharmacology,* 279(1):23-32. Accessed May20, 2014. doi.org/10.1016/j.taap.2014.05.008.

Jirovetza Leopold, Gerhard Buchbauera, Thomas Schweigera, Zapriana Denkovab, Slavchevb, Alexander, Stoyanovac, Albena, Schmidtd, Erich and Geissler, Margit. 2007. "Chemical Composition, Olfactory Evaluation and Antimicrobial Activities of *Jasminum grandiflorum* L. Absolute from India". *Natural Product Communications,* 2(4): 407-12. Accessed November 28, 2006.

Mohanasundari, P; T. Sivakumar; K. Krishna; Surendar and M. Ganga. 2018. "Prolonging the shelf life of jasmine (*Jasminum grandiflorum)* buds by chemical treatments under cold storage condition". *Journal of Agriculture and Ecology,* 6:85-93. Accessed November 27, 2018.

Pragadheesh, V.S., Chandan S. Chanotiya, Shubhra, Rastogi, Ajit K. Shasany. 2017. "Scent from *Jasminum grandiflorum* flowers: Investigation of the change in linalool enantiomers at various developmental stages using chemical and molecular methods". *Phytochemistry,*140:83-94. Accessed April 29, 2017.doi:10.1016/j.phytochem.2017.04.018.

Prakash, Om, Deeptanjali Sahoo and Prasant Kumar Rout. 2012. "Liquid CO2 Extraction of *Jasminum grandiflorum* and Comparison with Conventional Processes". *Natural Product Communications,* 7(1):89 - 92. Accessed December 5, 2011.

Sandeep Sachan, Padmaa. M. Paarakh and Usha Gavani. 2009. Antibacterial activity of *Jasminum grandiflorum* Linn leaves". *Journal of Pharmacy Research,* 2(7):1206-07 Accessed June 01, 2009.

Shekhar, Sushant and Prasad, M.P. 2015. "Evaluation of antimicrobial activity of Jasminum species using solvent extracts against clinical pathogenes". *World Journal of Pharmacy and Pharmaceutical Sciences*, 4 4(05):1247 7-56. Accessed April 16, 2015.

Tyagi Varun, Ranjeet Patel, Hemanga Hazarika, Piyali Dey, Diganta, Goswami and Chattopadhyay, P. 2017. "Chemical composition and bioefficacy for larvicidal and pupicidal activity of essential oils against two mosquito species". *International Journal of Mosquito Research,*4(4):112-18. Accessed June 14, 2017.

Biographical Sketches

Ghayth Rigane, PhD

Affiliation:Organic Chemistry Laboratory LR17ES08, Tunisia

Education: PhD Degree on Chemistry since 2013

Business Address: Sciences of Sfax Faculty, Chemistry Department, B.P. "1171" 3038, University of Sfax, Tunisia.

Research and Professional Experience: Supervisor for 6 Masters Degrees, 4 Co-supervisor of PhD students in Chemistry

Professional Appointments: Associate Professor

Publications from the Last 3 Years:

[1] Amira yahyaoui, Ghayth Rigane, Sami Mnif, Ridha Ben Salem, Ayşenur Acar, Derya Arslan. Ultrasound Technology Parameters: Effects on Phenolics in Olive Paste and Oil in Relation to Enzymatic

Activity. *European Journal of Lipid Science and Technology*, 2019, 121 (5), DOI: 10.1002/ejlt.201800295.

[2] Moufida A. Oueslati, Aynur Gunenc, Ghayth Rigane, Hanen Ghazghazi, Caroline Valencia, Ridha Ben Salem, Sadok Boukhchina, William G. Willmore and Farah Hosseinian. LC-MS AND ESI-MS QTOF-MS analysis of glycerophospholipid and triacylglycerol species in developing wild artichoke achenes. *Revue Roumaine de Chimie,* 2019, 64 (8), 733-742.

[3] Sondes Fkiri, Hanene Ghazghazi, Ghayth Rigane, Ridha Ben Salem, Faten Mezni, Abdelhamid Khaldi, M. Larbi Khouja and Zouhair Nasr. Chemical compositions and biological activities essential oil from the needles of north african *pinus pinaster* var. *Revue Roumaine de Chimie,* 2019, 64 (6), 511-517.

[4] Moufida A. Oueslati, Aynur Gunenc, Ghayth Rigane, Hanen Ghazghazi, Caroline Valencia, Ridha Ben Salem, Sadok Boukhchina, Williamn G. Willmore and Farah Hosseinian.Chemical composition, antioxidant and cytotoxic activities of onopordum acanthium L. crude oil and defatted meal. *Revue Roumaine de Chimie,* 2019, 64 (6), 503-510.

[5] Amira Yahyaoui, Moufida Oueslati Arfaoui, Ghayth Rigane, Achref Hkir, Kawther Amari, Ridha Ben Salem, Youssef Ammar. Investigation on the Chemical composition and antioxidant capacity of extracts from Crataegus azarolus L.: Effect of growing location of an important Tunisian medicinal plant. *Chemistry Africa,* 2019, 2, 361-365.

[6] Amira Yahyaoui, Olfa Khedher, Ghayth Rigane, Ridha Ben Salem and Younes Moussaoui. Chemical analysis of essential oil from *Echinops Spinosus* L. roots: antimicrobial and antioxydant activities. *Revue Roumaine de Chimie,* 2018, 63 (3), 199-204.

[7] Ghayth Rigane, Sami Mnif and Ridha Ben Salem. One step purification of 6-shogaol from *zingiber officinale* rosco, a phenolic compound having a high effectiveness against bacterial strains. *Revue Roumaine de Chimie,* 2018, 63 (1), 5-10.

[8] Amira Yahyaoui, Ghayth Rigane and Ridha Ben Salem. Oxidative stability of extra virgin olive oil with natural plant extracts during microwave heating. *Asian Journal of Chemistry*, 2017, 29 (12), 2655-2659.

[9] Ghayth Rigane, Moufida Oueslati Arfaoui, Moemen Chira, Hanene Ghazghazi, Amira Yahyaoui, Ridha Ben Salem, Sabiha Hamdi, Malek Hannachi, Hager Jouili and Youssef Ammari. Chemical compositions, antioxidantand antimicrobial activities of the essential oilof *Trachyspermum ammi*L. growing in Tunisia. *Revue Roumaine de Chimie,* 2016, 61(10), 807-813.

[10] Ghayth Rigane, Hanene Ghazghazi, Chedia Aouadhi, Ridha Ben Salem, Zouheir Nasr. Phenolic content, antioxidant capacity and antimicrobial activity of leaf extracts from *Pistacia atlantica.Natural Product Research,* 2016, 6, 696-699.

[11] Layla Mhamdi, Khemais Said, Ghayth Rigane, Ridha Ben Salem, Younes Moussaoui. Ultrasonic activation of Nozaki-Hiyama-Kichi reaction in the presence of phase transfer catalysis. *Journal of the Tunisian Chemical Society,* 2016, 18, 61-67.

[12] Moufida OueslatiArfaoui,Ghayth Rigane, HanenGhazghazi,Ridha Ben Salem, S. Hamdi, M. Hannachi, H. Jouili, Y. L'ammari. Phenoliccontent,antioxidantandantimicrobialactivitiesof *Trachyspermumammi*aerialpartsgrowingwildinthenorthof Tunisia. *Journal of New Sciences*, 2016, 25(4), 1151-1160.

Hajer Riguene

Affiliation: Organic Chemistry Laboratory LR17ES08, Tunisia

Education: PhD student in Chemistry

Business Address:Sciences of Sfax Faculty, Chemistry Department, B.P "1171" 3038, University of Sfax, Tunisia.

Publications from the Last 3 Years:

[1] Hanene Ghazghazi, Badiaa Essghaier, Hajer Riguene, Ghayth Rigane, Meriem El Aloui, Moufida A. Oueslati, Ridha Ben Salem, Najla Sadfi Zouaoui, Zouher Naser and Mouhamed Laarbi Khouja. Phytochemical analysis, antioxidant and antimicrobial activities of eucalyptus essential oil: a comparative study between eycalaptusmarginata L. and eucalyptus paucilora L. *Revue Romaine de Chimie,* 2019, in press.

[2] Ghayth Rigane, Jed Jebali, Hanen Ghazghazi, Hajer Riguene, Mohamed Laarbi Khouja, Ridha Ben Salem. Chemical composition and biological activities of pinushalepensis Mill. oil. *Revue Roumaine de Chimie,* 2019, in press.

Ridha Ben Salem, PhD

Affiliation: Organic Chemistry Laboratory LR17ES08, Tunisia

Education: PhD Degree on Chemistry since 1987

Business Address: Sciences of Sfax Faculty, Chemistry Department, B.P "1171" 3038, University of Sfax, Tunisia.

Research and Professional Experience: supervisor for 4 postdoctorate, 5 Masters Degrees, 12 PhD students in Chemistry

Professional Appointments: Full Professor and Head of Organic Chemistry Laboratory LR17ES08

Publications from the Last 3 Years:

[1] Amira yahyaoui, Ghayth Rigane, Sami Mnif, Ridha Ben Salem, Ayşenur Acar, Derya Arslan. Ultrasound Technology Parameters: Effects on Phenolics in Olive Paste and Oil in Relation to Enzymatic Activity. *European Journal of Lipid Science and Technology*, 2019, 121 (5), DOI: 10.1002/ejlt.201800295.

[2] Moufida A. Oueslati, Aynur Gunenc, Ghayth Rigane, Hanen Ghazghazi, Caroline Valencia, Ridha Ben Salem, SadokBoukhchina, Williamn G. Willmore and Farah Hosseinian. LC-MS AND ESI-MS QTOF-MS analysis of glycerophospholipid and triacylglycerol species in developing wild artichoke achenes. *Revue Roumaine de Chimie,* 2019, 64 (8), 733-742.

[3] Sondes Fkiri, Hanene Ghazghazi, Ghayth Rigane, Ridha Ben Salem, Faten Mezni, Abdelhamid Khaldi, M. Larbi Khouja and Zouhair Nasr. Chemical compositions and biological activities essential oil from the needles of north african *pinus pinaster* var. *Revue Roumaine de Chimie,* 2019, 64 (6), 511-517.

[4] Moufida A. Oueslati, Aynur Gunenc, Ghayth Rigane, Hanen Ghazghazi, Caroline Valencia, Ridha Ben Salem, Sadok Boukhchina, Williamn G. Willmore and Farah Hosseinian.Chemical composition, antioxidant and cytotoxic activities of onopordum acanthium L. crude oil and defatted meal. *Revue Roumaine de Chimie*, 2019, 64 (6), 503-510.

[5] Amira Yahyaoui, Moufida Oueslati Arfaoui, Ghayth Rigane, Achref Hkir, Kawther Amari, Ridha Ben Salem, Youssef Ammar. Investigation on the Chemical composition and antioxidant capacity of extracts from Crataegus azarolus L.: Effect of growing location of an important Tunisian medicinal plant. *Chemistry Africa*, 2019, 2, 361-365.

[6] Amira Yahyaoui, Olfa Khedher, Ghayth Rigane, Ridha Ben Salem and Younes Moussaoui. Chemical analysis of essential oil from *Echinops Spinosus* L. roots: antimicrobial and antioxydant activities. *Revue Roumaine de Chimie*, 2018, 63 (3), 199-204.

[7] Ghayth Rigane, Sami Mnif and Ridha Ben Salem. One step purification of 6-shogaol from *zingiber officinale* rosco, a phenolic compound having a high effectiveness against bacterial strains. *Revue Roumaine de Chimie*, 2018, 63 (1), 5-10.

[8] Amira Yahyaoui, Ghayth Rigane and Ridha Ben Salem. Oxidative stability of extra virgin olive oil with natural plant extracts during

microwave heating. *Asian Journal of Chemistry*, 2017, 29 (12), 2655-2659.

[9] Ghayth Rigane, Moufida Oueslati Arfaoui, Moemen Chira, Hanene Ghazghazi, Amira Yahyaoui, Ridha Ben Salem,Sabiha Hamdi, Malek Hannachi, Hager Jouili and Youssef Ammari. Chemical compositions, antioxidantand antimicrobial activities of the essential oilof *Trachyspermum ammi* L. growing in Tunisia. *Revue Roumaine de Chimie*, 2016, 61(10), 807 - 813.

[10] Ghayth Rigane, Hanene Ghazghazi, Chedia Aouadhi, Ridha Ben Salem, Zouheir Nasr. Phenolic content, antioxidant capacity and antimicrobial activity of leaf extracts from *Pistacia atlantica. Natural Product research,* 2016, 6, 696-699.

[11] Mhamdi Layla, Khemais Said, Ghayth Rigane, Ridha Ben Salem, Younes Moussaoui. Ultrasonic activation of Nozaki-Hiyama-Kichi reaction in the presence of phase transfer catalysis. *Journal of the Tunisian Chemical Society,* 2016, 18, 61-67.

[12] Moufida Oueslati Arfaoui, Ghayth Rigane, Hanen Ghazghazi, Ridha Ben Salem, Hamdi, S., Hannachi, M., Jouili, H., L'ammari, Y. Phenolic content, antioxidant and antimicrobial activitics of *Trachyspermumammi* aerial parts growing wild in the north of Tunisia. *Journal of New Sciences*, 2016, 25(4), 1151-1160.

In: What to Know about Essential Oils
Editor: Malene M. Kjeldsen
ISBN: 978-1-53617-986-6

Chapter 8

THE ROLE OF CHARACTERISED MOST ABUNDANT COMPOUNDS ON IMPACT NOTES IN ESSENTIAL OIL RESEARCH WITH BIOACTIVITY ASPECTS

Dorcas Olufunke Moronkola**, Emmanuel Onah Ojah, Clement Odunayo Ajiboye, Oluwafunmilola Elizabeth Akinpelu and Olusegun Ekundayo

Department of Chemistry, University of Ibadan, Ibadan, Nigeria

Abstract

We are giving a critical overview of the diverse roles of the most abundant compounds in essential oil (EO) samples as determinants of important features such as the influence of impact notes and biological activities displayed. It calls for genuine and reproducible characterisation of such dominant compounds. Essential oils (EOs) are complex odoriferous compounds, which are distillable exudates in natural products. Their ubiquitous content includes mono-terpenes, sesqui-terpenes and their oxygenated derivatives with varied functional groups such as esters, alcohols, ketones, carboxylic acids, and aromatic derivatives. Essential oils obtained from different parts (leaves, stem and stem bark, root and root bark, fruits parts, etc.) of the same plant do vary uniquely and significantly. They are important in medicine, perfumery, and flavouring which

*Corresponding Author's Email: funkemoronkola@gmail.com; do.moronkola@ui.edu.ng.

are commercially utilized in pharmaceutical, cosmetics, paints, petroleum and food industries as inhalants, germicides, stimulants, antiseptics, perfumes, toiletries, additives, preservatives and artificial flavours in foods and drinks. Characterised components have been reported to exhibit a broad spectrum of bioactivities such as larvicidal, anti-inflammatory and antimicrobial relevant for several therapeutic interventions. The values and importance of essential oils depend mainly on the type and quantity of impact compounds it contains. The dominance of some compounds in the essential oils has a great influence on the characteristics including bioactivity exhibited by the plant. They determine the nature of the EO and are usually responsible for impacting the characteristic notes of each EO sample. On the suitability of EOs, their most abundant compounds have characteristic impact notes, which are utilized on finished products industrially and for commercial purposes. There are earlier reports on dominant compounds in essential oils such as Limonene for the cashew fruity odour and β-caryophyllene for Hog plum fruity odour. Fragrances perceived and aroma exhibited by such abundant compounds play major roles in acceptability, accessibility (judging) and bioactivities expressed by the EOs. Most abundant compounds in EOs are important and reliable in chemotaxonomic studies of plants. Some of these we will be examining.

Keywords: essential oil, impact compound, notes, bioactivity, spectroscopic analyses

1. Essential Oils

1.1. Definition of Essential Oil

Essential oil (EO) is a natural product and concentrated liquid that is hydrophobic in nature containing volatile chemical compounds extracted from different parts of plants including the fruits, peels, flowers, leaves, rhizomes, wood, stem, stem bark and root especially from potentially beneficial plants [1]. EOs are insoluble in water but volatile with steam, rapidly evaporating at different rates of atmospheric pressure and room temperature. They are liquid mixtures of organic compounds that are considered necessary constituents of the plant, hence its Latin word esentia meaning the characteristic or the most important component of the natural substances. They are also referred to as ethereal oils which are suspensions and distillable exudates. EOs have pronounced odours, which could be detected even at low concentrations in air, though each of the volatile compounds has a varied range of sensory detection threshold [2],[3].

It occurs in extremely small amount in comparison with other compounds of the plants such as its water content [2]; it consists of odoriferous compounds which are responsible for the aroma and flavour of the various parts of a plant with its characteristic odour and taste depending on the plant from which it is derived [3]. The compositions of each essential oil differ, which is its characteristic feature and focus of its study.

The quality and quantity of essential oils depend mainly on genetic factors, drying method, botanical origin, harvesting season and geographical location [2], [4][9]. Essential oils can be made of a varied number of compounds ranging from one, though rare, to many. Cinnamaldehyde is the main compound in cassia essential [10] and methyl salicylate in wintergreen [11]. There are 140 compounds in Curuba (Passiflora mollissima) fruit pulp [12].

1.2. Classification of Essential Oil

Essential oils can be classified into the following four categories: terpenoids, phenylpropanoids, open-chain aliphatics, cyclic and hetero atoms [13], [14]:

1.2.1. Terpenes

Terpenes are primary constituents of essential oils, derived from isoprene (2-methyl-1,3-butadiene) units, which are formed from acetic acid and mevalonic acid; they are joined in head to tail fashions to form chains or rings. This is called isoprene rule [15]. Isoprene units are the building blocks of all terpenoids. Monoterpenes, sesquiterpenes and few diterpenes are ubiquitous EO compounds, which are usually responsible for its characteristic impact notes. Their oxygen-containing derivatives are known as terpenoids, although some literature uses terpenoids or isoprenoids.

Examples include pinenes found in pinewood and cannabis, it is a known anti-cancer agent and used for prevention of infections; myrcene a monoterpene in the bay, citrus fruits, cannabis, and lemongrass is known to treat peptic ulcer, insomnia and as pain-reliever. It is also utilised in perfumery [16], [17]. Limonene in limes, lemons, and oranges have antibacterial and antifungal activities; humulene which is in tobacco, hops and orange orchards is used in prevention of weight loss, as anti-inflammatory and anti-bacterial agent; camphene in turpentine, ginger, and camphor oil are known for reducing plasma cholesterol; linalool from rosewood and lavender is used to boost immunity, vitamin E formation, treatment of lung inflammation and often utilised as insecticides; caryophyllene from cloves, cinnamon, and black pepper treats arthritis, cancer, chronic and neuropathic pain.

1.2.2. Phenylpropanoids

Phenylpropanoids are benzene derivatives synthesized from amino acids phenylalanine and tyrosine [18]. Caffeic acid (in coffee), an anti-inflammatory and antioxidant agent; eugenol (in nutmeg, cloves, cinnamon, and wormwood) is a known anti-inflammatory, antioxidant and cardiovascular agent.

1.2.3. Open Chain Aliphatics

Open chain aliphatics are straight, or branch chain compounds. Examples are citral isolated from lemongrass which has perfumery and antimicrobial properties; geraniol found in rose, citronella, and lemongrass is known for antimicrobial, anti-inflammatory and antiseptic properties.

1.2.4. Cyclics and Heteroatoms

Essential oils can also be classified based on the presence of cyclic and heteroatom. For example borneol, a constituent of camphor, lavender, and rosemary relieves pain, treats coughs, colds, and bronchitis; carvacrol found in oregano and thyme cures cold and has antimicrobial activities.

1.3. Benefits of Essential Oil to Plant

The benefits of essential oils made them to be called the chemical weapons of the plant world because of the abilities of their chemical constituents to scare away insects or protect the plant against microbial attacks. They also act as plant pheromones to attract or seduce their pollinators. Likewise, their oxygenated molecules can serve as chemical messengers to the cells bringing life to plants, aiding growth, destroying infestation and stimulating healings [19].

2. Isolation and Extractions

2.1. Introduction

Extractions are methods utilized in obtaining a plants bioactive constituents that function as its life force. They are essentially the liquefied version of a plant and are produced when a botanical material is introduced to a solvent in which components of the plant material dissolve in. Likewise, their oxygenated molecules can serve as chemical messengers to the cells bringing life to plants, aiding growth, destroying infestation and stimulating healings [19]. The solution obtained at the end of the process is usually liquid, however, the liquid can be concentrated by removing the solvent to obtain the resultant solid extract. The solvents consequently act as preservatives or agents that aid plant cells to break down releasing their contents (compounds) into it [20]. The extraction method is one of the factors that determine the quality and quantity of essential oil extracted. Inappropriate extraction procedure can lead to total alteration of the chemical signature of essential oil, as well as artifact formation, resulting in a rapid change in bioactivity and natural characteristic features of the oils, hence rendering results of such studies unreliable [21], [22].

2.2. Methods of Extraction of Essential Oil

The extraction of essential oils from plant material can be achieved by various methods, of which hydro-distillation and steam distillation are the most common method of extraction [23][25]. Other methods include solvent extraction, aqueous infusion, cold or hot pressing, effleurage, supercritical fluid extraction and phytonic process [25][28]. The later process is newly developed, which uses refrigerant hydrofluorocarbon solvents at low temperatures (below room temperature), resulting in good quality of the extracted oils. Thus, the chemical composition of the oil, both quantitative and qualitative, may be influenced by the extraction techniques. For example, hydro-distillation and steam distillation methods yield oils rich in terpene hydrocarbons. While the super-critical extracted oils contained a higher percentage of oxygenated compounds [29][33].

2.2.1. Hydrodistillation

Hydrodistillation has become the standard method of essential oil extraction from plant materials and it is often used to isolate non-water-soluble natural products ranging from low to high boiling points. The process involves the complete immersion of macerated plant materials in water, with subsequent boiling at sufficiently elevated temperatures. This method protects the oil extracted since the surrounding water acts as a barrier to prevent it from overheating. The steam and essential oil vapours are condensed to an aqueous fraction at sufficiently low temperature under ice conditions. The main advantage of this method is that the required materials can be distilled at a considerably low temperature thereby preventing their loss and undesired chemical modifications. Okoh et al., 2010, studied different extraction processes on yield and properties of essential oils from rosemary (*Rosemarinus officinals* L.) by hydrodistillation and solvent-free microwave extraction (SFME). The total yield of the volatile fractions obtained through hydro-distillation and solvent-free microwave extraction was 0.31% and 0.39% respectively. Hydro-distilled oil contained more monoterpenes (28.6%)[34].

Delicate flowers such as roses and orange blossoms would clump together when introduced to steam in the distillation process, hence the most effective alternative method of extraction in this situation is to submerge the fragile plant material in pure boiling water (hydro-distillation). The condensed liquids in iced conditions cool down and separate from each other. The residual water, which contains some of the fragrance is referred to by several names including hydrolate, hydrosol, herbal water, essential water, floral water, or herbal distillate, which can also be utilized for other applications [35].

2.2.2. Expression

This method is accomplished either by sponge method, scarification, rasping or by a mechanical process. In the sponge method, the washed plant e.g. citrus (orange, lemon, grapefruit, etc.) is cut into halves to remove the juice completely, and turned inside out by hand, squeezed when the secretary gland rupture. The oozed volatile oil is collected by means of the sponge and subsequently squeezed in a vessel. Oil floating on the surface is carefully separated. For the rasping process, the outer surface of the peel of citrus fruits containing the oil gland is skillfully removed by a grater. The rasping is placed in horsehair bags and pressed strongly so as to ooze out the oil stored in the oil glands. Initially, the liquid has a turbid appearance but on allowing it to stand the oil separates out which may be decanted and filtered subsequently. For the scarification process, the apparatus Eucelle a Piquer (a larger bowl meant for pricking

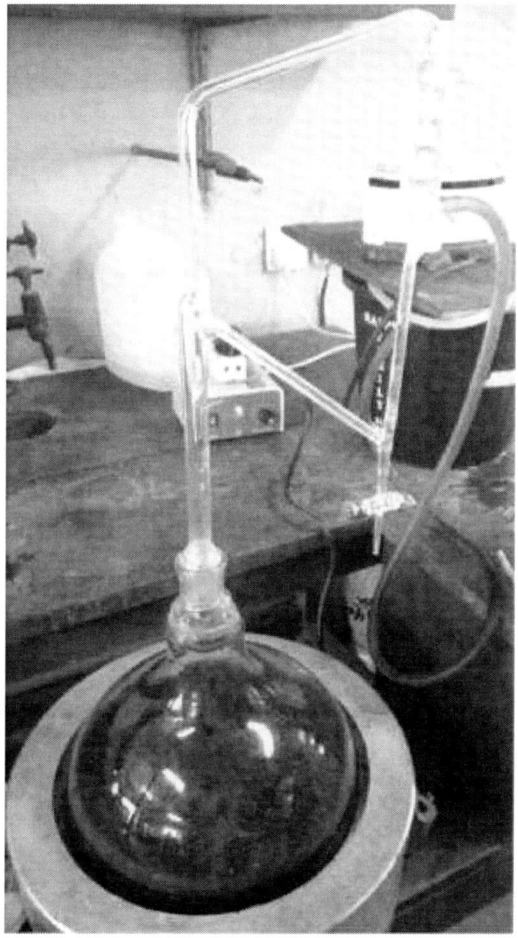

Figure 1. Hydrodistillation set up (Adapted Clevenger type).

the outer surface of citrus fruits) is used, the freshly washed lemons are placed in the bowl and rotated repeatedly when the oil glands are punctured thereby discharging the oil right into the handle. The liquid is then transferred to another vessel, where on keeping the clear oil may be decanted and filtered. The mechanical process involves the use of heavy-duty centrifugal devices so as to ease the separation of oil with water emulsions invariably formed. The advent of modern mechanical devices has impressively increased oil output. [36].

2.2.3. Effleurage

Effleurage is one of the oldest methods used for the extraction of essential oils. It is however rarely used today, probably because of its high cost. The effleurage process can be done either hot or cold. In both instances, the fat that is saturated with fragrance is called "effleurage pomade. The basic principles for both processes are explained below:

Cold Effleurage

1. Highly purified and odourless vegetable or animal fat, usually lard or tallow, is spread out over glass plates in a frame called a chassis and is allowed to set.

2. Fresh flower petals or fresh whole flowers are then placed on top of the layer of fat and pressed in. They are allowed to set for 1-3 days or for a couple of weeks depending on the flowers that are used. During this time, their scent seeps into the fat.

3. The depleted petals are replaced and the process is repeated until the fat reaches the desired saturation.

4. The final product is the effleurage pomade, which is the fat and the fragrant oil. This is washed with alcohol to separate the botanical extract from the remaining fat, hence utilized in soap making. When the alcohol evaporates from this mixture, the absolute is what is leftover.

Hot Effleurage

The main difference in this process is that the fats are heated. Despite the introduction of the modern process of extraction with volatile solvents, the old-fashioned method effleurage still plays an all-important role. Its principles are simple. Fat possesses a high power of absorption and when brought in contact with fragrant plant materials. This principle, methodically applied on a large scale, constitute eight to ten weeks, batches of freshly picked flowers are strewn over the surface of a specially prepared fat base (corps), left there and then replaced by fresh flowers. At the end of the harvest, the fat, which is not renewed during the process, is saturated with flower oil. Thereafter, the oil is extracted from the fat with alcohol and then isolated. The success of effleurage depends on a great extent upon the quality of the fat base employed. [20]

2.2.4. Solvent Extraction

Conventionally, solvent extraction has been implemented for plant materials that yield low amounts of essential oil, that are largely resinous, or that is delicate aromatics unable to withstand the pressure and distress of steam distillation. This method also produces a better fragrance than any type of distillation method. The extraction process can be carried out with volatile solvents (e.g. hexane and ethanol) resulting in the production of floral concretes-oils with solid consistency and partly soluble in non-volatile solvents, which results in the production of perfumes [37]. Usually, the solvent is mixed with plant materials and then heated to extract the essential oil, followed by filtration. Subsequently, the filtrate is concentrated by solvent evaporation. The concentrate is resin or concrete (a concentration of wax, fragrance and essential oil). From the concentrate, it is then mixed with pure alcohol to extract the oil and distilled at low temperatures. The alcohol absorbs the fragrance and when the alcohol is evaporated, the aromatic absolute oil remains. The solvent extraction method of extracting essential oil is dominated by perfume industries; used in shampoo, bath oils, toothpaste, fly sprays, and air fresheners. However, this method is a relatively time-consuming process, thus making the oils derived by this method more expensive than others.

2.2.5. Steam Distillation

Steam distillation is a separation process for temperature-sensitive materials like oils, resins, hydrocarbons, etc. which are insoluble in water. The fundamental nature of steam distillation is that it enables a compound or mixture of compounds to be distilled at a temperature substantially below that of the boiling point(s) of the individual constituent(s). Essential oils contain substances with boiling points ranging from low to high. In the presence of steam or boiling water, however, these substances are all volatilized. Fresh, or sometimes dried, the botanical material is placed in the plant chamber of the still and the steam is allowed to pass through the herb material under pressure which softens the cells and allows the essential oil to escape in vapour form, which is trapped under iced condition. The temperature of the steam must be high enough to vapourize the oil present, yet not so high that it destroys the plants or burns the essential oils [38], [39].

Steam distillation process involves the following:

1. A large container called a Still, which is usually made of stainless steel, containing the plant material has steam added to it.

2. Through an inlet, steam is injected through the plant material containing the desired oils, releasing the plants aromatic molecules and turning them into vapour.

3. The vaporized plant compounds travel to the condensation flask or the Condenser. Here, two separate pipes make it possible for hot water to exit and for cold water to enter the Condenser. This makes the vapour cool back into liquid form.

4. The aromatic liquid by-product drops from the Condenser and collects inside a receptacle underneath it, which is called a Separator. Because water and oil do not mix, the essential oil floats on top of the water. From here, it is siphoned off. (Some essential oils are heavier than water, such as clove essential oil, so they are found at the bottom of the Separator.)

The steam distillation process involves the following: Here essential oil vapours condense with the steam. Essential oil forms a film on the surface of the water. To separate the essential oil from the water, the film is then decanted or skimmed off the top. The remaining water, a by-product of distillation, is called floral water, distillate, or hydrosol. It retains many of the therapeutic properties of the plant, making it valuable in skincare for facial mists and toners (a solution containing chemicals that can change the colour of a photographic print). The advantage of Steam Distillation is that it is a relatively cheap process to operate at the basic level, also the properties of oils produced by this method are not altered. The steam involved in this method does not decompose the components of the EOs. This method apart from being economical is also relatively faster than other methods of obtaining EOs. Steam Distillation is the most popular method used to extract and isolate essential oils from plants in natural product studies [25], [27], [28].

2.2.6. CO_2 Extraction

Essential oils derived from the supercritical CO_2 extraction of herbs are similar to the oils produced through distillation in that they can be used in aromatherapy and natural perfumery. Oils derived from steam distillation vary in their qualities depending on the temperatures, pressures, and length of time applied for the process. The CO_2 extraction process might thus produce higher quality oils that have not been altered by the application of high heat.

The CO_2 extraction processes involve the following:

Pressurized carbon dioxide becomes liquid while remaining in a gaseous state, which means it is now "supercritical." In this state, it is pumped into a chamber filled with plant matter.

Because of the liquid properties of the gas, the CO_2 functions as a solvent on the natural plant matter, pulling the oils and other substances such as pigment and resin from the plant matter. The essential oil content then dissolves into the liquid CO_2.

The CO_2 is brought back to natural pressure and evaporates back into its gaseous state, while what is left is the resulting oil.

In CO_2 extraction, none of the constituents of the oil is damaged by heat. Thus, the difference between traditional distillation and supercritical extraction is that instead of heated water or steam, CO_2 is used as a solvent in the latter method. The supercritical extraction process operates at temperatures between 95 and 100 degrees F whereas steam distillation operates at temperatures between 140 and 212 degrees F. CO_2 extracts are usually thicker than their essential oil counterparts and often give off more of the aroma of the natural herb, spice, or plant than a distilled essential oil. CO_2 extracts have been said to contain more plant constituents than the amount extracted from the same plant using steam distillation. CO_2 is colourless, odourless and can be easily and completely removed by releasing the pressure in the extraction chamber. It is what we exhale and is needed by plants in order for them to thrive, which illustrates its harmlessness when employed in this extraction process. This absence of potentially harmful solvents in CO_2 extraction means neither the human body nor the environment is polluted [40]

2.2.7. Maceration

Macerated oils are also referred to as infused oils. They are created when carrier oils are used as solvents to extract therapeutic properties from plant material. Maceration process involves the following:

1. Plant material is finely cut, crushed, or ground into a moderately coarse powder.
2. Plant material is placed in a closed vessel.

3. Solvent is added.
4. The mixture is allowed to stand for 1 week and is shaken occasionally.
5. The liquid is strained.
6. Solid residue (Marc) is pressed to recover any remaining liquid.
7. Strained and expressed liquids are mixed.
8. Liquids are clarified through filtration or subsidence.

The benefit of macerated oil above distilled oil is that more of a plants essence is captured in the oil, because it captures heavier, larger plant molecules than the ones captured in the distillation process. This keeps the product closer to retaining more of the plants valuable offerings. The ideal plant material to be infused will be harvested so that it is as dry as possible, as any moisture will cause the oil to become rancid, thus encourage microbial growth. Adding 5% of Vitamin E oil or Wheatgerm oil (which is high in Vitamin E) will prevent rancidity. When the maceration process is complete, the base oil will likely have changed colour. The final maceration should be filtered off its plant material and poured into an airtight container to be stored in a cool, dry place. 5-10% of a macerated oil can be used as an active botanical in a cosmetic formula. Used in a larger quantity, it can also rcplace a plain base oil [22], [41], [42].

2.2.8. Cold-Press Extraction

This method is also called Expression or Scarification and is used for citrus peels in particular [41], [43].

1. Whole fruit is placed in a device that mechanically pierces it to rupture the essential oil sacs, which are located on the underside of the rind. Its essential oil and pigments run down into the devices collection area.
2. The whole fruit is pressed to squeeze out the juice and the oil.
3. Oil and juice that are produced still contain solids from the fruits, such as the peel and must be centrifuged to filter the solids from the liquids.
4. The oil separates from the juice layer and is siphoned off into another receptacle [41], [43].

3. Characterisations in Essential Oil Studies

3.1. Introduction

In essential oil studies, the active chemical compounds that have some medicinal applications must be identified. These compounds with many uses and high volatility require specialized analytical techniques for detailed characterisation in their identifications [43], [44].

Chromatography, especially gas chromatography (GC) and mass spectroscopy (MS) have been the most generally used analytical techniques for investigating the constituents of essential oils, which have proved reliable [44]. Other methods in sample preparation prior to injection have also been applied to improve characterisations in essential oil analyses. Such include Solid-Phase Matrix Extraction (SPME) [45], Headspace-GC [46] or coupling of analytical instruments to increase the separation power of one-dimensional techniques.

This section discusses some of the advancements in chromatography for essential oil analysis from gas chromatography to coupled techniques.

3.2. Essential Oil Analysis by Gas Chromatography

In GC analysis, essential oils are vaporised and then eluted through the column by the gas mobile phase, which are carrier gases such as He and H_2. Its constituents are separated based on their differential affinities for the stationary phase as well as their relative vapour pressure. This is a gradient elution method, where the separated constituents of the essential oil emerge from the outlet of the column with respect to time, which are detected and recorded in the form of a chromatogram. The chromatogram is a plotted signal against time where the peaks are a form of Gaussian distribution-curve shapes; its peak area and height indicate the amount of the compound present (% total ion concentration, TIC) with its width being a function of the band that is spread in the column. The retention time is characteristic of the solute (compound), the values obtained are utilised for detailed identification of the compound.

Capillary GC has strongly contributed to the advancement of the essential oil science from both academic research and industrial point of view (quality control, new sources for odoriferous compounds). Until the introduction of Golay columns and further improvement by Martin, which afforded higher sensitivity by suggesting a decrease in the diametre of the column, only metal columns packed with more or less inert support coated with a polar or non-polar liquid stationary phases were used in the early days [47].

Sample preparation, a significant stage in gas chromatography may include static headspace, SPME or direct thermal desorption. Headspace analysis is a powerful tool for solving problems such as detection of trace components, or for checking a wide variety of different materials [48]. The development of methods such as static headspace in GC, improves the sensitivity and allows the detection of lower concentration compounds. The improvements brought about by using SPME include the need for significantly less plant material, more rapid and reproducible sample preparation, less opportunity for the oxidation of volatiles to take place and no need for the use of organic solvents.

Another significant development of GC methods in essential oil analysis is the application of the GC-olfactometry (scent assessment) or GC-sniffing technique [49]. In the essential oil GC-sniffing method, the investigator writes notes on the GC chromatogram when the odour is perceived using his nose as a detector. In this way, he points out peaks and regions in the chromatogram where odours are detected. The method also has limitations because further work is required to identify the peaks for example by GC-MS.

Each of these developments has contributed a lot to improve the separation power of GC in terms of the number of peaks separated, as well as qualitative and quantitative information generated.

3.2.1. High-Speed Gas Chromatography

Instruments and techniques have been improved upon over the years to speed up capillary GC. A fast capillary should have an average peak width less than one second. It is a "super fast GC" when the average peak width is about 100 ms and "Ultra fast GC" when the peak width is less than 10 ms. Table 1 delineates the scopes of conditions for conventional, fast and ultra fast GC in terms of analysis time, heating rates, column length, internal diametre and peak width.

3.2.2. Fast Gas Chromatography in Essential Oils Analysis

The applicability of ultra-fast GC in essential oil investigation, when compared to conventional GC, is limited. A comparative study of ultra-fast GC with a resistively heated column and conventional GC with a decreased inner diametre column (0.25 mm) of various lengths (5 and 25 m long) was undertaken with

Table 1. Schematic representation of common requirements for reaching a high speed of analysis in GC [50]

Description	Heating rate (^{o}C/min)	Column length (m)	Column i.d. (μ m)	Analysis time (min)	Peak Width (s)
Ultra Fast	60 - 1200	5 2	100 - 50	$\sim$ 1	0.2 0.05
Fast	20-60	155	250 - 100	$\sim$ 10	5-0.5
Conventional	1-20	60-15	320 250	$\sim$ 30	105

different essential oils [48]. Essential oils studied were of different complexities (Chamomile, peppermint, rosemary, and sage). Comparable results of significant peaks expected in these oils were observed for both GC and ultra-fast GC techniques. Although ultra-fast GC has emerged as a powerful GC method to provide information in an extremely short time, the resolution is compromised by rapid heating and high flow rates in a short column. Because of the limited peak capacity in fast GC more of the peaks co-elute.

3.3. Multidimensional Chromatography

3.3.1. Concepts in Multidimensional Separation

Multidimensional chromatography is defined as the chromatographic procedure in which two or more analytical techniques are coupled together to improve their partition power [51]. The coupling can be either two chromatographic techniques or a chromatographic technique with spectroscopy.

The ultimate goal of chromatography has been to effectively separate sample mixtures with the largest number of compounds in the shortest time. The need to analyse samples of increasing complexity and at lower detection limits has placed more stringent requirements on the separating power required for analysis. A single chromatographic system is inadequate to handle very complex samples and attempts at analysing complex samples frequently lead to longer analysis times. The analysis of complex samples often requires the use of many separation mechanisms to minimise peak overlap and to obtain information on individual components [52].

Mass selective detectors that are capable of de-convoluting merged peaks have been utilised to aid the separating powers of single chromatographic systems and for the positive identification of compounds. However, selective detection is only successful when different responses are produced for the individual compounds represented by the merged peaks. An alternative solution appeared with the development of the special concept in separation science, known as Comprehensive Multidimensional Separations or Comprehensive Multidimensional Chromatography [53].

Two-Dimensional Liquid Chromatography (LCxLC)

Two-dimensional liquid chromatography was first demonstrated by Erni and Frei [54]. The framework involved a heart-cutting interface coupling the two liquid chromatographs, however, their data structure was not complete in nature. More enhancements were required for the system to meet the prerequisites of a comprehensive separation process. Their data structure being considered indicated correlation between the retention mechanisms of the two separations which lead to the inefficient generation of separation space that was not utilised. This ruled out its system data structure from being considered to be comprehensive.

Two-Dimensional Gas Chromatography (GCxGC)

A two-dimensional separation system, which met the comprehensive two-dimensional requirements, was first proposed by Guiochon and colleagues in the early 1980s [55]. Though the system had a few highlights of comprehensive multidimensional chromatography, more development of the system was needed. Liu and Phillips [56], pioneered the modern true GCxGC using an on-column thermal modulator interface to couple the two separation mechanisms. Fast sample transfer between columns was achieved using an on-column thermal modulator, which was an effective sample introduction device in fast GC.

Supercritical Fluid Chromatography and Gas Chromatography (SFCxGC)

The first comprehensive two-dimensional supercritical fluid chromatography and gas chromatography (SFCxGC) system were demonstrated by Lee and co-workers [57] using a thermal desorption modulator as the interface between the SFC and GC columns. The first dimension achieves molecular shape analysis

(SFC). This is followed in the second dimension by volatility analysis (GC). An integral flow restrictor was installed at the head of the GC column, and an on-column thermal desorption modulator was placed after the flow restrictor. Both columns of the SFC and GC were temperature programmed at the same rate and operated at the same temperature. CO_2 was the carrier gas in both dimensions.

SFCxGC with Independent Temperature Programming in the Second Dimension

A comprehensive two-dimensional supercritical fluid and independent temperature-programmed gas chromatography (SFCxGC) employs supercritical fluid chromatography to effect group type separation [58]. This is coupled on-line, through a modulating device, to a resistively heated, fast temperature-programmed gas chromatograph for volatility analysis. In SFCxGC, the arrangement of the separation mechanisms is the reverse of GCxGC [56], where volatility separation in the first dimension normally precedes polar separation in the second dimension.

This instrumentation was previously applied to the analysis of petrochemical samples [58]. The capabilities of the SFCxGC instrument to qualitatively differentiate oil samples of the same species but obtained in different geographical locations and distinguish two oils of the same species was an improvement shown by this method.

3.4. Coupled Techniques in Essential Oil Analysis

3.4.1. Gas Chromatography and Mass Spectrometry (GC-MS)

Gas chromatography-mass spectrometry (GC-MS) has probably been the best multidimensional method for the analysis and identification of essential oil components [59].

The GC works on the principle that the EOs will separate into individual compounds, after which the separated compounds are carried through the column with an inert gas such as He and H_2. Immediately separated compounds emerge from the column opening each fly into the mass spectrometer, MS. The MS identifies each compound by the charge to mass ratio of the positive ions, which is a plot referred to as a mass spectrum. The mass spectrum shows the characteristic fragmentation patterns, which afford direct information regarding chain length, degree of unsaturation, the position of branching, and nature and position of functional groups in the EO molecule.

The mass spectrometer may recognise overlaps from GC separations and apportion relative amounts to overlapping components. The availability of the accurate mass (high-resolution) MS is a valuable tool for confirmation of the molecular formula of detected unknown components [60]. Varieties of monoterpenes in essential oils, with similar or close spectra demands we know its accurate retention times for their identifications [61].

One of the newer methods that have been proposed to give an improved investigation of complex mixtures, especially for the deconvolution of overlapping GC peaks, is known as time-of-flight mass spectrometry coupled to fast GC (GC-TOF-MS) [62]. TOF-MS has the capability of generating instantaneous spectra. Due to this fact, there is no bias occurring from the mismatch between scan rates and the peak abundance changes in the ion source (mass spectral skewing). Unlike quadrupole mass spectrometers, TOF mass spectrometers provide uniform mass spectra across GC peaks, even for the narrow ones found in fast GC [61]. Recently, better separations of essential oils were accounted for with GC-TOF-MS [62], [63]. In TOF-MS fast spectral acquisition capabilities of 100+ mass spectra/second that are compatible with fast GC peaks have as of late pulled in a lot of consideration from specialists and routine research facilities [61].

3.5. Multidimensional GC and GCxGC

The application of multidimensional gas chromatography (MDGC) to essential oil analysis has been one of the most effective adopted technologies as a result of the improved resolving power the technique can offer when investigating complex mixtures. By effecting a heart-cut event of the analyte on a chosen region of a chromatogram (from the 1st dimension), the desired components are transferred into a second, more selective column, where components are better resolved. MDGC is focused on certain inadequately separated regions and provides increased resolution [51]. Quantitation or identification of components is significantly improved using this method. This may be important for essential oils and specific components whose relative abundance may be required to study a specific aspect of the sample quality, history, source, and biogenesis.

In spite of the fact that MDGC offers better separation, a significant part of the data is lost since it heart-cuts just chosen portions of the effluent from the first column. A portion of the MDGC applications to explicit parts for scent examination, for example, investigation of enantiomeric constituents of cold-squeezed and distilled fruits, have been reported [64], [65].

The recently described technique of comprehensive two-dimensional gas chromatography (GCxGC) [56] addresses a number of shortcomings of conventional MDGC when analysing very complex samples such as essential oils. So far there have been only a few reports of GCxGC application to essential oils analysis compared to MDGC. Marriott and co-workers [66] used GCxGC to characterise and compare the tea tree and lavender oils. A coupled column combination of non-polar (5% phenyl equivalent) and polyethylene glycol phase columns were used to attain the desired resolution. Dimandja and co-workers [67] reported work on the qualitative analysis of essential oils of peppermint (Mentha piperita) and spearmint (Mentha spicata) oils using GCxGC. High-resolution GC-MS and linear retention indices (LRI) results for the lavender oil samples were compared with GCxGC results and many compounds could be identified, even without MS [68].

The task of enantioselective analysis of essential oils is very challenging. The analysis of enantiomeric compositions of a number of monoterpene hydrocarbons and oxygenated monoterpenes in the Australian tea tree (Malaleuca alternifolia) by GCxGC was reported [66]. GCxGC as a new technique has a promising future in the analysis of essential oils and the enantiomeric arrangement of the oils.

3.6. High Performance Liquid and Gas Chromatography (HPLC-GC)

HPLC-GC (where the HPLC is coupled on-line to a GC) has been perceived as a separation technique providing a great deal of information in a single run. A compiled review of coupled HPLC-GC in food and essential oil analysis is accessible [69]. The HPLC step achieves isolation of components of similar chemical groups, primarily based on their polarity and as a result, oxygenates will be separated from the saturated and unsaturated/aromatic hydrocarbons.

Numerous papers report the application of HPLC-GC-MS to bergamot oil [70], the analysis of a wide range of oils [71] and also for chiral analysis [72]. Better results were obtained for the essential oils due to the efficient separation and reduced interference from overlapping peaks in the final GC. HPLC is a powerful technique that may be employed to obtain group separation; however, its interface to GC is hampered by problems normally associated with the removal of large volumes of HPLC eluent when introduced into the GC injection port.

3.7. Supercritical Fluid and Gas Chromatography (SFC-GC)

SFC is a separation technique that is often a compromise between GC and HPLC. SFC combines the group separation capabilities of HPLC with easy quantitation through the use of CO_2 mobile phase that is compatible with the universal flame ionisation GC detector. Yamauchi and Saito [73] used semi-preparative scale packed-column SFC to separate lemon-peel oil into different chemical classes.

An SFC/GC system was used for the group-type analysis of citrus essential oil [74]. The lemon-peel oil was fractionated on a silica-gel column into several compound types, namely, hydrocarbons, alcohols, aldehydes, esters and others using a stepwise pressure gradient and modifier added to the pure CO_2. The eluted groups from SFC were re-injected into a GC for further separation of individual compounds.

3.8. Identification of Essential Oil Components

GC is often coupled to a downstream analytical step, for example, MS, which quantifies and identifies those compounds based on their retention indices (determined with reference to a homologous series of n-alkanes), and by estimating mass-to-charge ratio in an ionized sample, thereby providing a molecular fingerprint that can be cross-referenced against mass spectral databases with standards for thousands of known compounds. Open-source databases include traditional reference tools operated by NIST National Institute for Standards and Technology (NIST) 2005database/Chemstation data system. Wiley GC-MS Library, Adams Library (Adams 2007), Mass Finder 3.1 Library [75], [76], in-house Baser Library of Essential Oil Constituents built up from genuine compounds and components of known oils, Mass Bank and next-generation collaborative libraries such as mzCloud. The complexity of data generated by GC-MS often requires another layer of deconvolution via interpretive software such as AMDIS, also provided by NIST.

4. Impact Notes of Abundant Compounds

4.1. Introduction

Essential oil aromas have the potential to enhance the mind, body, and atmosphere. While it can be confusing to make a selection when faced with the vast number of Essential Oil options due to their limitless impact notes, it can be easier to make a choice by narrowing down the options based on the characteristics of their "aroma families." Each Essential Oil aroma family exhibits a primary aromatic trait by which it is easily recognized (citrusy, floral, fruity, minty, etc.) and a corresponding effect (calming, cooling, energizing, clarifying, etc.), which can help to readily identify the ideal application for it. This section highlights the core aroma families, as families also have offshoots or sub-groupings in which several categories of Essential Oils overlap. One example is the Balsamic aroma family. Essential Oils in this group can be described as having soft, sweet, warm, earthy aromas with spicy and floral undertones. They are reminiscent of resins and exude the scent of the forest and especially of Balsam trees. Inhaling the scent of balsamic essential oils can produce a peaceful and soothing effect. Another example of a complex aroma family is Coniferous oils, which exude a woody and earthy pine scent, as they are generally distilled from cone-bearing trees. Their scents are characterized as sharp, biting, camphoraceous, and energizing, reminiscent of fresh outdoor air. Based on these descriptions, Essential Oils in these sub-groupings can fall into several of the eight main aroma families. The sub-group of lemony oils, too, can encompass not only oils with Lemon in their names Lemongrass, Lemon Balm, Lemon Eucalyptus but also oils like Ginger, Citronella, and Palmarosa [24], [77], [78]. The aroma can change from one batch to another, often for reasons based in nature, such as the source botanicals growing conditions. Thus, due to the complexity and subjectivity of scent profiles, this article focuses on the commonly-accepted and widely-recognized classes of aromas or aroma families. [79]

4.2. Essential Oil Aroma Notes

Aroma families can also be distinguished by their primary notes. An Essential Oils aroma note is the feature that distinguishes how long its scent will last. Notes are categorised as Top, Middle, or Base notes. Some oils can have multiple notes, which can give them a deep, full-bodied, and seemingly luxurious quality; however, oils are largely characterised by a sole defining note that overrides the others.

The reason that an oil blend changes over time, sometimes even over a short period of time, such as from the morning to the afternoon is because the Essential Oils that it comprises each have varying degrees of volatility, meaning they all have diverse rates of evaporation and it is the evaporation of each oil in its own time that causes a fluctuation in the strength of the fragrance.

In an Essential Oil blend, the oils with the smallest molecules the essential oils that are the most volatile are the first to evaporate. These are the Top notes. They are the first scent to be detected and the first to dissipate [79].

The oils with the largest and thus the heaviest molecules are the slowest or last to evaporate, thus they impart the longer-lasting scents. These are Base notes. Other Essential Oils the majority reveal their scents gradually and help to integrate the Top and Base notes for a harmonious fragrance, which is what makes them Middle notes [79].

4.3. Some Abundant Compounds in Essential Oil Research

The following table (Table 2) shows abundant and dominant compounds in some stated essential oils:

4.4. Eight (8) Essential Oil Aroma Families

The chart below depicts the most popular groupings of Essential Oils; however, keep in mind that many oils have more than one prevailing aroma and note.

5. Bioactivity and Industrial Applications of Essential Oils

5.1. Introduction

EOs have received scientists attention over the years due to many pharmacological activities attributed to them. Healing or soothing effects (aromatherapy) of EOs obtained from various parts are in varying degrees from plant to plant with inter and intra relationships across the family group. The biological activities of EOs largely depend on the major constituents of the oils and at the time the synergetic effects of the constituents in a particular EO.

Table 2. Some abundant compounds in essential oil research

S/N	Abundant Compound (% abundance)	Plant/Part	Reference
1	lauric and myristic acids (34%)	*Psidium guajava* L Fruits	[80]
2	α -farnesene (21.3%)	*Terminalia catappa* Fruits	[81]
3	dodecanoic acid (20.4%)	*Irvingia gabonensis* Fruits	[82]
4	β-caryophylene (19.99%)	*Spondias mombin* L. Leaf	[83]
	β -caryophylene	*Spondias mombin* L. Fruit	
5	α-pinene (34%)	*C. albidum* Root	[84]
6	α-pinene (32.9%)	*Tithonia diversifolia* Leaf	[85]
	Germacrene D (20.3%)	*Tithonia diversifolia* Flower	
7	limonene (85.9%)	*Anacardium occiden-tale* Leaf	[85]
8	(Z)-3-hexylnol (17.9%)	*Gmelina arborea* Roxb Fruit	[86]
9	Limonene (42.9%)	*Pinus Caribaea* Morelet Needle	[87]
10	(Z)-3-hexylnol (34.7%)	*Momordica charantia* L. Aerial shrubs	[88]
11	Linalool (36.4%)	*Phyllanthus Amarus* Aerial shrubs	[88]

Essential oils are widely used as components of drugs, biologically active additives, and dietary supplements. It is widely used in aromatherapy, food industry, and cosmetics. They have different applications locally, industrially and in religious settings. It is useful in pharmaceutical products, food, insecticides, perfumery, flavour, rituals and alternative medicine [90] and these applications depend on their chemical constituents. Impact compounds determine the characteristics and activities of the oil, although major and minor constituents of essential oils modify these activities to give significant synergistic or antagonistic effect [91].

Small sizes of molecules of essential oils allow them to easily penetrate

Table 3. Impact notes in essential oils

NOTES & CHARACTERISTICS	OILS IN THIS CATEGORY
Top This is the initial perceptible scent in an aroma blend and is usually the one fragrance that stands out to give the scent its distinctive essence. Despite the powerful and intense quality that makes it the first detected smell, it is also the first to quickly fade. Top notes can be classified as: Bright Refreshing Cheery Clarifying Inspiring and heartening Energizing	Bay Cardamom Citrus oils Cypress Eucalyptus Hyssop Mint oils Petitgrain Pine Ravensara Rosemary Sage Tagetes Vanilla Oleoresin (10 Fold) Yarrow
Middle These notes become noticeable just as Top notes fade. Smooth and soft, Middle notes unify the Top and Base notes, helping to reduce the intensity of any disagreeable or piercing scents and to promote roundedness to aromas, making them softer. These notes are generally more enduring than Top notes, lasting up to an hour after the blend has been applied. We can classify their effect as Balancing Warming Grounding	Black Pepper, Cajeput Cedarwood, Chamomile Cinnamon, Clove Bud Geranium, Ho Wood Jasmine, Juniper Berry Marjoram, Myrtle Myrrh, Niaouli Nutmeg, Palmarosa Rose Absolute
Base Not to be mistaken for a Base Oil, which is meant to dilute an Essential Oil, a Base note emerges after the Heart note and is the longest-lasting scent in a blend. Base notes often have strong, provocative aromas with earthy nuances and ascend gradually, remaining for a longer time than the other notes, all the while helping to reduce the rate of the other oils evaporation and subsequently enabling the fragrance of the blend to persist. Calming Emotionally grounding and soothing Relaxing Lend a richer aroma to blends	Copaiba Balsam Frankincense Patchouli (Light & Organic) Sandalwood Spikenard Valerian Vetiver

through cell walls and affect various biochemical processes. The biological activity of essential oils depends on their composition. Essential oils that contain substituted phenols (eugenol, thymol, carvacrol, and guaiacol) exhibit strong antibacterial and antioxidant effects. The eucalyptus has been known for hundreds

Table 4. Eight aroma families

AROMA FAMILY	ESSENTIAL OILS	NOTE	REPUTED BENEFITS
CITRUS These light oils often have fruity scents that are characteristic of the rinds from which they are extracted. They can be described as tangy or tart, fresh, clean, vibrant, invigorating, exciting, energizing, and uplifting.	Lemon Orange Grapefruit Bergamot Lime Tangerine Citronella Lemongrass Mandarin Litsea Cubeba Tagetes	Most often top notes	Energizing Uplifting Emotionally balancing to reduce feelings of stress and anxiety Deodorizing Cleansing; popular addition to antibacterial oil blends Refreshing Stimulating for mental and spiritual vigor
FLORAL These scents are often reminiscent of the flowers from which they are extracted and can be described as being feminine, powdery, subtle, modest, romantic, and even poetic. They are often sweet-smelling and create a feeling of cheerfulness. Floral scents are considered to be classic and timeless	Chamomile Geranium Jasmine Lavender Neroli Rose Rosewood Ylang-Ylang Petitgrain	Most often middle notes	Comforting Promotes rest Sometimes sleep-inducing Mood balancing
HERBACEOUS Essential Oils, that have herbaceous scents can be further described as smelling green or grassy. These Essential Oils often have mild floral yet invigorating spring-like scents that are associated with lush, wet foliage. They are reminiscent of the aroma of fresh leaves, moss, mown grass, herbs, and trees.	Chamomile Angelica Root Clary Sage Eucalyptus Radiata Fennel Hyssop, Marjoram Melissa, Rosemary Thyme, Oregano Bay Laurel, Catnip Sage Dalmatian, Parsley Tea Tree, Yarrow	Most often middle notes	Calming Promotes positivity Encouraging Emotionally balancing Grounding

of years as antibacterial, fungicidal and antiseptic in nature. The essential oil from Eucalyptus species is among the worlds top traded oils. Also, Eucalyptus oil ranks superior in quality and has advantages over essential oil from others, since it has multipurpose uses in perfumery, pharmaceutical, and other indus-

Table 4. (Continued)

CAMPHORACEOUS These Essential Oils have strong scents and are known to be beneficial for clearing the respiratory system due to their clarifying, penetrating, energizing, purifying, and almost medicinal aromas.	Camphor Cajeput Eucalyptus Pennyroyal Laurel Leaf Lavandin	Most often middle notes	Stimulating Refreshing Focus-enhancing
MINTY Essential Oils with a minty scent are strong-scented and are distinctly known for their bracing, fresh fragrances. They are reputed to be clearing and cooling when used in aromatherapy and topical applications.	Spearmint Wintergreen Peppermint	Can be top, middle, or base Notes	Motivating Cooling Invigorating Mentally clarifying
SPICY These Essential Oils have exotic, warm, intense aromas that are often reminiscent of baking and other warm memories. With strong scents, they are commonly used to stimulate energy and focus.	Aniseed Basil Black Pepper Cardamom Cinnamon Coriander Cumin Ginger Nutmeg Allspice Cassia Clove Bud	Middle or base notes	Bracing Rousing Crisp and penetrating Lively
RESINOUS/MUSKY These Essential Oils exude deep, rich scents that are smoky, woody, earthy, sweet, leather-like, and warm. Their mellow, alluring, and long-lasting fragrances lend a reassuring quality that makes them ideal for use in spiritual practices.	Benzoin Elemi Frankincense Myrrh Peru Balsam	Middle or base notes	Grounding Promotes relaxation and a sense of inner calm Emotionally balancing Uplifting Known to be commonly used for intimacy enhancement Tend to be associated with a casual feeling

Table 4. (Continued)

WOODY/EARTHY These Essential Oils have deep, warm, lingering scents. Often described as smelling brown, these oils are reminiscent of the scents of a forest floor or damp soil. Their fragrances are soft, masculine, musky, and sensual. Their alluring, seductive, and hypnotic qualities create an atmosphere of mystery.	Cypress Juniper Berry Pine Sandalwood Fir Cedarwood (Atlas & Virginian) Palo Santo Rosewood Patchouli Vetiver Valerian Carrot Seed	Most often middle or base notes	Grounding Uplifting Emotionally balancing Promote feelings of comfort, security, and well-being Often considered being aphrodisiacs

tries. The oil has therapeutic, perfumery, flavoring, antimicrobial and biopesticide properties. Lavender oil has been used as a healing agent for burns for half a century, and it has been appreciated as an antiseptic. Lavender essential oil is one of the most appreciated oils in the perfume and soap industry. EOs have equally been reported to increase leather resistance to the actions of bacteria [92].

5.2. Bioactivities Established in Essential Oils

Biological activities established in essential oils make it useful as chemopreventive, antioxidant, antibacterial, antifungal, antiviral, anticancer and antimutagenic agents [93][96]. Essential oils of various sources have been reported to possess these activities.

5.2.1. Chemopreventive Activity of Essential Oil

A chemopreventive agent is a substance that intervenes in different stages of carcinogenesis by reduction of tumorigenesis. Chemopreventive activity which include antimutagenic activity using strains and known mutagens with and without microsomal activation and anticarcinogenic activity using topical application of 7, 12 dimethylbenz[a]anthracene (DMBA) as initiator and 1% croton oil as promoter for the induction of skin papillomas in mice was established in turmeric essential oil for example [97]. The major chemical constituent of turmeric essential oil is ar-turmerone (61%) which was reported to possess anticancer property [97], [98].

5.2.2. Antioxidant Activity of Essential Oil

Antioxidants are substances that inhibit oxidation or scavenge free radicals that can cause damage on the cells of organisms. There are different methods to establish antioxidant activity [99]. These are hydrogen atom transfer (HAT) and Electron Transfer methods (ET). HAT is lipid peroxidation inhibition capacity (LPIC), oxygen radical absorbance capacity (ORAC), scavenging of superoxide radical formation by alkaline (SASA), hydroxyl radical scavenging activity by p-NDA (p-butrisidunethyl aniline), total radical trapping antioxidant parameter (TRAP), ABTS radical scavenging, scavenging of H2O2 radicals, crocin bleaching nitric oxide radical inhibition activity and inhibited oxygen uptake (IOC) while ET is 2,2-diphenyl-1-picrylhydrazyl (DPPH) free radical scavenging, Trolox equivalent antioxidant capacity (TEAC) decolourization, N,N-dimethyl-p-phenylenediamine (DMPD), copper(II) reduction capacity, total phenols by Folin-Ciocalteu and ferric reducing antioxidant power (FRAP). For example, antioxidant activity of *Valeriana jatamansi* essential oil was established using DPPH radical scavenging and chelation power activity and the major constituents are are β-vatirenene (28.07%), β-patchoulene (20.18%), dehydroaromadendrene (15.92%), β-gurjunene (13.0%), patchoulic alcohol (11.72%), β-guaiene (5.88%), and α-muurolene (5.20%) (Sakshima et al., 2004). Likewise, antioxidant activity of *Blighia sapida* essential oils was established using DPPH radical-scavenging activity [100]. The dominating constituents of leaf, leaf stalk, stem bark, root, fruit pulp, fruit husk and fruit seed essential oils are butyl cyclobutyl phthalate (9.11%), pentadecanal (5.18%), (E)-1,10-dimethyl-trans-9-decalol(6.31%), 4,8,12,15,15-pentamethylbicyclo[9,3,1]pentadeca-3,7-den-12-ol (7.92%), tributyl-1-propene-1,2,3-tricarboxylate (12.69%), 4,8,12,15,15-penta methylbicyclo[9,3,1]pentadeca-3,7-den-12-ol (29.10%) and (Z)-vaccenic acid (14.24%) respectively. Farnesol (3.93%), a known antioxidant agent is present in stem bark [101].

5.2.3. Antimicrobial Activity of Essential Oil

Antimicrobial is the substance that stops the growth of microbes or kills the organism. It can be antibacterial, antifungal or antiviral. There are different methods to test for the antimicrobial activity [102] namely diffusion method which are antimicrobial gradient method (Etest), agar disk-diffusion method, cross streak method, agar well diffusion method, agar plug diffusion method and poisoned food method; thin-layer chromatography (TLC) bioautography which are agar diffusion, agar overlay bioassay and direct bioautography; dilution methods which are agar dilution and broth dilution method; time-kill test and ATP bioluminescence assay.

Antibacterial and anti-Candida albicans activity of aromatic plants of various chemical constituents were tested against Staphylococcus aureus, Enterococcus faecium, Salmonella cholerasuis and Candida albicans. The results showed inhibition of the essential oils against these organisms [103].

Another example is the antimicrobial activity of Blighia sapida essential oils that was established against Staphylococcus aureus, Escherichia coli, Bacillus subtilis, Pseudomonas aeruginosa, Klebsiella pneumoniae, Salmonella typhi, Candida albicans, Aspergillus niger, Rhizhopus stolonifer and Penicillium notatum [100]. The major constituents of *Blighia sapida* were reported as mentioned above and known antimicrobial agents were detected from this Blighia sapida, they are germacrene (0.48%) in fruit seed; (Z)-1,8(2H,5H)-hexahydro-8a-methyl-naphthalenedione (3.34%), farnesylacetate (0.65%), 1-Dodecanol (0.15%), geranylgeraniol (0.59%) from leaf; pentadecanal from leaf stalk (5.18%), stem bark (4.83%), fruit husk (0.41%) and fruit seed (0.15%); farnesol (3.93%) from stem bark and α -cardinal (2.01%) from root [101]

5.3. Some Industrial Influences of Essential Oils

Grandview research report in 2019 established on the basis of product, due to the increasing therapeutic application of essential oils for various disease conditions, consumables held the largest share of the aromatherapy market in 2018. These products possess tremendous healing properties in a natural way, thereby, making them a lucrative segment. For instance, Aura Cacia Lavender Harvest Essential Oil manufactured by Frontier Natural Products is a blended oil used for relaxation [104].

Consumables are divided into essential and carrier oils. Essential oils are sub-divided into singles and blends. For example, Evening Primrose is a carrier oil, manufactured by Edens Garden. It is used for skincare and treatment of cardiovascular diseases [104].

Diffusers are emerging products that are likely to pose huge growth opportunities. For instance, Bamboo Diffuser by Young Living Essential Oils used for relaxation is an innovative one. The introduction of novel and innovative diffusers is anticipated to propel their demand in the next couple of years [104].

Orange oil was the most significant and fastest-growing product segment, with a demand of 52.1 kilotons in 2018. Major end-use industries, such as cosmetics, are increasingly utilising orange essential oils to improve product value and sensory appeal. This oil is believed to firm up the skin, promote elasticity, and tone up the skin as well as treat acne, dermatitis, and stretch marks. They also contribute to improving the quality of hair, nails, and skin, boosting their appeal among women and female teenage consumers. Widening base of the working women population and rising disposable income are poised to supplement the growth of the segment during the forecast period [104].

The demand for lavender oil is also projected to witness a significant rise over the coming years owing to rising interest among the populace of developing countries in products of natural origin. Surging solvent demand in developed countries and an extensive range of end-users of the plant are also anticipated to spur the growth of the lavender oil segment [104].

Shifting preference of consumers in developed countries towards natural products manufactured through environmentally sustainable processes is stirring up the demand for lavender oil. In addition, rising consumption of premium products and upgraded standard of living of consumers, especially in developing countries, are creating ample growth opportunities for lavender oil manufacturers [104].

In 2018, spa and relaxation emerged as the largest application segment in terms of revenue for cedarwood essential oil. Cedarwood essential oil is of four types, namely Himalayan cedarwood (Cedrus deodora), Atlas cedarwood (Cedrus atlantica), Texas cedarwood (Juniperus mexicana), and Virginian cedarwood (Juniperus virginia). The most commonly used types are Himalayan and Atlas cedarwood oils. The personal care industry widely utilizes these oils for formulating haircare and skincare products [104].

REFERENCES

[1] Hyldgaard M., Mygind T. and Meyer R. L., Essential oils in food preservation: mode of action, synergies and interactions with food matrix components, *Front. Microbiol.*, vol. 3, pp. 124, 2012.

[2] Moronkola D. O., *Essential oils from the fruits of six Nigerian plants and syntheses of fragrant terpenoids,* PhD Thesis, Department of Chemistry, University of Ibadan. 1-10, 2001.

[3] Burdock G. A., Handbook of flavor ingredients. *Fenarolis handbook of flavor ingredients*, 5th ed. New York: CRC Press, 2005.

[4] Di Cesare L. F., Forni E., Viscardi D. and Nani R. C., Changes in the chemical composition of basil caused by different drying procedures, *J. Agric. Food Chem.*, no. 51, pp. 35753581, 2003.

[5] Burt S., Essential oils: their antibacterial properties and potential applications in foods-a review, *Int. J. Food Microbiol.*, vol. 94, pp. 223253, 2004.

[6] Figueiredo A. C., Barroso J. G., Pedro L. G. and Scheffer J. J. C., Factors affecting secondary metabolite production in plants: volatile components and essential oils, *Flavour Fragr. J.*, vol. 23, pp. 213226, 2008.

[7] Hussaina A. I., Anwar F., Sherazi S. T. and Przybylski R., Chemical composition, antioxidant and antimicrobial activities of basil (Ocimum basilicum) essential oils depends on seasonal variations, *Food Chem.*, vol. 108, pp. 986995, 2008.

[8] Karakaya S., El S. N., Karagzl N. and Sahin S., Antioxidant and antimicrobial activities of essential oils obtained from oregano (Origanum vulgare spp. hirtum) by using different extraction methods, *J. Med. Food*, vol. 14, pp. 645652, 2011.

[9] Jos-Luis R., Essential Oils in Food Preservation, Flavor and Safety, *Sci. Direct*, vol. 1, pp. 310, 2016.

[10] Siddig I. A. et al., Chemical composition and antioxidant properties of the essential oil of Cinnamomum altissimum Kosterm. (Lauraceae), *Arab. J. Chem.*, vol. 10, no. 1, pp. 131135, 2017.

[11] Botma M., Colquhoun-Flannery W. and Leighton S., Laryngeal oedema caused by accidental ingestion of Oil of Wintergreen, *Int. J. Pediatr Otorhinolaryngol.*, vol. 58, no. 3, pp. 229232, 2001.

[12] Froehlich O., Duque C. and Schreifr P., Volatile constituents of Curuba Passiflora mollissima fruit, *J. Agric. Food Chem.*, vol. 37, no. 2, pp. 421425, 1989.

[13] Mohamed A. A., El-Emary G. A. and Ali H. F., Influence of some citrus essential oils on cell viability, glutathiones, transferase and lipid peroxidation in Ehrlich ascites carcinoma cells, *J. Am. Sci.*, vol. 6, pp. 820826, 2010.

[14] Schmidt E., Production of essential oils. In: Baser KHC, Buchbauer G, editors. *Handbook of essential oils. Science, technology and applications*. New York: Taylor & Francis, 2010.

[15] Ruika L., The isoprene rule and the Biogenesis of terpenic compounds, *Cell. Mol. Life Sci.*, vol. 9, no. 10, pp. 357367, 1953.

[16] Behr A. and Johnen L., Myrcene as a Natural Base Chemical in Sustainable Chemistry: A Critical Review, *Chem Sus Chem*, vol. 2, no. 12, pp. 10721095, 2009.

[17] Chyau C. C., Mau J. L. and Wu C. M., Characteristics of the Steam-Distilled Oil and Carbon Dioxide Extract of Zanthoxylum simulans Fruits, *J. Agric. Food Chem.*, vol. 44, no. 4, pp. 10961099, 1996.

[18] Barros J., Serrani-Yarce J. C., Chen F., Baxter D., Venables B. J. and D. R. A., Role of bifunctional ammonia-lyase in grass cell wall biosynthesis, *Nat. Plants*, vol. 2, p. 16050, 2016.

[19] Hamid A. A, Aiyelaagbe O. O. and Usman L. A., Essential oils: its medicinal and pharmacological uses, *Int. J. Curr. Res.*, vol. 3, no. 2, pp. 8698, 2011.

[20] Harborne J., Phytochemical Methods, *A guide to modern techniques of plant analysis*. 1998.

[21] Sarker S. D., Latif Z. and Gray A. I., *Natural Products Isolation*. New Jersey: Humana Press, 2006.

[22] Handa S., An Overview of Extraction Techniques for Medicinal and Aromatic Plants. In: Handa, S. S., Khanuja, S. P. S., Longo, G. and Rakesh,

D. D. (eds.) *Extraction Technologies for Medicinal and Aromatic Plants*. Trieste: International Centre for Science and High Technology, 2008.

[23] Bowles E. J., *The Chemistry of Aromatherapeutic Oils*, 3rd ed. Griffin Press, 2003.

[24] Margaris N., Koedam A. and Vokou D., *Aromatic Plants: basic and applied aspects*. The Hague, London, Boston: Martinus Nijhoff Publishers., 1982.

[25] Surburg H. and Panten J., *Common Fragrance and Flavor Materials. Preparation, Properties and Uses*, 5th ed. Weinheim: WILEY-VCH, 2006.

[26] Da Porto C., Decorti D. and Kikic I., Flavour compounds of Lavandula angustifolia L. to use in food manufacturing: Comparison of three different extraction methods, *Food Chem.*, vol. 112, pp. 10721078, 2009.

[27] Martinez J. L., *Supercritical Fluid Extraction of Nutraceuticals and Bioactive Compounds*. NW: CRC Press, 2008.

[28] Pourmortazavi S. M. and Hajimirsadeghi S. S., Supercritical fluid extraction in plant essential and volatile oil analysis, *J. Chromatogr. A,* vol. 1163, pp. 224, 2007.

[29] Donelian A., Carlson L. H. C., Lopes T. J. and Machado R. A. F., Comparison of extraction of patchouli (Pogostemon cablin) essential oil with supercritical CO_2 and by steam distillation, *J. Supercrit. Fluids*, vol. 48, pp. 1520, 2009.

[30] Eikani M. H., Golmohammad F. and Rowshanzamir S., Subcritical water extraction of essential oils from coriander seeds (Coriandrum sativum L.), *J. Food Eng.*, vol. 80, pp. 735740, 2007.

[31] Reverchon E., Supercritical fluid extraction and fractionation of essential oils and related products, *J. Supercrit. Fluids*, vol. 10, pp. 137, 1997.

[32] Wenqiang G., Shufen L., Ruixiang Y., Shaokun T. and Can Q., Comparison of essential oils of clove buds extracted with supercritical carbon dioxide and other three traditional extraction methods, *Chem. Essent. oils. Food Chem.*, vol. 101, pp. 15581564, 2007.

[33] Seenivasan P., Manickkam J. and Savarimuthu I., In vitro antibacterial activity of some essential oils, *BMC Complement Alter Med.*, vol. 6, p. 39, 2006.

[34] Okoh O. O., Sadimenko A. P. and Afolayan A. J., Comparative evaluation of the antibacterial activities of the essential oils of Rosmarinusofficinalis L. obtained by hydrodistillation and solvent free microwave extraction methods, *J. Food Chem.*, vol. 120, no. 1, pp. 308312, 2010.

[35] Golmakani M. and Rezaei K., Comparison of microwave-assisted hydrodistillation with the traditional hydrodistillation method in the extraction of essential oils from Thymus vulgaris, *J. Food Chem.*, vol. 109, pp. 2530, 2008.

[36] Schmeiser H. H., Gminski R. and Mersch-Sunderman V., Evaluation of health risks caused by musk ketone, *Int. J. Hyg. Environ. Heal.*, vol. 203, pp. 293299, 2001.

[37] Areias J., Valentao P., Andrade P. B., Ferreres F. and Seabra R. M., Flavonoids and phenolic acids of sage: influence of some agricultural factors, *J. Agric. Food Chem.*, vol. 5, no. 48, pp. 60816084, 2000.

[38] Baker G. R, Lowe R. F. and Southwell I. A., Comparison of oil recovered from tea tree by ethanol extraction and steam distillation, *J. Agric. Food Chem.*, vol. 48, pp. 40414043, 2000.

[39] Masango P., Cleaner production of essential oil by steam distillation, *J. Clean. Prod.*, vol. 13, pp. 833839, 2004.

[40] Wood J. A, Bernards W. W. and Charpentier P. A., Extraction of ginsenosides from North American ginseng using modified supercritical carbondioxide, *J Supercrit. Fluids*, vol. 39, pp. 4047, 2006.

[41] Harbone J. B., A Guide to Modern Techniques of Plants Analysis, *Phytochemical*, vol. 3, pp. 4660, 1993.

[42] Seidel V., *Natural Products Isolation, Initial an.* New Jersey: Humana Press., 2006.

[43] Yeung A., *Encyclopedia of common Natural Ingredients*. New York: John Willey and Sons, 1980.

[44] Masada Y., *Analysis of essential oils by GC and MS*. Chichester: John Willey and Sons, 1976.

[45] Pham-Tuan H., Vercammen J. and Sandra P., *LC.GC Europe, coupling matters*, pp. 18, 2001.

[46] Kolb B., *J. Chromatogr. A*, no. 842, p. 163, 1999.

[47] Golay M. J. E., *Theory and Practice of gas liquid partition chromatography with coated capillaries in gas chromatography*. New York: Academic Press, 1958.

[48] Bicchi C., Sandra P., Cordero C., Iori C. and Rubiolo P., , 23, 90(2000), *J. High Resol. Chromatogr.*, vol. 23, no. 90, pp. 539546, 2000.

[49] Jirovetz L., Buchbauer G., Ngassoum M. B. and Geissler M., J. Chromatogr A, *J. Chromatogr A*, vol. 976, pp. 265275, 2002.

[50] Blumberg L. M. and Klee M. S., *Proceedings of 20th International symposium of Capillary Chromatography* 26-29 May, 1998, pp. 2629.

[51] Giddings J. C., in *Multidimensional Chromatography, Chromatographic Science Series*, vol 50. New York: Marcel Dekker, 1990.

[52] Davis J. M. and Giddings J. C., *Anal. Chem.*, vol. 57, pp. 21682177, 1985.

[53] Huber J. F., Kenndler E. and Reich G., *J Chromatogr.*, vol. 172, p. 15, 1979.

[54] Erni F. and Frei R. W., (1978), *J. Chromatog.*, vol. 149, pp. 561569, 1978.

[55] Guiochon G., Gonnord M. F. and Zakaria M., 3 (1983), *Chromatographia*, vol. 3, pp. 121124, 1983.

[56] Liu Z. and Phillips J. B., 29 (1991), *J. Chromatogr. Sci.*, vol. 29, pp. 227231, 1991.

[57] Liu Z., Ostrovsky I., Farnsworth P. B. and Lee M. L., 35, *Chromatographia*, vol. 35, no. 912, pp. 567573, 1993.

[58] Venter A., *Comprehensive two-dimensional supercritical fluid and gas chromatography (SFCxGC)*, PhD Thesis, University of Pretoria, 2003.

[59] Fornacek A. and Kubeczka K. H., *Essential Oils by Capillary Gas Chromatography and Carbon-13NMR Spectroscopy*. Chichester, UK: John Willey and Sons, 1982.

[60] Claude S. G. and Tabacchi R., (1988), *J. High Resol. Chromatogr.*, vol. 11, p. 187, 1988.

[61] Marriott P. J., Shellie R. and Cornwell C., *J. Chromatogr.*, vol. 936, pp. 122, 2001.

[62] Song J., Gardines B. D., Holland J. F. and Beaudry R. N., 45 (1997) 1801, *J. Agric. Food Chem.*, vol. 45, p. 1801, 1997.

[63] Song J., Fan L. and Beaudry R. M., , 46 (1997) 3721., *J. Agric. Food Chem.*, vol. 46, p. 3721, 1997.

[64] Mondello L., Catalfamo M., Cotroneo A., Dugo G., Dugo P. and McNair H., 22 (1999) 350., *J. High Resol. Chromatogr.*, vol. 22, p. 350, 1999.

[65] Mondello L., Catalfamo M., Cotroneo A., Dugo G. and Dugo P., 10 (1998) 203., *J. Microcol.*, vol. 10, p. 203, 1998.

[66] Marriott P., Shellie R. and Cornwell C., 23,9 (2000) 554-560, *J. High Resol. Chromatogr.*, vol. 23, no. 9, pp. 554560, 2000.

[67] Dimandja, J.-M.D., Stanfill, S.B., Grainger, J. and Patterson, D.G., Jr. (2000), "Application of Comprehensive Two-Dimensional Gas Chromatography (GCGC) to the Qualitative Analysis of Essential Oils." *J. High Resol. Chromatogr.*, 23: 208-214.

[68] Shellie R., Mondello L., Marriott P. and Dugo G., 970 (2002) 228-234., *J. Chromatogr.*, vol. 970, pp. 228-234, 2002.

[69] Mondello L., Dugo G. and Bartle K. D., Sep., 8 (1996) 275, *J. Microcol.*, vol. 8, p. 275, 1996.

[70] Mondello L., Dugo P., Bartle K. D., Dugo G., and Gans P., Sep., 6 (1994) 237, *J. Microcol.*, vol. 6, p. 237, 1994.

[71] Mondello L., Dugo P., Bartle K. D., Dugo G., and Cotroneo A., 10 (1995) 33, *Flav. Fragr. J.*, vol. 10, p. 33, 1995.

[72] Mondello L., Dugo P., Bartle K. D., Dugo G., and Lewis A., (1999, *J. Chromatogr.*, vol. 842, p. 373, 1999.

[73] Saito M. and Yamauchi Y., (1990) 237, *J. Chromator.*, vol. 505, p. 237, 1990.

[74] Yarita T., Nomura A. and Horimoto Y., 10 (1994) 25-29, *Anal. Sci.*, vol. 10, pp. 2529, 1994.

[75] Joulain D. and Koenig W. A., *The atlas of spectra data of sesquiterpene hydrocarbons: In mass finder 3.1 library*. Hamburg, Germany.: E. B Verlag, publishers, 1998.

[76] Daniel Joulain W. A. K., The atlas of spectral data of sesquiterpene hydrocarbons, *Phytochemistry*, vol. 52, no. 7, pp. 13851386, 1999.

[77] Baris O. et al., Biological activities of the essential oil and methanol extract of Achillea biebersteini Afan Afan (Asteraceae), *Turkish J. Biol.*, vol. 30, pp. 6567, 2006.

[78] Tisserand R. B., In *The Art of Aromatherapy*. Rochester, VT.: Healing Arts Press, 1997.

[79] Martin G., *Dragoco report: Fruity Notes in perfumery*, 1991.

[80] Ekundayo O, Ajani F., Seppanen-Laakso T. and Laakso I., Volatile constituents of Psidium guajava L. (Guava) Fruits., *Flavour Fragr. J.*, vol. 6, pp. 233236, 1991.

[81] Moronkola D. O. and Ekundayo O., Chemical constituents in the fruit essential oil of Terminalia catappa Linn (Almond Fruits), *J. For. Trop. Resour.*, vol. 16, pp. 7279, 2000.

[82] Moronkola D. O. and Ekundayo O., Volatile Constituents of Irvingia gabonensis Aubry-Lecomte ext ORorke Baillon Fruits (African Native Mango), *J. For. Trop. Resour.*, vol. 18, no. 1, pp. 5663, 2002.

[83] Moronkola D. O., Adeleke A. K. and Ekundayo O., Constituents of the Spondias mombin Linn and the Comparison between its Fruit and Leaf essential oils, *J. Essent. oil Bear. plants*, vol. 6, no. 3, pp. 148152, 2003.

[84] Moronkola D. O., Oyedeji O. A., Ekundayo O. and Ogunbinu O. A., Composition of the root essential oil of Chrysophyllim albidum G. Don, *Bowen J. Agric.*, vol. 3, no. 1, p. 53, 2006.

[85] Moronkola D. O. and Ogunwande I. A., Identification of the main volatile compounds in the leaf and flower of Tithonia diversifolia (Hemsl) Gray, *J. Nat Med.*, vol. 61, pp. 6366, 2007.

[86] Moronkola D. O. and Ogunwande I. A., Essential Oil Composition of Gmelina arborea Roxb., Verbenaceae from Nigeria, *J. Essent. Oil Res.*, vol. 21, pp. 264266, 2009.

[87] Moronkola D. O., Ogunwande I. A. and Oyewole I. O., The Needle Oil of Pinus caribaea Morelet from Nigeria, *J. Essent. Oil Res.*, vol. 21, pp. 342344, 2009.

[88] Moronkola D. O., Ogunwande I. A. and Oyewole I. O., Studies on the Volatile Oils of Momordica Charantia L.(Cucurbitaceae) and Phyllanthus Amarus She. Et Thonn (Euphorbiaceae), *J. Essent. Oil Res.*, vol. 21, pp. 393399, 2009.

[89] Moss M., Cook J., Wesnes K. and Duckett P., Aromas of rosemary and lavender essential oils differentially affect cognition and mood in healthy adults, *Int. J. Neurosci.*, vol. 113, pp. 1538, 2003.

[90] Buchbauer G., The detailed analysis of essential oils leads to the understanding of their properties, *Perfum. flavourist*, vol. 25, pp. 6467, 2000.

[91] Pandey A. K., Singh P. and Tripathi N. N., Chemistry and bioactivities of essential oils of some Ocimum species: an overview, *Asian Pac. J. Trop. Biomed.*, vol. 4, pp. 682694, 2014.

[92] Sirvaityte J., Siugzdaite J. and Valeika V., Application of Commercial Essential Oils of Eucalyptus and Lavender as Natural Preservative for Leather Tanning Industry, *Rev. Chim.*, vol. 62, no. 9, pp. 884893, 2011.

[93] Bakkali F., Averbeck S., Averbeck D. and Idaomar M., Biological effects of essential oilsa review,*Food Chem. Toxicol.*, vol. 46, pp. 446475, 2008.

[94] Bassol I. H. and Juliani H. R., Essential oils in combination and their antimicrobial properties, *Molecules*, vol. 17, pp. 39894006, 2012.

[95] Iqbal T., Hussain A. I., Chatha S. A., Naqvi S. A. and Bokhari T. H., Antioxidant activity and volatile and phenolic profiles of essential oil and different extracts of wild mint (Mentha longifolia) from the Pakistani Flora, *J. Anal. Methods Chem.*, vol. 2013, p. 536490., 2013.

[96] Victoria F. N. et al., Essential oil of the leaves of Eugenia uniflora L.: antioxidant and antimicrobial properties, Food Chem. Toxicol., vol. 50, pp. 26682674, 2012.

[97] Liju V. B., Jeena K. and Kuttan R., An evaluation of antioxidant, anti-inflammatory and antinociceptive activities of essential oils from curcuma longa, *Indian J. Pharmacol.*, vol. 43, pp. 526531, 2011.

[98] Baik K. U., J. S. H. and Ahn B. Z., Recognition of pharmacophore of ar-turmerone for its anticancer activity.,*Arch Pharmacal Res*, vol. 16, pp. 254256, 1993.

[99] Moharram H. A. and Youssef M. M., Methods for Determining the Antioxidant Activity: A Review. Alex., *J. Food, Sci. Technol.*, vol. 11, no. 1, pp. 3142, 2914.

[100] Akinpelu O. E., Moronkola D. O. and Dawodu F. A., Antibacterial, Antifungal and Antioxidant Activities of Seven Essential Oils from Blighia sapida (K. Koenig), *J. Chem., Biol. Phys. Sci.*, vol. 6, no. 4, pp. 11791187, 2016.

[101] Akinpelu O. E., Moronkola D. O., Dawodu F. A. and Sichilongo K., Chemical compositions of seven essential oils from Blighia sapida (K. Koenig), (Sapindaceae), *Int. J. Biol. Chem. Sci.*, vol. 10, no. 5, pp. 23512367, 2016.

[102] Mounyr B., Moulay S. and Saad K. I., Methods for in vitro evaluating antimicrobial activity: A review, *J. Pharm. Anal.*, vol. 6, pp. 7179, 2016.

[103] Sartoratto A., Machado A. L., Delarmelina C., Figueira G. M., Duarte M. C. and Rehder V. L., Composition and antimicrobial activity of essential oils from aromatic plants used in Brazil, *Brazilian J. Microbiol.*, vol. 35, pp. 275280, 2004.

[104] Grand View Research, *Essential Oils Market Size and Share Industry Growth Report*, 2019-2025, 2019.

In: What to Know about Essential Oils
Editor: Malene M. Kjeldsen
ISBN: 978-1-53617-986-6

Chapter 9

INCREASE OF ESSENTIAL OIL YIELD IN *MENTHA PIPERITA* BY INOCULATION WITH PLANT GROWTH-PROMOTING RHIZOBACTERIA

Lorena del Rosario Cappellari[1], Maricel Valeria Santoro[2], Julieta Chiappero[1], Tamara Belén Palermo[1] and Erika Banchio[1,*]

[1]INBIAS Instituto de Biotecnología Ambiental y Salud (CONICET-Universidad Nacional de Río Cuarto), Río Cuarto, Argentina

[2]Department of Biochemistry, Max Planck Institute for Chemical Ecology, Jena, Germany

ABSTRACT

Peppermint (*Mentha piperita*) is one of the most important EO (essential oil crops) and is cultivated worldwide. It is composed primarily of monoterpenes, whose medicinal properties are mainly due to their EO

* Corresponding Author's Email: ebanchio@exa.unrc.edu.ar.

composition, accumulated in glandular trichomes. Nowadays, agriculture relies heavily on the use of synthetic chemicals, such as fertilizers and pesticides, to achieve high yields but without taking into account their deleterious effects on the environment. However, there is an interesting biotechnological alternative using microorganisms to increase the availability and intake of nutrients by crops and to control phytopathogenic organisms and herbivorous insects. The group of bacteria termed plant growth-promoting rhizobacteria (PGPR) colonizes the rhizosphere and stimulates plant growth and development by direct or indirect mechanisms. Thus, in the search for new strategies of plant production to optimize essential oil (EO) yield, inoculation with PGPR is an interesting candidate. We present here an integrated summary of our experimental findings from an analysis of the community of fluorescent Pseudomonas strains in the rhizosphere of commercially grown *Mentha piperita*, including the effects of inoculation and co-inoculation with different PGPR strains (native and wild type) on total EO yield and glandular trichome density. The qualitative and quantitative compositions of the main monoterpenes (menthol, menthone, pulegone, limonene and linalool) were also determined to analyze the effects of the volatiles emitted by PGPR rhizobacteria on EO production. The various PGPR strains (*Bacillus amyloliquefaciens* GB03, *Pseudomonas fluorescens* WCS417r, *Azospirillum brasilense* SP7, *Pseudomonas putida* SJ04-SJ25-SJ48) and co-inoculations evaluated produced significant increases in the production of EO in peppermint plants, but at different magnitudes. Bacterial inoculants are thus an effective biotechnological tool for stimulating the secondary metabolism in plants. Application of these techniques may contribute to environmental conservation, increased crop productivity and sustainable agricultural practices.

Keywords: *Mentha piperita*, essential oil, rhizobacteria, PGPR, glandular trichome, menthol, menthone

INTRODUCTION

Aromatic plants have been cultivated by man since time immemorial and include a great diversity of plant species whose common characteristic is the production of essential oils (Güenther, 1948). In contemporary agriculture, traditional food crops, fodder and fiber are no longer the only commercially significant crops. Nowadays, there are crops cultivated involving plants whose secondary metabolites are valued for their aromatic characteristics and therapeutic attributes, as natural compounds, which are utilized mainly in the food industry, but also in perfumery and chemistry (Arizio and Curioni, 2014).

We are also now in the presence of a growing and sustained trend of consumption and demand for healthy, organic and natural products, which has generated worldwide an attractive and expanding market for the commercialization of aromatic plants (Informe Sectorial sobre Infusiones y Especias [Sectorial Report on Infusions and Spices] 2010). The main regional destinations of these plants are distilleries of non-alcoholic bitters and snacks, medical specialty laboratories, perfumery ingredients, cosmetology, aromatherapy, and pharmacies. Demand is also growing rapidly for hygiene and health care formulations (Muñoz López de Bustamante, 1996).

The international trade of aromatic products is currently undergoing a constant increase at a pace double that of world population growth (Paunero, 2012; Mathe, 2015). This expansion of demand can be explained by: a) changes in consumption habits, with an increase in pre-prepared foods and a greater demand for condiments with antioxidant properties; b) Trends towards a healthier life imposing the use of flavorings, supplements and preservatives of natural origin; c) A clear trend of substitution of industrial synthetic medicines for others of a natural origin (Sangwan et al., 2001; Arizio and Curioni, 2014); d) The rise in ethnic foods, a product of large migrations to industrialized countries (Arizio and Curioni, 2014; Mathe 2015).

The genus *Mentha* is a highly diverse and very important taxon in the family Lamiaceae, and includes 25–30 species that grow worldwide (Dorman et al., 2003). Mints are fast growing, invasive and can tolerate a wide range of agro-climatic conditions (Božovićet al., 2015). The species belonging to the genus *Mentha* form an irreplaceable resource of essential oils, which as a result of their chemical diversity, are a target of human exploitation. Currently, these are used in a wide range of industries; for example, in pharmaceutical and perfume products, as flavorings, as food supplements in the form of vitamins or sweeteners, in pesticides and for medicinal purposes (Bohlmann and Keeling, 2008). In addition, they contain a large number of antioxidant compounds, such as polyphenols, terpenoids, flavonoids, carotenes, α-tocopherol, betaine and choline, which can have beneficial effects in the prevention of various degenerative diseases (Sharafi et al., 2010; Farnad et al., 2014). In fact, *Mentha* spp. has been used as a folk remedy for the aliments anorexia, nausea, flatulence, bronchitis, liver complaints and colitis due to its stimulant, antiemetic, diaphoretic, carminative, anti-inflammatory, analgesic, emmenagogue, antispasmodic and anti-catarrhal activities (Iscan et al., 2002; Moreno et al., 2002). Commercially, the most important mint species are spearmint (*Mentha spicata*), peppermint (*M. x piperita*) (Askary et al., 2016) and corn mint (*M. canadensis*) (Singh and Pandey 2018), with peppermint being a natural sterile hybrid between the species *Mentha spicata* and *Mentha aquatica*. It is very aromatic, with branched stems of between 30 and 70 cm high and a quadrangular section, and is grown from an underground rhizome. The leaves are petiolated, opposite and oval with sharp margins. Both leaves and stems are usually slightly hairy. From the leaf axils, flower stem shoots grow at the beginning of summer, which appear as terminal spike-shaped inflorescences. The flowers are small, up to 8 mm, with the tetra lobed corolla being purple or pink. Given its sterility, it reproduces almost exclusively by vegetative propagation, by underground rhizomes and also by cuttings obtained from dividing young bushes (Shah and Mello, 2004).

Essential oils are responsible for the characteristic odour of plants and are formed by complex mixtures of volatile constituents. Specifically, EO are composed primarily of monoterpenes with smaller amounts of sesquiterpenes (Gershenzon et al., 2000). The amount and number of components of EO varies depending on the region, soil type, climate, agronomic conditions (Burt, 2004), harvesting season, technique of oil extraction and drying method (Singh et al., 2012; Gavahian et al., 2015), with the EO yield of *M. piperita* being about 1 to 3%. The menthol and pulegone present in the essential oil of Mentha species are the substances that give the mints their characteristic aromas and flavors (Lubbe and Verpoorte, 2011, Singh and Pandey 2018). Peppermint oil is applied to flavor pharmaceuticals and many of the oral preparations (toothpastes, dental creams, and mouth washes). This plant is also used as a flavoring agent in confectionery, cough drops, chewing gums, and in some alcoholic liqueurs. It is also used used in medicines, with its pleasant taste making it an excellent gastric stimulant (Dorman et al., 2003; MIRC 2010).

The rhizosphere has been defined by Hiltner (1904) as the volume of soil influenced by the presence of roots of a living plant. Its extent can vary according to the type of soil, plant species and their age, among other factors (Foster, 1998). Live roots provide a source of nutrients for soil organisms from radical exudates, which are chemical compounds released by exudation, secretion or autolysis of old roots. These contain abundant low molecular weight compounds including sugars, amino acids, organic acids, vitamins and various secondary metabolites, as well as high molecular weight compounds such as proteins and polysaccharides, in addition to inorganic ions, water and electrons (Pérez-Montaño et al., 2014; Rasmann and Turlings, 2016). Among the different microbial populations present in this area of the soil, bacteria are by far the most abundant microorganisms, with a density of up to 10^9 cells per gram of soil (Nadeem et al., 2013).

Interaction and communication between roots and microorganisms is a highly regulated process used to control and alter the activities of the organisms involved. Fungi and bacteria are able to detect host plants and initiate the rhizosphere colonization strategy. Moreover, plants are capable of recognizing compounds synthesized by microorganisms, thereby regulating their defense lines according to the species found. This molecular dialogue results in a relationship that goes from pathogenicity to symbiosis through a highly coordinated cellular process (Walker et al., 2003; Bais et al., 2004; Ortiz-Castro et al., 2009; Babalola, 2010).

PGPR (*Plant Growth Promoting Rhizobacteria*) are beneficial bacteria of soil-free life that play a significant role in promoting growth and plant development by colonizing the root system through different mechanisms (Kloepper 1993; Lucy et al., 2004; Pérez Montaño et al., 2014; Shrivastava et al., 2015). The benefits to the plant that result from host-PGPR interaction include increases in the germination rate of the seeds, stronger growth of the root and leaf area, higher chlorophyll and protein content and nutrient absorption, tolerance to abiotic stress, the suppression of diseases caused by pathogens and a decrease in senescence (Yang et al., 2009; Pérez Montaño et al., 2014; Glick 2012; Verbon and Liberman, 2016; Etesami and Maheshwari, 2018).

The mechanisms by which PGPR promote plant growth depend on each microorganism-plant interaction. Therefore, it is necessary to determine the particular effects of a certain PGPR strain on the physiology and development of a specific plant species (Santoro et al., 2015). These mechanisms can be either direct or indirect. The direct ones include the biological fixation of nitrogen, phosphate solubilization, siderophore production, phytohormone production (auxin, giberelin and citokinin), regulation of the ethylene level, and production of volatile organic compounds (mVOCs) (Gupta et al., 2017). Among the indirect ones are siderophore production, the production of antibiotics and antifungal compounds, lithic activity, competition for substrates, inhibition of enzymes or toxins produced by phytopathogens, and hydrocyanic acid production (Kloepper 1993; van Loon 2003, Lucy et al., 2004; Shrivastava et al., 2015, Vejan et al., 2016; Etesami and Maheshwari, 2018).

In the search for new strategies of plant production with high yield, but without undesirable effects or compounds being created, it is important to investigate unconventional alternatives such as inoculation with PGPR. However, to date, very little is known regarding the effects of inoculation with this type of bacteria on aromatic and medicinal plants. Thus, the purpose of the present chapter is to present and discuss results regarding the responses to the inoculation with various PGPR strains on *M. piperita*, considering in particular the effect on Essential Oil yield and composition of the main compounds of *M. piperita*. Related to this, the effects of PGPR volatile organic compounds (VOCs) emission and the combined effect of phytohormone application and PGPR inoculation under controlled conditions were also considered.

PLANT GROWTH PROMOTION RHIZOBACTERIA INDUCED ESSENTIAL OIL PRODUCTION BY DIRECT INOCULATION

For the aromatic plant studied (*M. piperita*), increases were recorded for different parameters of growth and development after the inoculation and co-inoculation with strains capable of promoting plant growth (Santoro et al., 2011; 2015; 2016; Cappellari et al., 2017), as has been reported for other plant species (Vessey, 2003; van Loon, 2007; Pérez Montaño et al., 2014; Vejan et al., 2016). The dimension of the changes registered was found to depend on the bacterial strain inoculated (Santoro et al., 2015; Cappellari et al., 2017).

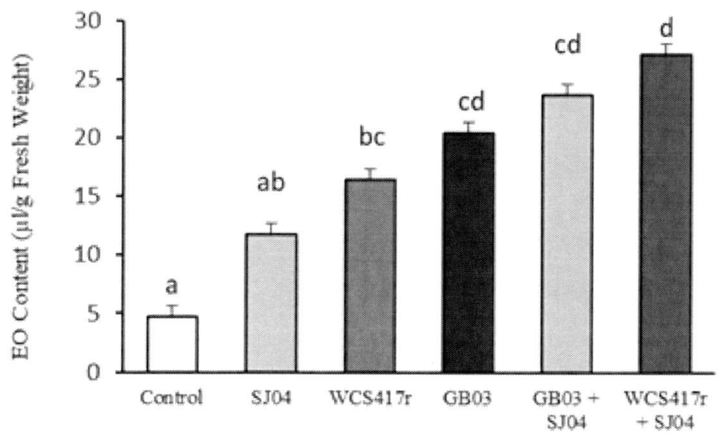

Figure 1. Essential Oil (EO) yields in the *Mentha piperita* control and treatment groups. Different letters above bars indicate significant differences according to Fisher's LSD test ($p < 0.05$).

Yields of the major EO components ((+) pulegone, (−) menthone, (−) menthol, 1,8-cineole and linalool) were higher for all five treatment groups compared to the control group (Figure 2). Menthol yield increased to 2.09 µg/g fresh weight ($p < 0.05$) in the WCS417r+SJ04 group in comparison with 0.22 µg/g fresh weight in the control group and 1.1–1.2 µg/g fresh weight in the other treatment groups. Similar trends were observed for menthone, 1,8–cineole, linalool and pulegone, with the yield always being higher for the WCS417r+SJ04 group than for the other treatment groups. Generally, when plants were inoculated individually, the yields for each of the major EO components were higher for the GB03 group than for WCS417r or SJ04, but the differences between these three singly-inoculated groups were generally not significant (Cappellari et al., 2015).

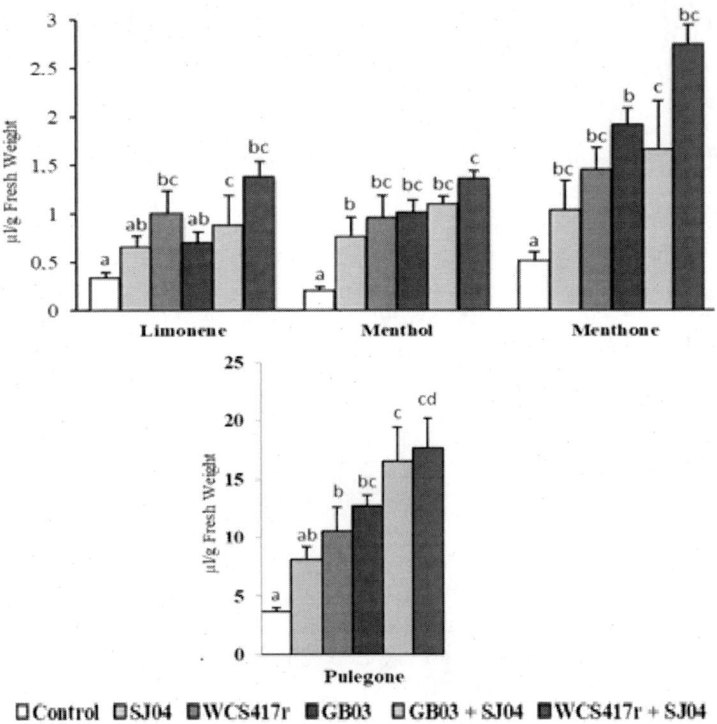

Figure 2. Concentrations of major essential oil (EO) components in *Mentha piperita* control and treatment groups. Different letters above bars indicate significant differences according to Fisher's LSD test ($p < 0.05$).

To determine which factors contributed to the increase in essential oil content, we measured the density of the glandular trichomes, which are the structures that synthesize and store monoterpene-rich essential oil. Peppermint (*M. piperita*) has single glandular capitate trichomes and peltate glandular trichomes on the adaxial and abaxial leaf surfaces, with a small capitate glandular trichome consisting of a globose unicellular head attached to the leaf by a two- or three-celled uniseriate stalk. The peltate glandular trichomes consisted of a large eight-celled head with an enlarged secretory cavity attached to a one-celled short stalk, with these trichomes being present on both surfaces of the plants, but with their density being higher on the abaxial surface (Rios-Estepa et al., 2010). The increased EO yield was associated with the larger number of peltate glandular trichomes, the primary site of EO synthesis. The average numbers of trichomes recorded per mm^2 for the control group and the five treatment groups are shown in Figure 3. Trichomes were significantly more abundant on the abaxial than the adaxial surface. Peltate trichomes were present on both surfaces of the treatment groups, but their density was lower on the adaxial surface, with the density of peltate trichomes on both surfaces being higher for the treatment groups than the control group (Figure 3). Differences in peltate trichome density among the five treatment groups were not significant (Cappellari et al., 2015).

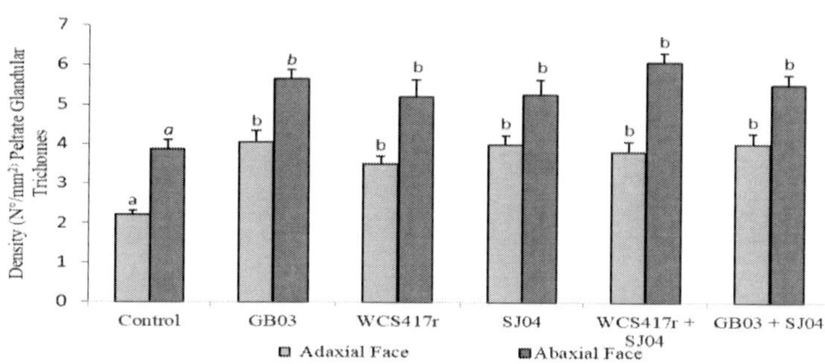

Figure 3. Density (per mm^2) of peltate glandular trichomes in *M. piperita* control and treatment groups. Different letters above bars indicate significant differences according to Fisher's LSD test ($p < 0.05$).

Other experiments with *M. piperita* grown in *in vitro* conditions and inoculated with native strains were carried out. Peppermint plants were grown in Petri dishes coated with MS semisolid medium (0.5% agar) and inoculated with three native pseudomonad strains (*Pseudomonas putida* SJ04, *P. putida* SJ25, *P. putida* SJ48) isolated from the rhizosphere soil of *M. piperita* plants in a commercial agricultural field in San Jose, Villa Dolores, Cordoba province, Argentina, and a reference strain (*P. fluorescens* WCS417r) bacteria was used at a concentration 10^6 CFU $dish^{-1}$. The total essential oil content in plants inoculated with three of the tested bacterial strains was significantly ($p < 0.05$) higher than in controls (Figure 4), with this increase being ~two-fold for native strain SJ25, and ~60% for reference WSC417r and native SJ04. Essential oil content in native SJ48 was not significantly different from that of controls (Santoro et al., 2015).

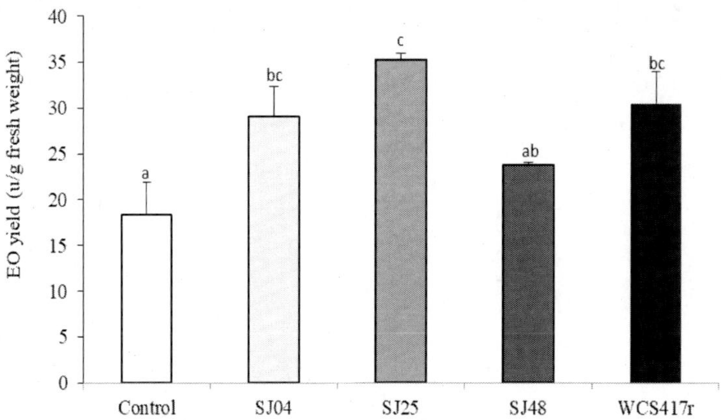

Figure 4. Total essential oil yield in *M. piperita* plants grown in vitro inoculated with native PGPR strains. Letters above bars indicate significant differences according to Fisher's LSD test ($p < 0.05$).

The effects of direct bacterial inoculation in the *in vitro* condition on the major monoterpenes present in *M. piperita* EOs were variable (Table 1). Terpineol content increased significantly after treatment for all four strains, and by up to four-fold for SJ25. The increase in menthone was similar (~50%) for the four strains. Menthol revealed the largest increases for the treatments with SJ04 (~seven-fold) and SJ25 (~six-fold). The levels of limonene, menthofuran and pulegone were not significantly different ($p > 0.05$) for any of the strains (Santoro et al., 2015).

Regarding the trichomes, their number increased significantly after treatment with each of the strains (Figure 5), which was ~2.5-fold higher for SJ25 and ~60% higher for the other strains in comparison with controls. SJ25 also produced the greatest increase in the EO yield (Santoro et al., 2015).

Table 1. Variation in content (µg/mg FW) of major essential oils of *M. piperita* inoculated with bacterial strains

Treatment	**limonene (µg/mg FW)**	**terpineol (µg/mg FW)**	**menthone (µg/mg FW)**	**menthofuran (µg/mg FW)**	**menthol (µg/mg FW)**	**pulegone (µg/mg FW)**
control	0.20 ±0.03 a	0.13 ±0.01 a	0.13± 0.05 a	0.20 ±0.09 a	0.55 ±0.08 a	17.13 ±3.15 a
SJ04	0.17 ±0.02 a	0.23 ±0.03 b	0.23 ±0.03 b	0.20 ±0.04 a	4.20 ±0.45 c	15.73 ±4.91 a
SJ25	0.26 ±0.08 a	0.63 ±0.09 c	0.18 ±0.04 b	0.17 ±0.05 a	3.55 ±0.67 bc	17.21 ±3.46 a
SJ48	0.26 ±0.09 a	0.40 ±0.10 b	0.19 ±0.05 b	0.16 ±0.02 a	2.68 ±0.06 b	19.46 ±0.72 a
WCS417r	0.20 ±0.01 a	0.33 ±0.07 b	0.22 ±0.06 b	0.37 ±0.11 a	0.70 ±0.12 a	27.18 ±3.43 a

Data shown are mean ± SE. Values within a column followed by the same letter are not significantly different according to Fisher's LSD test ($p < 0.05$).

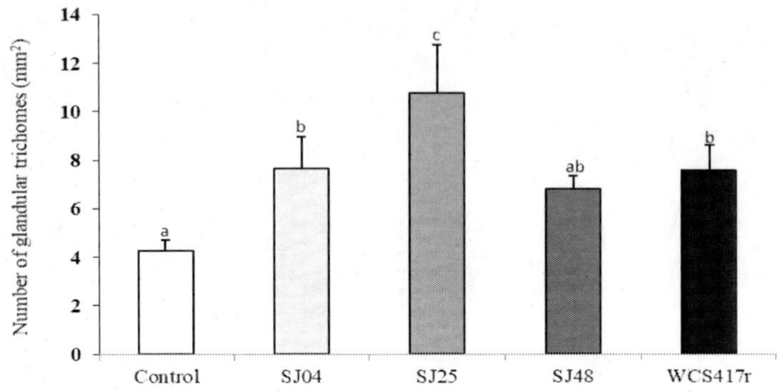

Figure 5. Number of glandular trichomes per mm^2, at day 30, in *M. piperita* plants inoculated with five PGPR strains. Letters above bars indicate significant differences according to Fisher's LSD test ($p < 0.05$).

Volatile Organic Compounds Emitted by Plant Growth Promoting Rhizobacteria Induced Essential Oil Yield

Treatment of plants with PGPR has been shown to increase shoot growth, total biomass, seed weight, early flowering, and the yields of grain, fodder, fruit, etc. (van Loon 2007). Numerous mechanisms have been proposed to explain how rhizobacteria promote plant growth, including increased nitrogen fixation, the production of auxin, gibberellins, cytokinins and ethylene, solubilization of phosphorus, oxidation of sulfur, increased availability of nitrates, extracellular production of antibiotics, lytic enzymes and hydrocyanic acid, increased root permeability, competition for available nutrients and root sites, suppression of harmful rhizobacteria, and the enhanced uptake of essential nutrients (Vessey 2003; Niranjan et al., 2006; Vejan et al., 2016). In addition to the above mechanisms, studies over recent years have shown that rhizobacteria are capable of releasing functional volatile organic compounds (VOCs) (Fernando et al., 2005; Kai et al., 2007; Vespermann and Piechulla 2007; Kai et al., 2009), which are characterized by their relatively low molecular mass (<300 Da), low boiling point and lipophilic properties. Various rhizobacteria have a great variability in the qualitative and quantitative complexity of their VOC profiles, and the number of different compounds produced and emitted by a particular strain may be as high as 60 (Kai et al., 2007). However, for most VOCs, their exact chemical structure still remains to be elucidated (Kai et al., 2009). The manifestation of a characteristic volatile compound or profile is attributable to specific metabolic pathways being active in the bacterium. Thus, depending on the growth conditions or medium, the "bouquet" of released VOCs can vary for each species (Fincheira and Quiroz 2018).

To evaluate the effect of volatile organic compounds (VOCs) emitted by rhizobacteria, one node of *M. piperita*, from an aseptically cultured plantlet, was placed on one side of a specialized plastic Petri dish (90 x15 mm) containing a center partition (I-plate, Fisher Scientific), with both sides of the dish containing 50% strength MS solid medium. Then, a 20 ml suspension culture of various PGPR strains in sterile distilled water was applied drop-wise to the side of the dish opposite the plant node. By this method, plants were exposed to bacterial VOCs without any actual physical contact. The dishes were sealed with parafilm and placed in a growth chamber with controlled conditions of light, temperature and relative humidity, and plants were harvested after 30 days.The three strains *P. fluorescens* WCS417r, *B. subtilis* GB03, *A. brasilense* SP7, previously reported as PGPR, were then assessed for their effects (Santoro et al., 2011).

Regarding the effect of rhizobacterial VOCs on the formation of plant secondary compounds, we observed an almost 2-fold increase in the accumulation of EOs in plants treated with *P. fluorescens*, compared to *B. subtillis*, *A. brasilensis*, or control (Figure 6). In *P. fluorescens*- and *Azospirillum brasilense*-treated plants, the EO yields were 4.46 and 3.22 mg/mg fresh weight, respectively, which were 2-fold higher than in controls (Figure 6). *B. subtilis* did not produce any increase in EO yield, in contrast with our previous study, whereas *O. basilicum* plants exposed to *B. subtilis* VOCs showed an increased accumulation and content of major EOs (Banchio et al., 2009; Santoro et al., 2011).

Yields of the major EOs (+) pulegone, (-) menthone, (-) menthol and (+) menthofuran were generally higher in plants exposed to rhizobacterial VOC emission compared to controls (Figure 7). The pulegone concentration was only significantly increased (3.14-fold; $p < 0.05$) *by P. fluorescens* treatment, while Menthone was increased 15.4- and 13.5-fold ($p < 0.05$) in *P. fluorescens*- and *A. brasilense*-treated plants, respectively. Also, menthofuran was increased significantly in *P. fluorescens* treated plants. In fact, the only decreases in EO yield (5-fold) were observed for menthol and menthofuran in *A. brasilense*-treated plants, compared to control plants (Santoro et al., 2011).

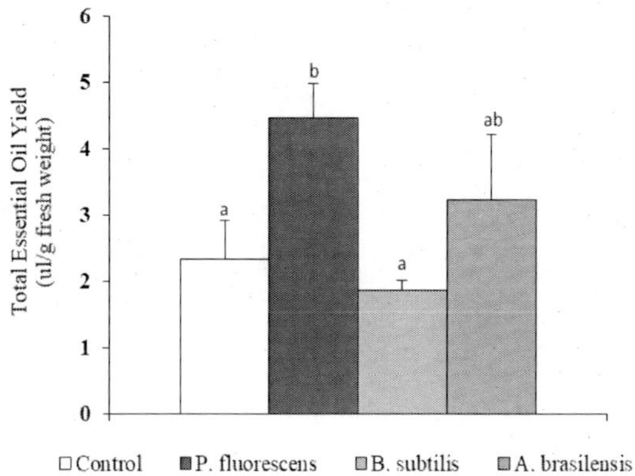

Figure 6. Essential oil (EO) yield in *M. piperita* exposed to VOCs from three PGPR species. Letters above bars indicate significant differences according to Fisher's LSD test ($p < 0.05$).

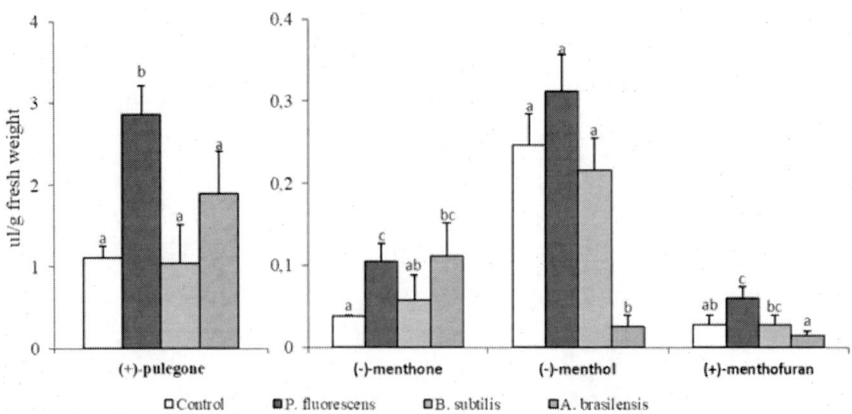

Figure 7. Concentrations of major EO components in *M. piperita* exposed to VOCs from three PGPR species. Letters above bars indicate significant differences according to Fisher's LSD test ($p < 0.05$).

The observed changes in the EO levels suggest that VOCs from soil bacteria, as well as inducing biosynthesis of secondary metabolites in *M. piperita*, can also influence the pathway flux or specific parts of the monoterpene metabolism. An increased pulegone content in EOs may enhance pulegone reductase enzyme activity, and favor the reduction of pulegone to menthone rather than oxidation to menthofuran (Santoro et al., 2011).

It has also been observed that full interaction of bacteria with plants (inoculation) may induce secondary metabolite responses (Tabanca et al., 2004; Banchio et al., 2008; 2010). The inoculation of peppermint with *P. fluorescens* increased the yield and accumulation of major EOs. In fact, plant growth can be promoted by bacterial effects including growth hormone production, VOC production, solubilization of phosphates, oxidation of sulfur, increased nitrate availability, increased root permeability or bacterial volatiles, or by a combination of these effects (Kai et al., 2009; Liu and Zhang 2015).

It is noteworthy that *A. brasilense* VOCs did not significantly affect the EO yields, and caused a decrease in the menthol level. *B. subtilis* VOCs revealed a growth promoting effect in both *O. basilicum* and *M. piperita,* but caused an increased yield of EOs only in the former species. These findings suggest that the effects of bacterial VOCs on plants are species-specific, so VOCs from a given bacterial strain do not cause the same effects, or at least not to the same degree, in all plant species, with responses being characteristic of a specific plantebacteria combination. Possible explanations for this phenomenon are: (i) different plants respond to different components of VOC mixtures; (ii) reactive sites are different; (iii) plant differ in their ability to metabolize VOCs (Santoro et al., 2011).

The VOCs from bacteria show a diversity and complexity comparable to those from plants and fungi, and are rich sources for new natural compounds. However, the biological functions of most bacterial VOCs are still not well understood. Using an analogy to VOCs from plants and fungi, we may expect that bacterial VOCs may serve as: (a) "infochemicals" for communication within and among organisms; (b) cell-to-cell communication signals; (c) carbon release valves; (d) growth-promoting or growth-inhibiting agents. The present results indicate that the VOCs from soil bacteria released underground play a crucial role in rhizosphere interactions (Fincheira and Quiroz 2018). Investigation into the structural elucidation and biological activities of these volatile compounds should now be the subjects of ongoing and future studies.

Plant Growth Promotion Rhizobacteria Inoculation Combined with Exogenous Phytohormones, as Elicitor, Increased Essential Oil Yield

To evaluate the effect of the phytohomones methyl Jasmonate (MeJa) and salicylic acid (SA) combined with PGRR inoculation, the following procedure was carried out. Plants growing in sterile vermiculite were first inoculated with 1000 μL bacterial suspension, with sterile water being applied to the control seedlings. After 7 days of inoculation, plants were sprayed until run-off with 1, 2 or 4 mM MeJA solution or 1, 2 mM SA solution. After 14 days of applied phytohormone treatment, the plants were removed from their pots and different parameters were evaluated (Cappellari et al., 2019).

The gas chromatographic (GC) analysis of EO revealed that spraying with MeJA increased the EO yield. In addition, plants treated with 1 or 2 mM MeJA increased their EO yield approximately three-fold with respect to the control (similar to that of PGPR) ($p < 0.05$), while using 4mM MeJA led to a five-fold increase (Figure 8). After spraying with SA, the EO yield rose approximately two-fold in comparison to the control, similar to the increase observed in PGPR-inoculated plants (Figure 9) (Cappellari et al., 2019).

The response of plants treated with PGPR in addition to MeJA depended on the concentration of MeJA applied. The strongest effect was observed when plants were treated with 2 mM, with an increase in EO yield of nearly 8-fold being observed compared to controls without MeJA or PGPR, which was also much greater than that observed for either treatment alone. In addition, plants treated with 2 mM MeJA + WCS417r revealed the greatest increase, followed by SJ04 (~7 times) and then WCS417r (~5 times). In plants inoculated with PGPR and then sprayed with 1mM or 4 MeJA, the EO yield was similar to that in plants which had only been inoculated (Figure 8). Finally, the EO content was similar to that of control plants only for plants treated with 1 mM MeJA+GB03 and 4 mM MeJA + SJ04, and this value was less than that of the inoculated plants. (Cappellari et al., 2019).

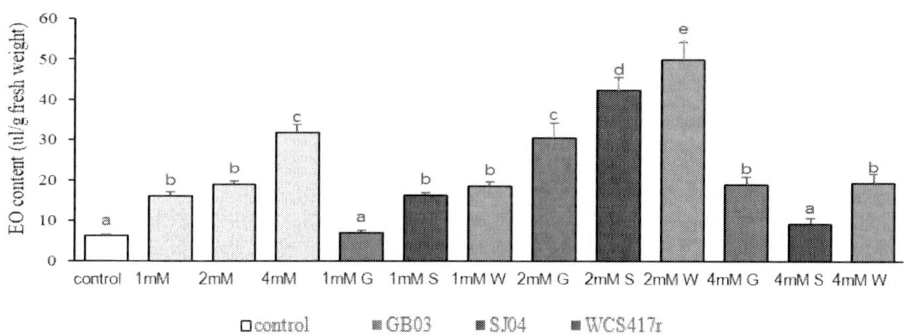

Figure 8. Inoculation with PGPB and MeJA treatments increased the essential oil concentration in shoots of *M. piperita* plants. Different letters above bars indicate significant differences according to Fisher's LSD test ($p < 0.05$).

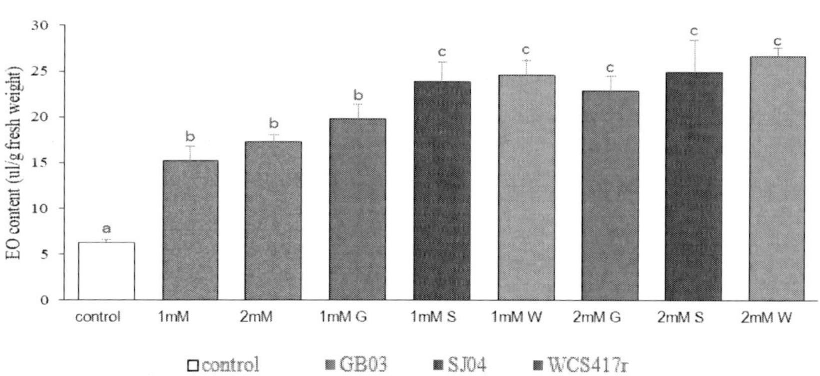

Figure 9. Inoculation with PGPB and SA treatments increased the essential oil concentration in shoots of *M. piperita* plants. Different letters above bars indicate significant differences according to Fisher's LSD test ($p < 0.05$).

Table 2. Inoculation with PGPB and MeJA or SA treatments increased the density of peltate glandular trichomes on the abaxial (lower) surface of the *M. piperita* leaves (units of trichomes per mm^2)

Treatment	Density (N°/mm^2)
Control	4.07 ± 0.2 a
GB03	4.35 ± 0.22 a
SJ04	4.98 ± 0.18 b
WCS417r	5.07 ± 0.2 b
MeJA 1 mM	6.16 ± 0.24 b
MeJA 1 mM + GB03	6.47 ± 0.35 b
MeJA 1 mM + SJ04	6.69 ± 0.27 b
MeJA 1 mM + WCS417r	6.73 ± 0.41 b
MeJA 2 mM	5.98 ± 0.15 b
MeJA 2 mM + GB03	6.47 ± 0.35 b
MeJA 2 mM + SJ04	5.94 ± 0.46 b
MeJA 2 mM + WCS417r	6.21 ± 0.58 b
MeJA 4 mM	6.71 ± 0.26 b
MeJA 4 mM + GB03	5.76 ± 0.34 b
MeJA 4 mM + SJ04	8.88 ± 0.36 c
MeJA 4 mM + WCS417r	8.39 ± 0.26 c
SA 1 mM	5.92 ± 0.26 bc
SA 1 mM + GB03	6.89 ± 0.74 c
SA 1 mM + SJ04	6.14 ± 0.39 bc
SA 1 mM + WCS417r	6.13 ± 0.28 bc
SA 2 mM	7,11 ± 0,6 c
SA 2 mM + GB03	9,41 ± 0,29 d
SA 2 mM + SJ04	7,29 ± 0,33 c
SA 2 mM + WCS417r	7,83 ± 0,31 cd

Data shown are mean ± SE. Different letters above bars indicate significant differences according to Fisher's LSD test ($p < 0.05$).

The EO yield of plants treated with PGPR in addition to 1 and 2 mM concentrations of SA showed an increase of approximately three-fold in comparison to untreated uninoculated controls, which was generally higher than for either treatment alone (Figure 9), irrespective of the inoculated strain.

The density of the peltate glandular trichomes was increased by JA and SA treatments. PGPR alone induced a 20–25% rise in the peltate glandular trichome density, with spraying with MeJA also significantly increasing the peltate trichome density on the abaxial surface ($p < 0.05$). The MeJA treatment produced an increase in peltate trichomes of approximately 50% in plants sprayed with respect to control or PGPR inoculated plants (Table 2). However, the combination of MeJA spraying and PGPR inoculation resulted in higher densities, with the highest values being observed for plants inoculated with SJ04 and WCS417r and sprayed with 4mM MeJA. The SA applications led to a significantly increased density of peltate trichomes on the abaxial surface (Table 2) compared to control or PGPR inoculated plants, with plants treated with 2mM and inoculated with GB03 and WCS417r producing the highest increase in the number of peltate trichomes. As the control with solvent for MeJA and SA did not differ statistically from the control ($p > 0.05$), this is not shown in the Table 2.

Our finding that the endogenous levels of SA and JA increase after PGPR inoculation (Cappellari et al., 2019), suggests that both phytohormones are involved in the signaling pathways elicited by rhizobacteria. PGPR inoculation has been shown to increase the EO yield in *M. piperita* plants (Cappellari et al., 2015), but the promotion of growth and the increased EO production induced by PGPR cannot be replaced by the external application of phytohormones (as JA causes an increase in EO yield, but a decrease in growth). In the present study, we observed that in addition to inoculation, the external application of MeJA at 2mM increased the EO production by up to 8-fold, indicating that there is synergy between PGPR and MeJA. Thus, from a biotechnological standpoint, our findings could be useful to help improve the production of EOs (Cappellari et al., 2019). Nevertheless, further studies are still required in order to identify the main molecular mechanisms driving the increase in essential oil after PGPR inoculation.

CONCLUSION

Essential oil in plants plays several key roles in plant-environment interactions and plant-plant communication, which depend on the EO composition and concentrations. Terpenoids are crucial components in plant defensive responses to abiotic and biotic stresses (Unsicker et al. 2009;

Vickers et al. 2009), in signaling among plant organs (Heil and Silva Bueno 2007), and in plant-plant communication (Baldwin et al. 2006; Lange and Ahkami 2013). The increases in EO synthesis observed in various investigations presumably represent defensive responses to colonization by microorganisms. In previous studies, we have observed a significant rise in free jasmonic acid, the active form JA-Ile and SA, in *M. piperita* plants inoculated with different rhizobacteria strains (Cappellari et al., 2019). While the induction of SA and JA by PGPR may have various benefits for their host plants, the increase of these two defense hormones suggests that plants may perceive these bacteria as a threat and thereby initiate a defensive response. Related to this, several EO compounds in *M. piperita* exert insecticidal, antifungal, and/or antibacterial effects (Sangwan et al. 2001).

Induction of systemic resistance, which can be elicited not only by pathogens and herbivores but also by beneficial microorganisms and certain synthetic compounds, provides plants with an enhanced capacity for rapid and effective activation of cellular defensive responses against pathogen or insect attack (Conrath 2011). The induction of systemic resistance against herbivores also involves the priming of jasmonate-dependent responses and also some other as yet unidentified mechanisms (Pineda et al. 2010; van Oosten et al. 2008). Priming of plant defenses by beneficial microorganisms has been proposed to be a consequence of the modulation of the plant immune systems associated with the establishment of symbiosis, and other related changes in defense-related signaling (Pozo and Azcón- Aguilar 2007; Zamioudis and Pieterse 2012).

The higher monoterpene concentrations we observed in inoculated plants may have resulted in addition to the increase in defensive phytohormones, from growth-promoting substances, secreted by PGPR, which affect the plant metabolic processes. Increases in stomatal density and chlorophyll content in inoculated plants can be reflected in a higher rate of carbon assimilation and result in an increased terpenoid biosynthesis, requiring carbon fixation through photosynthesis (Ghirardo et al., 2011; Cappellari et al., 2015).

Terpenoid biosynthesis depends on the primary metabolism (photosynthesis) and oxidative pathways for carbon and energy supplies

(Singh et al. 1991). Giri et al. (2003) found that net photosynthesis of PGPR-hosting plants is correlated with nutritional status. Moreover, factors that increase dry matter production affect the interrelationship between the primary and secondary metabolisms, leading to increased biosynthesis of secondary products (Shukla et al. 1992). In our studies, the trichome density was higher in the treatment groups than in the control group. Related to this, oil yield is strongly correlated with the total number and developmental distribution patterns of glandular trichomes, the biosynthetic machinery that quickly and efficiently converts imported carbohydrates into EOs (Lange et al. 2011; Lange and Turner 2012). Rios-Estepa et al. (2010) proposed a mechanism whereby the increased expression of a biosynthetic gene induces production of glandular trichomes, thereby facilitating the production and storage of EOs.

In summary, we have described a novel approach for evaluating the effects of specific PGPR strains on *M. piperita* using bacterial inoculants, which are an effective biotechnological tool for stimulating the secondary metabolism in plants. Future studies of the activities of these inoculants will help clarify certain adaptive processes that are poorly understood at present.

There is a steadily increasing demand for environmentally safe and sustainable organic agricultural practices that can reduce the negative environmental effects associated with food and feed production (Lind et al. 2004). In fact, a worldwide shift is currently underway, moving from traditional inorganic farming methods toward ecofriendly, organic farming methods. Indeed, for the numerous medicinal and aromatic plant species that are consumed without further processing, it is important that no synthetic compounds be present in the harvested crop. Thus, these type of crop plants are ideal candidates for the development of growth-promoting strategies involving PGPR and biofertilizers.

ACKNOWLEDGMENTS

This study was supported by a grant from Consejo Nacional de Investigaciones Científicas y Tecnológicas. TBP, JC and LC have fellowships from Consejo Nacional de Investigaciones Científicas y Técnicas of Argentina (CONICET). EB is Career Member of CONICET. The authors are grateful to Dr. Paul Hobson, native speaker, for editorial assistance.

References

Arizio, O. P., Curioni, A. O. (2014). Global and regional exchange of spices in terms of value 1992-2011. *Revist. Col. de Cs. Hortíc.* 8 (1):142-154.

Askary, M., Talebi, S. M., Amini, F., Bangan, A. D. B. (2016). Effects of stress on foliar trichomes plasticity in *Mentha piperita*. *Nusantara.* 8:32-38.

Babalola, O. O. (2010). Beneficial bacteria of agricultural importance. *Biotechnol. Lett.,* 32: 1559-1570.

Baldwin, I. T., Halitschke, R., Paschold, A., von Dahl, C. C., Preston, C. A. (2006).Volatile signaling in plant-plant interactions: Talking trees in the genomics era. *Science,* 311:812-815.

Banchio, E., Xie, X., Zhang, H., Paré, P. W. (2009). Soil bacteria elevate essential oil accumulation and emissions in sweet basil. *J. Agric. Food Chem.*, 57: 653-657.

Banchio, E., Bogino, P., Zygadlo, J., Giordano, W. (2008). Plant growth promoting rhizobacteria improve growth and essential oil yield in *Origanum majorana* L. *Biochem. Syst. Ecol.* 36: 766-771.

Banchio, E., Bogino, P. C., Santoro, M., Torres, L., Zygadlo, J., Giordano, W. (2010). Systemic induction of monoterpene biosynthesis in *Origanum × majoricum* by soil bacteria. *J. Agric. Food Chem.* 58: 650-654.

Bohlmann, J., Keeling, C.I. (2008). Terpenoid biomaterials. *Plant J.*, 54: 656-669.

Božović, M., Pirolli A., Ragno, R. (2015). *Mentha suaveolens* Ehrh. (*Lamiaceae*). Essential oil and its main constituent piperitenone oxide: biological activities and chemistry. *Molecules* 20: 8605-8633Lange, B. M., Ahkami, A. (2013). Metabolic engineering of plant monoterpenes, sesquiterpenes and diterpenes—current status and future opportunities. *Plant Biotech. J.,* 11:169-196.

Burt, S. (2004) Essential Oils: Their Antibacterial Properties and Potential Applications in Foods—A Review. *Int. J. Food Microbiol*, 94, 223-253.

Cappellari, L., Chiappero, J., Santoro, M., Giordano, W., Banchio, E. (2017). Inducing phenolic production and volatile organic compounds emission by inoculating Mentha piperita with plant growth-promoting rhizobacteria. *Scientia Horticulturae,* 220: 193-198.

Cappellari, L., Santoro, M., Reinoso, H., Travaglia, C., Giordano, W., Banchio, E. (2015). Anatomical, morphological, and phytochemical effects of inoculation with plant growth promoting rhizobacteria on peppermint (*Mentha piperita*). J. Chem. Ecol. 41: 149-158. DOI: 10.1007/s10886-015-0549-y.

Cappellari, L., Santoro, V.M., Schmidt, A., Gershenzon, J., Banchio, E. (2019). Induction of essential oil production in Mentha x piperita by plant growth promoting bacteria was correlated with an increase in jasmonate and salicylate levels and a higher density of glandular trichomes. *Plant Physiol. Biochem.*, 141: 142–153. doi:10.1016/j. plaphy.2019.05.030.

Choi, S.K.; Jeong, H.; Kloepper, J.W.; Ryu, C.M. (2014). Genome sequence of Bacillus amyloliquefaciens GB03, an active ingredient of the first commercial biological control product. *Genome Announc.,* 2, e01092–14. doi:10.1128/genomeA.01092-14.

Dorman, H.D., Kosar, M., Kahlos, K., Holm, Y., Hiltunen, R. (2003). Antioxidant properties and composition of aqueous extracts from Mentha species, hybrids, varieties, and cultivars. *J Agric Food Chem*, 51:4563–4569.

Etesami, H., Maheshwari, D.K., 2018. Use of plant growth promoting rhizobacteria (PGPRs) with multiple plant growth promoting traits in stress agriculture: action mechanisms and future prospects. *Ecotoxicol. Environ. Saf.* 156, 225–246.

Farnad, N., Heidari, R., Aslanipour, B. (2014). Phenolic composition and comparison of antioxidant activity of alcoholic extracts of Peppermint (*Mentha piperita*). *J. Food Meas. Charact.* 8:113–121.

Fernando, W. G. D., Nakkeeran, S. y Zhang, Y. (2005). Chapter 3: Biosynthesis of antibiotics by PGPR and its relation in biocontrol of plant diseases. En: Sidiqqui, Z. A. (Ed.) *PGPR: Biocontrol and Biofertilization.* (pp: 67-109). Netherlands:Springer.

Fincheira P, Quiroz A (2018) Microbial volatiles as plant growth inducers. Microbiol Res 208:63-75.

Foster, R. C. (1998). Microenvironments of soil microorganisms. *Biol. Fert. Soils,* 6: 189- 203.

Gavahian, M., Farahnaky, A., Farhoosh, R., Javidnia, K., Shahidi, F. (2015). Extraction of essential oils from Mentha piperita using advanced techniques: microwave versus ohmic assisted hydrodistillation. *Food Bioprod Process.* 2015;94:50–58. doi: 10.1016/ j.fbp.2015.01.003

Gershenzon, J., Mc Conkey, M. E., Croteau, R. B. (2000). Regulation of monoterpene accumulation in leaves of peppermint. *Plant Physiol,* 122: 205-213.

Ghirardo, A., Gutknecht, J., Zimmer, I., Brüggemann, N., Schnitzler, J. P. (2011). Biogenic volatile organic compound and respiratory CO2 emissions after 13C-labeling: online tracing of C translocation dynamics in poplar plants. *PLoS One* 6:e17393

Giri, B., Kapoor, R., Mukerji, K. G. (2003). Influence of Arbuscular mycorrhizal fungi and salinity on growth, biomass and mineral nutrition of *Acacia auriculiformis*. *Biol. Fert. Soils,* 38:170-175.

Glick B. R. (2012). Plant growth-promoting bacteria: mechanisms and applications. *Scientifica* 2012: 1-15. DOI: org/10.1016/j.jksus. 2013.05.001.

Güenther E. 1948. *The essential oil,* Vol. 1. D. Nostrand Co. Londres. 342 p.

Gupta, P. y Kumar, V. (2017). Value added phytoremediation of metal stressed soils using phosphate solubilizing microbial consortium. *World J. Microbiol. Biotechnol.* 33 (1): 9. DOI: 10.1007/s11274-016-2176-3.

Heil, M., Silva Bueno, J. C. (2007). Within-plant signaling by volatiles leads to induction and priming of an indirect plant defence in nature. *Proc. Natl. Acad. Sci. USA,* 104:5467-547.

Hiltner, L. (1904). Über neurer erfahrunger und problem auf dem gebeit der boden akteriologie und unter besonderer beruck sinchtingung der grundungung und brache. *Arbeiten Deutscher Landwirtschafts Gesellschaft* 98: 59-78.

Informe Sectorial sobre Infusiones y Especias. [Sectorial Report on Infusions and Spices] (2010). Argentina.

Iscan, G., Kirimer, N., Kurkcuoglu, M., Baser, K. H., and Demirci, F. (2002). Antimicrobial screening of Mentha piperita essential oils. *J. Agric. Food Chem.* 50:3943–3946. doi: 10.1021/jf011476k.

Kai, M., Effmert, U., Berg, G., Piechulla B. (2007) Volatiles of bacterial antagonists inhibit mycelial growth of the plant pathogen *Rhizoctonia solani, Arch. Microbiol.*, 187:351-360.

Kai, M., Haustein, M., Molina, F., Petri, A., Scholz, B., Piechulla, B. (2009). Bacterial volatiles and their action potential, *Appl. Microbiol. Biotechnol.*, 81:1001-1012.

Kloepper, J.W.E. 1993. Plant-growth-promoting rhizobacteria as biological control agents". In: Metting, F.B. (Ed.), *Soil Microbial Ecology: Applications in Agricultural and Environmental Management.* Marcel Dekker Inc., New York, pp. 255–273.

Lange, B. M., Turner, G. W. (2012). Terpenoid biosynthesis in trichomes current status and future opportunities. *Plant Biotech. J.*, 11:2-22.

Lange, B. M., Mahmoud, S. S., Wildung, M. R., Turner, G. W., Davis, E. M. (2011). Improving peppermint essential oil yield and composition by metabolic engineering. *Proc. Natl. Acad. Sci. USA*, 108:16944–16949.

Lind, K., Lafer, G., Schloffer, K., Innerhoffer, G., Meister, H. (2004). *Organic fruit growing.* UK. CABI Publishing, Wallingford.

Liu, X. M. y Zhang, H. (2015). The effects of bacterial volatile emissions on plant abiotic stress tolerance. *Front. Plant Sci.* 6: 774.DOI: 10.3389/fpls.2015.00774.

Lubbe, A., Verpoorte, R. (2011). Cultivation of medicinal and aromatic plants for specialty industrial materials. *Ind. Crops Prod,* 34, 785–801. doi: 10.1016/j.indcrop.2011.01.019

Lucy. M., Reed. E., Glick. B. R. (2004). Application of free living plant growth-promoting rhizobacteria. Antonie van Leeuwenhoek. *Int. J. Gen. Mol. Microbiol.,* 86: 1-25.

Mathe A. (Ed.). 2015. *Medicinal and aromatic plants of the world.* doi:10.1007/978-94-017-9810.

MIRC, 2010. *Mint Industry Res. Council.* Great Falls, MT Available at: http://usmintindustry.org/ (accessed March 2014).

Moreno, L., Bello, R., Primo-Yúfera, E., Esplugues, J. (2002). Pharmacological properties of the methanol extract from Mentha suaveolens Ehrh. *Phytother. Res.* 16:10–13. doi: 10.1002/ptr.744.

Muñoz López de Bustamante, F. (1996). *Plantas medicinales y aromáticas. Estudio, cultivo y procesado.* [Medicinal and aromatic plants. Study, cultivation and processing] Ed. Muni-Prensa, Madrid Paván M.F., Furlan V., Caminos S., Ojeda M.S. 2017. Las personas y las plantas medicinales en el noroeste de Córdoba, Argentina. Reconocimiento y valoración de los recursos naturales locales Boletín Latinoamericano y del Caribe de Plantas Medicinales y Aromáticas 16: 78 – 87.

Nadeem, S. M., Ahmad, M., Ahmad Zahir, Z., Javaid, A., Ashraf, M. (2013). The role of mycorrhizae and plant growth promoting rhizobacteria (PGPR) in improving crop productivity under stressful environments. *Biotechnol. Adv.*, 32: 429-448.

Niranjan, R. S., Shetty, H.S., Reddy, M. S. (2006). *Plant growth promoting rhizobacteria:bpotential green alternative for plant productivity.* In: Z. A. Siddiqui (Ed.), PGPR:vBiocontrol and Biofertilization. Springer, Netherlands, pp. 197-216.

Ortiz-Castro R., Valencia-Cantero E., López-Bucio J. (2008). Plant growth promotion by Bacillus megaterium involves cytokinin signaling. *Plant Signal Behav.,* 3: 263-265.

Paunero, I. E. (2012). *Mejoramiento genético en plantas aromáticas* [*Genetic improvement in aromatic plants*]. EEA San Pedro, INTA.

Pérez-Montaño, F., Alías-Villegas, C., Bellogín, R. A., del Cerro, P., Espuny, M. R., Jiménez-Guerrero, I., López-Baena, F. J., Ollero, F. J., Cubo, T. (2014). Plant growth promotion in cereal and leguminous agricultural important plants: from microorganism capacities to crop production. *Microb. Res.,* 169: 325:336.

Pineda A, Zheng SJ, Van Loon JJA, Pieterse CMJ, Dicke M (2010). Helping plants to deal with insects: the role of beneficial soil borne microbes. *Trends Plant Sci.,* 15:507-514.

Pozo, M. J., Azcón-Aguilar, C. (2007). Unravelling mycorrhiza-induced resistance. *Curr. Opin. Plant Biol.,* 10:393-398.

Rasmann, S., Turlings, T. C. (2016). Root signals that mediate mutualistic interactions in the rhizosphere. *Curr. Opin. Plant Biol.*, 32: 62-68.

Rios-Estepa, R., Lange, I., Lee, J. M, Lange, M. (2010). Mathematical modeling-guided evaluation of biochemical, developmental, environmental, and genotypic determinants of essential oil composition and yield in peppermint leaves. *Plant Physiology*, 152: 2105-2119.

Sangwan, N. S., Farooqi, A. H. A., Shabih, F., Sangwan, R. S. (2001). Regulation of essential oil production in plants. *Plant Growth Regul,* 34: 3–21.

Santoro, M. V., Zygadlo, J., Giordano, W. y Banchio, E. (2011). Volatile organic compounds from rhizobacteria increase biosynthesis of essential oils and growth parameters in peppermint (Mentha piperita). *Plant Physiol. Biochem.* 49: 1177- 1182.DOI: 10.1016/j.plaphy. 2011.07.016.

Santoro, M., Cappellari, L., Giordano, W. y Banchio, E. (2015). Plant growth promoting effects of native Pseudomonas strains on *Mentha piperita* (peppermint): an in vitro study. *Plant Biol.*, 17: 1218-1226. DOI: 10.1111/plb.12351.

Santoro, V. M., Bogino, P. C., Nocelli, N., Cappellari, L., Giordano, W. F., Banchio, E. (2016). Analysis of plant growth-promoting effects of fluorescent Pseudomonas strains isolated from *Mentha piperita* rhizosphere and effects of their volatile organic compounds on essential oil composition. *Front. Microb.*, 7: 1085.

Shah, P. P., D`Mello, P. M. (2004). A review of medicinal uses and pharmacological effects of *Mentha piperita. Nat. Product Radiance*, 3: 214-221.

Sharafi, S.M., Rasooli, I., Owlia, P., Taghizadeh, M., Astaneh, S.D.A. (2010). Protective effects of bioactive phytochemicals from *Mentha piperita* with multiple health potentials. *Neuropsychopharmacol. Hung*, 6:147–153. https://doi.org/10.4103/0973-1296.66926.

Shrivastava, S., Egamberdieva, D., Varma, A. (2015). Chapter 1: Plant growthpromoting rhizobacteria (PGPR) and medicinal plants: the state of the art. In: Egamberdieva, D., Shrivastava, S. y Varma, A. (Eds.) *Plant Growth-Promoting Rhizobacteria (PGPR) and Medicinal Plants.* (pp. 1-16). New York, USA: Soil Biology Series. Springer Books.

Shukla, A., Farooqi, A, H., Shukla, Y. N., Sharma, S. (1992). Effect of triacontanol and chlormequat on growth, plant hormones andartemisinin yield in *Artemisia annua* L. *Plant Growth Regul.,* 11:165-171.

Singh, P., Pandey, A. K. (2018). Prospective of Essential Oils of the Genus Mentha as Biopesticides: A Review. *Front. Plant Sci*. 9:1295. doi: 10.3389/fpls.2018.01295

Singh, N., Luthra, R., Sangwan, R. S. (1991). Mobilization of starch and essential oil biogenesis during leaf ontogeny of lemongrass (Cymbopogon flexuosus Stapf.). *Plant Cell Physiol.* 32:803-811.

Singh, R., Shushni, M.A.M., Belkheir, A. (2015). Antibacterial and antioxidant activities of Mentha piperita l. *Arabian J.Chemi.* 128:322–328.

Tabanca, N., Ozek, T., Baser, K. H. C., Tumen, G. (2004) Comparison of the essential oils of *Origanum majorana* L. and *Orignaum majoricum* Cambess, J. *Essent. Oil Res.*, 16: 248-252.

Unsicker, S., Kunert, G., Gershenzon, J. (2009) Protective perfumes: the role of vegetative volatiles in plant defense against herbivores. *Curr Opin Plant Biol.,* 12:479-485.

van Loon L.C.(2007). Plant response to plant growth-promoting rhizobacteria. *Eur.J. Plant Pathol.*. 119: 243–254.

Van Oosten, V. R., Bodenhausen, N., Reymond, P., Van Pelt, J. A., Van Loon, L. C., Dicke, M. (2008) Differential effectiveness of microbial induced resistance against herbivorous insects in Arabidopsis. *Mol. Plant Microbe Interact.,* 21:919-930.

Vejan, P., Abdullah, R., Khadiran, T., Ismail, S., Boyce, A. N. (2016). Role of plant growth promoting rhizobacteria in agricultural sustainability - A review. *Molecules,* 21:573. DOI: 10.3390/molecules21050573

Verbon, E. H., Liberman, L. M. (2016). Beneficial microbes affect endogenous mechanisms controlling root development. *Trends Plant Sci.*, 21: 218-229.

Vespermann, M., Kai, M., Piechulla, B. (2007). Rhizobacterial volatiles affect the growth of fungi and *Arabidopsis thaliana. Appl. Environ. Microbiol.*, 73:5639-5641.

Vessey, J. K. (2003). Plant growth promoting rhizobacteria as biofertilizers. *Plant Soil,* 255: 571-586. DOI: 10.1023/A: 102603 7216893.

Vickers, C. E, Gershenzon, J., Lerdau, M. T, Loreto, F. (2009) A unified mechanism of action for volatile isoprenoids in plant abiotic stress. *Nat Chem Biol.,* 5:283-291.

Walker S.T., Bais H.P., Grotewold E., Vivanco J.M. (2003). Root exudation and rhizosphere biology. *Plant Physiol.,* 132: 44-51.

Yang, J., Kloepper, J. W., Ryu, C. M. (2009). Rhizosphere bacteria help plants tolerate abiotic stress. *Trends Plant Sci.*,14: 1-4.

Zamioudis, C., Pieterse, C. M. (2012). Modulation of host immunity by beneficial microbes. *Mol. Plant Microbe.,* 25:139-150.

In: What to Know about Essential Oils
Editor: Malene M. Kjeldsen
ISBN: 978-1-53617-986-6

Chapter 10

TAKING ADVANTAGE OF SOME ESSENTIAL OILS CONTAINING PHENYLPROPANOIDS/ TERPENOIDS AS RENEWABLE CHEMICAL REAGENTS FOR FINE SYNTHESIS OF HETEROCYCLES

Vladimir V. Kouznetsov[1,*], Amner Muñoz-Acevedo[2], Martha Cervantes-Díaz[3], María C. González[2] and Leonor Y. Vargas-Méndez[1]

[1]Laboratorio de Química Orgánica y Biomolecular, CMN, Universidad Industrial de Santander, Parque Tecnológico Guatiguará, Piedecuesta, Colombia
[2]Departamento de Química y Biología, Universidad del Norte, Barranquilla, Colombia
[3]Grupo de Investigaciones Ambientales para el Desarrollo Sostenible – GIADS, Facultad de Química Ambiental, Universidad Santo Tomás, Seccional Bucaramanga, Colombia

[*] Corresponding Author's Email: kouznet@uis.edu.co, vkuznechnik@gmail.com.

Abstract

Certain plants produce some essential oils containing phenylpropanoids/terpenoids (e.g., (*E*)-anethole, estragole, eugenol, (E)-isoeugenol, safrole, (*E*)-/(*Z*)-citral, (*R*)-/(*S*)-citronellal, (*E*)-/(*Z*)-geraniol and carvacrol) as main constituents (relative amounts >50%), which are isolated of different parts from star anise/aniseed, winter tarragon/Mexican tarragon, clove tree, sassafras, lemongrass, lemon balm, citronella grass, palm rose, and Cuban oregano. These EO/molecules have many and different bioactivities (e.g., antimicrobial, antiparasitic, antioxidant, anti-inflammatory, anticancer/chemopreventive, cytotoxic/toxic, anesthetic/analgesic, antinociceptive, antispasmodic, pro-cholinergic, anticonvulsant, hypotensor/vasorelaxant, antidiabetic, insecticidal, larvicidal, fumigant and repellent, among other) and are used as flavoring/preserving/active ingredients in foods and beverages, personal care and cosmetics, perfumery, etc., as well as raw materials. Since the 1950s, the EO have been sources of substances as starting materials for different chemical synthesis; however, with the emergence of green chemistry, the EO and their main constituents (as biomass) have become attractive to the scientific community, as starting/raw material for fine chemical synthesis. Some examples are the preparation/obtaining of tetrahydroquinoline, isoindoloquinolinone, dihydrobenzofuranol, iridoid, octahydroacridine, trioxane, oxirane and benzochrome derivatives, from EO isolated of star anise fruit, clove bud, citronella and palm rose grasses, and Cuban oregano leaves. These hemisynthetic derivatives showed interesting biological properties, e.g., antiparasitic, antimicrobial, antiviral, antioxidant, and anticancer.

Keywords: essential oils, renewable resources, phenylpropanoids, terpenoids, chemical reagents, fine synthesis, heterocycles

Introduction

Some essential oils (EO) produced by certain plants contain phenylpropanoid or terpenoid molecules such as (*E*)-anethole [(*E*)-1-methoxy-4-(1-propenyl)-benzene], estragole (4-allyl-1-methoxy-benzene), eugenol (4-allyl-2-methoxy-phenol), (*E*)-isoeugenol [(*E*)-2-methoxy-4-(1-propenyl)-phenol], safrole (4-allyl-1,2-(methylenedioxy)-benzene), (*E*)-/(*Z*)-citral [(*E*)-/(Z)-3,7-dimethyl-2,6-octadienal], (*R*)-/(*S*)-citronellal [(*R*)-

/(*S*)-3,7-dimethyl-6-octen-1-al], (*E*)-/(*Z*)-geraniol [(*E*)-/(*Z*)-2,6-dimethyl-2,6-octadien-8-ol] and carvacrol (5-isopropyl-2-methyl-phenol), as major constituents (relative amounts >50%).

These EO have been isolated of useful parts (flowers, buds, fruits, seed, leaves, stem or trunk/wood/bark) from *Illicium verum* L. (star anise)/*Pimpinella anisum* L. (aniseed), *Artemisia dracunculus* L. (winter tarragon)/*Tagetes lucida* L. (Mexican tarragon), *Syzygium aromaticum* L. (clove tree), *Sassafras albidum* L. (sassafras), *Cymbopogon citratus* L. (lemongrass), *Melissa officinalis* L. (lemon balm), *Cymbopogon nardus* L. (citronella grass), *Cymbopogon martinii* L. (palm rose) and *Plectranthus amboinicus* L. (Cuban oregano), and, both EO and the constituent major molecules have many, different and interesting biological properties e.g., antimicrobial, germicidal, antioxidant, antiulcer, anti-inflammatory, anticancer, pro-cholinergic, anesthetic/analgesic, antiseptic, sedative/ anxiolytic, stimulant, skin irritant, enzyme inhibitors, ion channel modulators, antiviral, anti-*quorum* sensing, insecticidal, anti-feedant, mosquitocidal, nematicidal, anthelmintic, fumigant and repellent, among other) and are used as flavoring/preserving/active ingredients in foods and beverages, personal care and cosmetics, perfumery, and agriculture/ pharmaceuticals; as well as raw materials, etc.

Since the 1950s, the EO have been sources of substances as starting materials for different chemical synthesis or isolation of pure molecules, particularly, fixative and flavor/fragrant agents. Nonetheless, with the advent of green chemistry as a tool for sustainable development, three decades ago, researchers have turned their attention to the use of biomass as a renewable carbon resource, which is one of the most important principles of this chemical science. Thenceforth, the EO and their main constituents have become attractive as starting/raw material for fine chemical synthesis, because they could efficiently replace those chemical reagents based on fossil resources.

It is worth mentioning some interesting examples: the EO from star anise, clove bud, citronella grass, palm rose, and Cuban oregano were used for obtaining tetrahydroquinoline, isoindoloquinolinone, dihydrobenzofuranol, iridoid, octahydroacridine, trioxane, oxirane and benzochromene derivatives which showed biological properties such as antiparasitic, antiprotozoal, antimalarial, antimicrobial, anti-tubercular, antiviral, antioxidant, and anticancer. Therefore, the use of EO mentioned above in the preparation of these pharmacologically important molecules is the central subject of this chapter. Its goal is to highlight the advances in the synthetic efforts to construct new heterocyclic compounds using basic principles of sustainable chemistry.

Text Mining about Essential Oils as Renewable Reagents for Fine Synthesis

In order to identify the use of essential oils as renewable reagents for fine synthesis, the following search equation was structured in the Scopus database (Elsevier, VB; 2020): (*TITLE-ABS-KEY ("essential oil * "OR" volatile oil * "OR phenylpropanoid * OR terpenoid * OR biomass OR derivative *) AND TITLE-ABS-KEY (tetrahydroquinoline OR isoindoloquinolinone OR dihydrobenzofuranol OR iridoid OR octahydroacridine OR trioxane OR oxirane OR benzochromene) AND NOT TITLE-ABS-KEY (ABS) biosynthesis AND NOT glycosid * AND NOT sugar)) AND DOCTYPE (ar) AND PUBYEAR > 1999 AND (LIMIT-TO (SUBJAREA, "CHEM") OR LIMIT-TO (SUBJAREA, "PHAR"))*, which linked the keywords related with essential oils and the compounds of interest obtained by organic synthesis. Consequently, 3025 indexed registers were found in the database during the 2000-2020 timeline.

The obtained data were processed/analyzed by using *VantagePoint* software (Search Technology, Inc, version 12) with which the scientometric indicators (article number published per year) were obtained, representing the scientific dynamic in the subject of interest (Figure 1) whose general trend was increasing. Thus, the year with greatest science activity was 2014 with 212 registers, followed by 2018 and 2016 with 206 and 203 records, respectively. In addition, the growth rate (percentage value/year) of the publications was 16.0% per year (R^2 0.8812), calculated by means of De Solla Price's law [1].

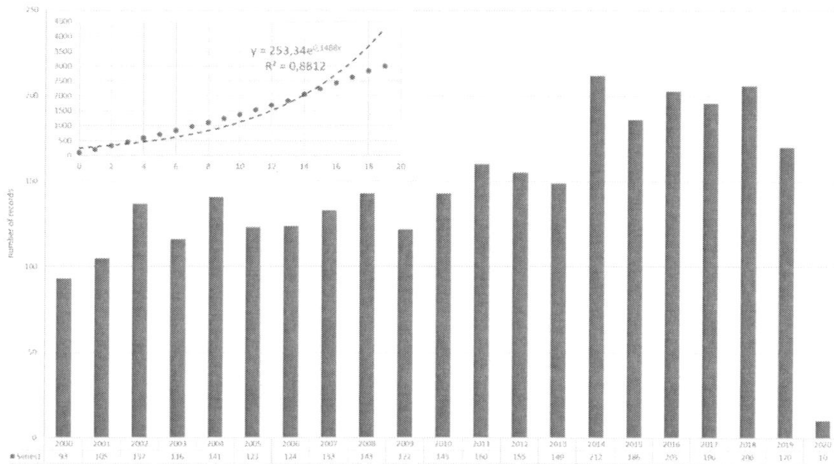

Source: Bibliometry Unit - CRAI-Library, Universidad Santo Tomás (Bucaramanga). Data based on Scopus information (Elsevier, 2020) and processed with VantagePoint software (*Search Technology*).

Figure 1. Scattering of science articles by number of records per year (2000-2020 timeline) correlating the main constituents of EO with hemisynthetic derivatives along with the growth rate of publications by De Solla Price law.

The most important knowledge areas of research/application (as interdisciplinary teamwork) on this topic were *Chemistry* (2442 records), *Pharmacology*, *Toxicology* and *Pharmaceutics* (1482 records), and *Biochemistry*, *Genetics* and *Molecular Biology* (1223 records). As well as, the top five (highest number of articles) of scientific Journals were Tetrahedron (139), Journal of Organic Chemistry (129), Tetrahedron Letters (128), Bioorganic and Medicinal Chemistry Letters (88) and Synlett (68). In addition, the register distribution by countries was mainly headed by China (674) followed by the USA (370), India (295), Japan (271), among others. If Latin America is taken into account, Brazil, Argentina, Colombia, Mexico and Chile, were the countries with highest register numbers, each one with 61, 39, 34, 21 and 13 registers, individually.

On the other hand, from the general search equation described in the first paragraph of this topic, a new more specific search equation was proposed in the Scopus database to correlate the main constituents of EO with compound derivatives: *(TITLE-ABS-KEY (anethole OR estragole OR eugenol OR safrole OR citral OR citronellal OR geraniol OR carvacrol) AND TITLE-ABS-KEY (tetrahydroquinoline OR isoindoloquinolinone OR dihydrobenzofuranol OR iridoid OR octahydroacridine OR trioxane OR oxirane OR benzochromene)) AND DOCTYPE (ar) AND PUBYEAR > 1999*. The evaluated timeline was ranged between 2000-2020.

The science behavior based on the indexed record number, according to the last search equation, is represented in Figure 2, in which a generalized growth trend can be observed, although with some variability/distribution in maximums and minimums. Therefore, 84 published articles were indexed during the observation window, and 2018 and 2019 were the years with the highest number of records (14 and 11, respectively). The growth rate of the publications, calculated with De Solla Price's law, was 16.4% per year (R^2 0.967).

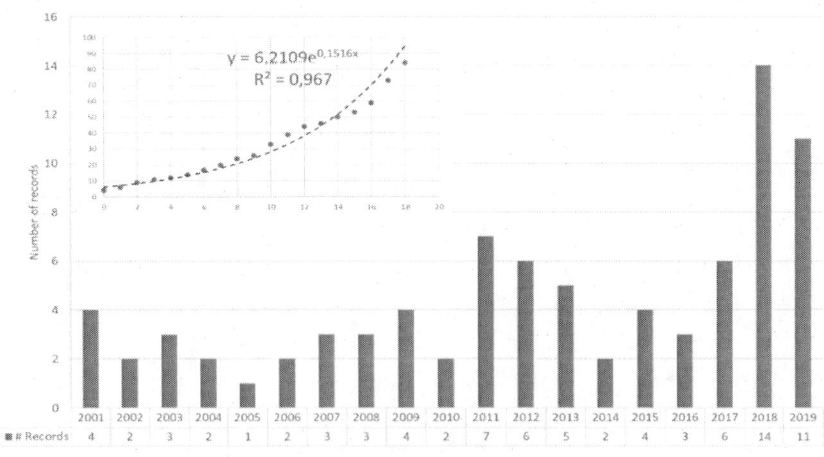

Source: Bibliometry Unit - CRAI-Library, Universidad Santo Tomás (Bucaramanga). Data based on Scopus information (Elsevier, 2020) and processed with VantagePoint software (*Search Technology*).

Figure 2. Distribution of science articles by number of registers per year (2000-2020 timeline) related to the use of essential oils as renewable reagents for fine synthesis; besides, the growth rate by De Solla Price law is included.

Some of the most important areas of research or application were *Biochemistry*, *Genetics* and *Molecular Biology* (48 registers), *Chemistry* (42 registers), and *Pharmacology*, *Toxicology* and *Pharmaceutics* (28 registers). Whilst among the Journals stood out Tetrahedron Letters (7 articles), Industrial Crops and Products/Insect Biochemistry and Molecular Biology (each one 4 articles), Organic Letters/Synthetic Communications (each one 3 articles), etc. When considering the distribution of publications by countries, in the first place is China (15) followed by India/USA (each one 11 registers), among others. At the Latin American level, Colombia (7) and Brazil (6) were between the 10 main countries in which the topic is studied.

As a deduction based on the scientometric measurement, the topic related to the essential oils and their main constituents, as renewable reagents for synthesis of heterocycle compounds, is still a relevant subject for the sciences of natural product and organic synthesis.

SOME PLANTS CONTAINING ESSENTIAL OILS RICH IN PHENYLPROPANOIDS/TERPENOIDS

The production of volatile mixtures such as essential oils (consisting of terpenoids and phenylpropanoids) from the secondary metabolism of some plants is well-kown. Many of them (EO and their components) fulfill different functions, f.i., reproductive or defense mechanisms (inter-/intraspecies attractants), as alerting or signaling of food sources. Furthermore, they have showed certain therapeutic (i) and non-therapeutic (ii) biological properties: (i) *external* - antiphlogistic/antiinflammatory, antiseptic/disinfectant, deodorant, etc.; *internal* - antinociceptive, antiinflammatory, anticancer, antimicrobial, antiviral, antispasmodic, antioxidant, sedative, carminative, expectorant, penetration-enhancer, etc.; (ii) antiseptic/disinfectant, absorption enhancer, preservative and spice, repellent/pesticide, toxic, etc [2-5].

Chemical and Biological Importance

Pursuant to the reviewed science literature, 11 plants were selected (star anise/aniseed, winter tarragon/Mexican tarragon, clove tree, sassafras, lemon grass, lemon balm, citronella grass, palm rose and Cuban oregano) which produce EO containing phenylpropanoids or terpenoids as the most abundant components [e.g., (*E*)-anetol (1), estragole (2), eugenol (3), (E)-isoeugenol (4), safrole (5), (*E*)-/(*Z*)-citral (6/7), (*R*)-/(*S*)-citronellal (8/9), (*E*)-/(*Z*)-geraniol (10/11) or carvacrol (12)]. These EO were associated with renewable chemical reagents for synthesis of particular heterocycle compounds. The location of these plants along with the plant parts producing EO, yields, chemical compositions (main constituents, including relative amounts) and demonstrated bioactivities are reported in Table 1.

According to this Table, the content of (*E*)-anethole, as well as the EO yield from star anise fruits of different locations, varied between 77-94% and 2-7.5%, in that order. Nonetheless, some EO from China did not contain (*E*)-anethole but foeniculin (48-50%) or anisole (71%) [134, 135]. Among the most significant biological properties determined for star anise EO could be mentioned: antimicrobial (against bacterium [*Escherichia coli* (0.5-5%, ϕ inh. 6-9 mm)] and fungi [*Alternaria alternate* (MIC/MFC 2.5 μL/mL), *A. solani* (IC_{50} 90 μg/mL), *Aspergillus parasiticus* (MIC 2 μL/mL; 73% inh. at 100 μg/mL), *A. flavus* (MIC 1 μL/mL; 83% inh. at 100 μg/mL), *Aureobasidium pullulans* (MIC/MFC 2.5 μL/mL), *Bipolaris maydis* (IC_{50} 70 μg/mL), *Candida albicans* (MIC/MFC 5 μL/mL), *Cladosporium cladosporioides* (MIC/MFC 2.5 μL/mL), *C. fulvium* (MIC/MFC 2.5/5 μL/mL), *Fusarium graminearum* (IC_{50} 80 μg/mL), *F. sporotrichioides* (MIC/MFC 5 μL/mL), *F. tricinctum* (MIC/MFC 5 μL/mL), *F. verticillioides* (89% inh. at 200 μg/mL), *Mucor mucedo* (MIC/MFC 5/10 μL/mL), *Phoma magdonaldii* (MIC/MFC 2.5/5 μL/mL), *Phomopsis helianthi* (MIC/MFC 2.5 μL/mL), *Pythium aphanidermatum* (IC_{50} 90 μg/mL), *Rhizoctonia solani* (IC_{50} 80 μg/mL) and *Trichphyton mentografites* (MIC/MFC 5/10 μL/mL)] strains), larvicidal [*Culex pipiens* (LC_{50}/LC_{90} 18/23 μg/mL)]/adulticidal [*Aedes aegypti* (KC_{50} 7.3 μg/$mg_{fem.}$ and LC_{50} 10.3 μg/$mg_{fem.}$)]/repellent [*Brevicoryne brassicae* (effect at 0.5%)]/fumigant [*Callosobruchus chinensis* (LC_{50} 7 μg/mL)] and antiproliferative [HCT116 (IC_{50} 50 ± 1 μg/mL)]. Lastly, the antimicrobial effectiveness of (*E*)-anethole isolated from star anise EO against yeast/fungi/bacterium strains (*Agrobacterium tumefaciens*, *Bacillus cereus*, *B. licheniformis*, *B. megatarium*, *B. subtilis*, *Escherichia coli*, *Helminthosporium oryzae*, *Macrophomina phaseolina*, *Myrothecium roridum*, *Penicillium cryogenum*, *Rhizobium leguminosarum*, *Saccharomyces cerevisiae*, *Sarcina lutea*, *Sclerotium rolfsii*, etc.) was verified by means of the MIC values, which were between 5-50 μg/mL [136].

Other EO rich in (*E*)-anethole come from the aerial parts/fruits/seeds of *P. anisum*; the content of (*E*)-anethole has been reported between 38-98%, and the EO yields varied among 0.5-3.9%. This plant and its EO did not have great variability in terms of the majority component. The main bioactivities of these EO were insecticidal [*C. quinquefasciatus* (LC_{50} 0.6-27 μL/mL, LC_{90} 1-34 μL/mL) and *Daphnia magna* (LC_{50} 31 μL/mL)]/larvicidal [*C. pipiens* (LC_{50}/LC_{90} 15/24 μg/mL)]/fumigant [*Lycoriella ingenua* (93% mortal. at 1.2 μL/mL)], antifungal [*A. alternate* (10-100 μg/mL, ϕ inh. 15 ± 1 - 20 ± 3 mm), *A. niger* (10-100 μg/mL, ϕ inh. 24 ± 3 - 38 ± 4 mm; 4.8 mg, 20.0 ± 0.5 - 40.0 ± 0.7 mm), *A. parasiticus* (10-100 μg/mL, ϕ inh. 8 ± 2 - 15 ± 2 mm), *Trichophyton rubrum* (4-16 μg/mL, ϕ inh. 20-38 mm), *Botrytis cinerea* (600 μL/mL, inh. radial growth <1 cm)], and anticancer [A549 (IC_{50} 334 μg/mL), HepG2 (EC_{50} 0.39 ± 0.03 mg/mL), Caco2 (EC_{50} 0.25 ± 0.04 mg/mL), MCF-7 (EC_{50} 0.30 ± 0.01 mg/mL) and THP-1 (EC_{50} 0.1100 ± 0.0007 mg/mL)].

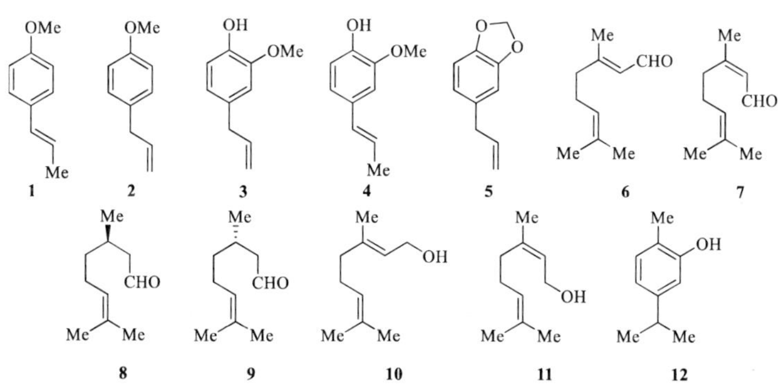

Table 1. General information (e.g., useful parts, yields, main constituents and bioproperties) on 11 selected plants that produce EO (as renewable resources) used as fine synthesis reagents

Species	Location	Useful part	Yield, %	Main constituent (relative amounts %)	Biological properties
I. verum	Brazil	Fruits	NR	(*E*)-Anethole (90)	Repellent [6]
					Antimicrobial [7]
			3.1		Larvicidal/adulticidal, anti-AChE [8]
	China		6.1	(*E*)-Anethole (77)	Antimicrobial [9]
			7.5	(*E*)-Anethole (90)	Antifungal [10]
	Colombia		2.0	(*E*)-Anethole (83)	Antioxidant [11]
	Egypt		NR		Antioxidant/antifungal, antimycotoxigenic [12]
	Greece		2.4	(*E*)-Anethole (86)	Larvicidal [13]
	India		NR	(*E*)-Anethole (94)	Antioxidant [14]
	Malaysia			(*E*)-Anethole (7)	Antioxidant/anticancer [15]
	Serbia			(*E*)-Anethole (91)	Antifungal [16]
	Vietnam				Fumigant [17]
P. anisum	Czech Republic	Seeds-Fruits	3.3	(*E*)-Anethole (81)	Insecticidal [18]
	Greece		1.2	(*E*)-Anethole (94)	Larvicidal [13]
			NR	(*E*)-Anethole (88)	Antifungal/cytotoxic [19]
	India		NR	(*E*)-Anethole (90)	Antioxidant [20]
	Iraq			(*E*)-Anethole (19)	Antifungal/cytotoxic [21]
	Korea			(*E*)-Anethole (90)	Fumigant [22]
	Iran			(*E*)-Anethole (91)	Antifungal [23, 24]
	Turkey		1.9	(*E*)-Anethole (94)	
		Aerial parts	2.1	(*E*)-Anethole (83)	Antimicrobial [25]
A. dracunculus	Canada		NR	Methyleugenol (36), terpinolene (19)	Antibacterial/antioxidant [26]
	China		0.7	Sabinene (19)	Antimicrobial [27]
	Egypt		1.0	Methyleugenol (73)	Antifungal [28]
	France		NR	Estragole (77)	AChE inhibition [29]
	Hungary			Estragole (77-83)	
	Iran			Estragole (76-83)	Antioxidant [30-32]
			NR	(*Z*)-Anethole (52)	
				Estragole (85)	
				(*E*)-Anethole (21), α-*trans*-ocimene (21)	Anticonvulsant [33]
				Estragole (68)	Larvicidal [34]
				Estragole (85)	Antibacterial [35]

Species	Location	Useful part	Yield, %	Main constituent (relative amounts %)	Biological properties
	Italy			Estragole (80-82)	AChE inhibition [29]
				(*E*)-Anethole (53)	Antibacterial [36]
	Poland			Methyleugenol (31), elemicin (27)	Larvicidal/antimicrobial [37]
	Russia		0.24	Sabinene (42)	Antioxidant [38]
	Turkey		NR	(*Z*)-Anethole (81)	Antimicrobial/antioxidant [39]
	USA			Estragole (89) [28]	AChE inhibition [29]
T. lucida	Colombia	Flower	0.5	Estragole (93)	Antioxidant [11]
		Leaves	0.9	Estragole (94)	
		Whole plant	0.4	Estragole (92)	Insecticidal [40]
		NR	NR	Estragole (94)	Cytotoxic/antiinflammatory (inhibitions NO/iNOS, PGE-2/COX-2, TNF-α) [41]
				Estragole (96)	Cytotoxic/antioxidant [42]
	Cuba		0.8	Estragole (97)	Antibacterial/antiparasitic, antioxidant [43]
	Mexico	Whole plant	NR	Estragole (36), methyleugenol (27)	Insecticidal/repellent [44]
		Aerial part	0.3	Estragole (49), (*E*)-anethole (36)	Antifungal [45]
S. aromaticum	Brazil	Buds	NR	Eugenol (62-69)	Antibacterial [46]
	Cameroon		4.1	Eugenol (60)	Antioxidant [47]
	Chad		1.9	β-Caryophyllene (44), eugenol (43)	Antibiotic [48]
	China		NR	Eugenol (87)	Antioxidative [49]
			1.5	Eugenol (77)	Larvicidal [50]
	Colombia		12	Eugenol (60)	Antioxidant [51]
	Croatia		NR	Eugenol (92)	Antioxidant [52, 53]
	Egypt		extract	Eugenol (72)	
			NR	Eugenol (80)	Antioxidant/antibacterial [54]
	India		NR	Eugenol (75)	Antifungal [55]
	Korea		NR	Geranial (28), neral/citronellal (21)	Antifungal [56]
	Malaysia		3.0	Eugenol (49)	Antibacterial [57]
	Mexico		2.7	Eugenol (75)	Antifungal [58]
	Nigeria		NR	Eugenol (80)	Larvicidal [59]
			21	Eugenol (75)	Antimicrobial [60]
	Pakistan		8.5	Eugenol (19)	Antidiabetic [61]
	Saudi Arabia		0.6	Eugenol (75), chavibetol (20)	Antifungal [16, 62-64]
	Serbia		NR	Eugenol (79)	
	Spain			Eugenol (89)	

Table 1. (Continued)

Species	Location	Useful part	Yield, %	Main constituent (relative amounts %)	Biological properties
	Sri Lanka			Eugenol (79)	
	Togo		14	Eugenol (83)	Antimicrobial [65, 66]
	Tunisie		NR	Eugenol (89)	
	UK			Eugenol (78)	Cytotoxic [67]
S. albidum	Serbia	NR		Safrole (82)	Antifungal [68]
C. citratus	Algeria	Leaves	0.6	Geranial/neral (42/32)	Antifungal/antiinflamm. [69]
	Benin		0.7	Geranial/neral (40/36)	Antiparasitic/cytotoxic [70]
			0.9	Geranial/neral (27/20), myrcene (28)	Analgesic/antiinflammatory [71]
	Brazil	NR	NR	Geranial/neral (43/33)	Cytotoxic [72]
		Leaves		Geranial/neral (44/34)	Repellent [6]
		NR		Geranial/neral (26/32)	Insecticidal, effect respir. rate, locomotory behavior [73]
		Leaves	0.4	Geranial/neral (41/36)	Anticonv./neurobehavior [74]
		NR	1.0	Geranial/neral (50/38)	Insecticidal [75]
		Leaves	0.3	Geranial/neral (25/60)	Antinociceptive [76]
			NR	Geranial/neral (43/32)	Hypotensive/vasorelaxant [77]
				Geranial/neral (53/36)	Insecticidal/larvicidal [78]
	Burkina Faso		1.5	Geranial/neral (48/35)	Antimicrobial [79]
			1.4	Geranial/neral (45/33)	Antioxidant [80]
	Cameroon	NR	0.8	Geranial/neral (38/21)	Antifungal [81]
	Colombia	Whole plant	0.5	Geranial/neral (26/29), myrcene (20)	Insecticidal [40]
			NR	Geranial/neral (34/28)	Repellent [82]
	Cuba	Leaves		Geranial/neral (51/35)	Insecticidal/larvicidal [78]
	Ethiopia		0.8	Geranial/neral (41/31)	Skin irritation/toxicity [83]
	France	Leaves	0.5	Geranial/neral (33/29)	Antiparasitic [84]
	India		NR	Geranial/neral (42/30)	Antidiabetic [85]
				Geranial/neral (29/18)	Insecticidal [86]
	Iran			Geranial/neral (39/31)	Antifungal [87, 88]
	Kenya	Whole plant	0.8	Geranial/neral (40/33)	
	Malaysia		0.3	Geranial/neral (45/30)	Antioxidant/cytotoxic, antiangiogenic [89]
	Netherlands	NR	NR	Geranial/neral (46/35)	Antifungal [90]
	Nigeria	Leaves	0.6	Geranial/neral (27/20), myrcene (28)	Antioxidant/antibacterial [91]
	Togo	Arial parts	1.6	Geranial/neral (45/32)	Cytotoxic [92]

Species	Location	Useful part	Yield, %	Main constituent (relative amounts %)	Biological properties
C. martinii	Brazil	NR	NR	Geraniol (81)	Anthelmintic [93]
		Whole plant	2.0	Geraniol (64), geranyl acetate (29)	Antibacterial [94]
			NR	Geraniol (58)	Cytotoxic/antiinflammat. [95]
	India	Leaves	0.2	Geraniol (61)	Antimicrobial [96]
	Taiwan	Leaves	0.7	Geraniol (52)	Antimicrobial/antioxidant, antiinflammatory [97]
	UK	NR	NR	Geraniol (65), geranyl acetate (20)	Antimicrobial [98]
C. nardus	Benin	Leaves	1.1	Citronellal (36), nerol (24)	Antiparasitic [70]
			NR	Citronellal (41), geraniol (23)	Analgesic [99]
	Brazil	NR	NR	Citronellal (28), citronellol (25), nerol (22)	Antimicrobial/cytotoxic [100]
	Colombia			Citronellal (31-42)	Toxic/antioxidant [42]
	Congo	Leaves	NR	Citronellal (38), geraniol (29)	Analgesic [99]
	France		1.4	Elemol (26), citronellal (13)	Antioxidant/antibacterial [101]
		NR	NR	Citronellal (42), geraniol (21)	Antifungal [102]
	India	Leaves	3	Geranial/neral (39/31)	Antimicrobial [103, 104]
	Malaysia	Whole plant		Citronellal (30)	
		Leaves	NR	Citronellal (33), geraniol (24)	Toxic/antitermite/repellent [105]
	Thailand	Aerial parts	0.1	Geraniol (36), geranial (23)	Antifungal [106]
	Togo		1.3	Citronellal (36), geraniol (28)	Cytotoxic [92]
M. officinalis	Argelia	Leaves	0.3	Geranial/neral (44/30)	Antimicrobial [107]
	Brazil		1.0	Geranial/neral (47/39)	Antitumoral/antioxidant [108]
	Germany	NR	NR	Geranial/neral (20/14)	Antiviral [109]
				β-Caryophyllene (24), geranial/neral (20/15)	Antibacterial/cytotoxic [110]
	Greece	Aerial parts	0.2	Terpinen-4-ol (16), caryophyllene oxide/sabinene (13)	Larvicidal [111]
	Iran		0.1	Geranial/neral (35/24)	Antispasmodic [112]
	Korea	Leaves	NR	Geranial/neral (65/25)	Antidiabetic [113]

Table 1. (Continued)

Species	Location	Useful part	Yield, %	Main constituent (relative amounts %)	Biological properties
	Morocco		0.5	Nerol (30), citral (27), isopulegol (22)	Antiinflammatory [114]
		Aerial parts	1	*p*-Mentha-1,2,3-triol (13)	Antifungal [115]
	Serbia		0.09	Geranial/neral (24/18), citronellal (21-22)	Toxicity [116]
			0.2	Geranial/neral (23/16) citronellal (14)	Antimicrobial/antioxidant [117]
	Turkey		NR	β-Cubebene (15), β-caryophyllene (14)	Antiviral [118]
P. amboinicus	Brazil	Leaves	0.1	Carvacrol (89)	Allelophatic [119]
			NR	Carvacrol (90-98)	Antibacterial [120-122]
			0.2	Germacrene D (39), β-caryophyllene (19)	
		Leaves stem	0.07	Carvacrol (88)	
		Leaves	0.01	Thymol (64)	Antimicrobial [123, 124]
			0.1	Carvacrol (38)	
	Colombia		0.1	Carvacrol (54)	Antioxidant [11]
	India		0.2	Carvacrol (29), thymol (22)	Larvicidal [125]
			NR	Carvacrol (70)	Antifungal/antioxidant [126]
				Carvacrol/thymol (NR)	Chemopreventive [127]
	Malaysia	Whole plant	0.2	3-Carene (21), carvacrol (19), camphor (18)	Antimicrobial [128]
	Marocco	Leaves	1.2	Carvacrol (23), camphor (22)	Antibacterial [129, 130]
	Philippines		0.04	Carvacrol (51)	
	Taiwan	Whole plant	0.6	Carvacrol (62)	Larvicidal [131]
	Venezuela		0.05	Carvacrol (65)	Antibacterial [132]
	Yemen		1.4-1.6	Thymol (37-79)	Antibacterial/antioxidant [133]

NR - not reported.

For its part, EO from *A. dracunculus* presented a certain chemical variability, i.e., they were rich in estragole (68-89%), (*E*)-anethole (21-53%), (*Z*)-anethole (52-81%), methyleugenol (25-76%) or sabinene (19-

42%). In addition, EO yields were found between 0.01-1%. Astonishing activities such as antimicrobial [*Acinetobacter* spp. (0.6-1.2 mg/disk, ϕ inh. 7-11 mm), *A. niger* (ϕ inh. 13 ± 1 mm), *B. subtilis* (10 μg/mL, ϕ inh. 13.6 ± 0.1 mm), *C. albicans* (ϕ inh. 10.0 ± 0.7 mm), *Cryptococcus neoformans* (ϕ inh. 13 ± 1 mm), *E. coli* (ϕ inh. 8 mm), *Fonsecaea pedrosoi* (ϕ inh. 15 ± 1 mm), *Klebsiella pneumoniae* (10 μg/mL, ϕ inh. 11.00 ± 0.09 mm; 0.6-1.2 mg/disk, ϕ inh. 7-8 mm), *K. oxytoca* (MIC 7.8 mg/mL), *Listeria monocytogenes* (MIC 15.6 mg/mL), *Micrococcus luteus* (10 μg/mL, ϕ inh. 10.6 ± 0.2 mm), *Microsporum canis* (ϕ inh. 15 ± 1 mm), *M. gypseum* (ϕ inh. 16 ± 1 mm), *Proteus vulgaris* (0.6-1.2 mg/disk, ϕ inh. 7-15 mm), *Pseudomonas aeruginosa* (10 μg/mL, ϕ inh. 10.5 ± 0.2 mm; 0.6-1.2 mg/disk, ϕ inh. 7-13 mm), *P. syringae* (0.6-1.2 mg/disk, ϕ inh. 7-15 mm), *Salmonella paratyphi* (10 μg/mL, ϕ inh. 13.0 ± 0.1 mm), *S. typhimurium* (0.6-1.2 mg/disk, ϕ inh. 7-9 mm), *Serratia marcescens* (MIC/MBC 3.8/7.8 mg/mL), *Shigella dysenteriae* (MIC/MBC 3.8/7.8 mg/mL), *S. cerevisiae* (10 μg/mL, ϕ inh. 12.3 ± 0.1 mm), *Staphylococcus aureus* (10 μg/mL, ϕ inh. 10.0 ± 0.1 mm; 1-4 μl/disk, 20 ± 1 - 35 ± 2 mm), *S. aureus* MRSA (ϕ inh. 10 mm), *S. epidermidis* (ϕ inh. 10.0 ± 0.7 mm), *T. rubrum* (ϕ inh. 20 ± 2 mm), *Vibrio* spp. (0.6-1.2 mg/disk, ϕ inh. 7 mm), *Xanthomonas axanopodas* (0.6-1.2 mg/disk, ϕ inh. 8-14 mm)], AChE inhibition [IC_{50} 0.06 ± 0.03 - 1.9 ± 0.1 mg/mL], anticonvulsant/sedative [(ED_{50} 0.84 mL/kg (MES) and 0.26 mL/kg (PEM)] and larvicidal [*Anopheles stephensi* (LC_{50}/LC_{90} 11/18 μg/mL)] were reported for these EO. It is worth noting that in the Indian EO was identified capillene (56%) as main constituent [137]; as well as other terpenes (from Russia and USA) have been reported such as β-pinene (24-32%) and terpinolene (25%) [138, 139].

A Latin American source of estragole is *T. lucida* (both leaves and flowers); their EO have contained it between 36-97%. Into the bargain, the EO yields have been relatively moderate (0.3-0.9%). Among the biological properties could be highlighted insecticidal [*A. aegypti* (LC_{50}/LC_{90} 65-66/94-95 μg/mL)]/repellent [*Diaphorina citri* (20-40 mg/mL, 45-99% repellency)], cytotoxic, anti-inflammatory (0.2 mg/mL, 100% inh. production of prostaglandins E_2, production of $NO^{\cdot}$ > 100%, cytokine TNF-α production > 2000 pg/mL), antiparasitic [*Plasmodium berghei* (IC_{50} 72 ± 4 μg/mL)] and antimicrobial [*A. niger* (2%, 27% mycelial red., ϕ inh. 6.6 ± 0.6 mm), *F. oxysporum* (2%, 48% mycelial red., ϕ inh. 4.7 ± 0.2 mm), *Penicillium janthinellum* (2%, 24% mycelial red., ϕ inh. 6.8 ± 0.6 mm), *R. solani* (2%, 57% mycelial red., ϕ inh. 3.9 ± 0.6 mm)].

Regarding clove (*S. aromaticum*), these plant/EO are well-known and widely distributed in the world; and, eugenol (its main molecule) is a *quasi*-biomarker for this species. The relative amounts of eugenol in the EO have varied amid 19-92% and the percentage yields of EO were ranged between 0.6-14%. Aside from the wide distribution of clove, eugenol and EO that contain it are powerful antimicrobials [*Actinomyces* spp. (MIC/MBC 30-40/100 μL/L), *Aeromonas* spp. (MIC 0.015-0.031 μg/mL), *A. alternate* (MIC/MFC 0.25 μL/mL), *A. flavus* (MIC 1 μL/mL; MIC/MFC 1/2.5 μL/mL), *A. niger* (MIC/MFC 0.5 μL/mL), *A. ochraceus* (MIC/MFC 1 μL/mL), *A. pullulans* (MIC/MFC 0.25 μL/mL), *A. terreus* (MIC/MFC 2.5 μL/mL), *A. versicolor* (MIC/MFC 0.5/1 μL/mL), *B. cereus* (MIC 2.5 mg/mL), *B. megaterium* (MIC 2.2 mg/mL), *B. subtilis* (MIC 2.8 mg/mL), *Botrytis cinerea* (MIC 93 μL/L), *C. albicans* (MIC 1 μL/mL; MIC/MFC 1.25-2.5/2.5-5.0 μL/mL; MIC/MFC 0.5/1 μL/mL), *Citrobacter freundii* (MIC 0.015 μg/mL), *C. cladosporioides* (MIC/MFC 0.1/0.25 μL/mL), *C. fulvium* (MIC/MFC 0.1 μL/mL), *Colletotrichum musae* (MIC/MLC 0.04/0.065%), *Edwardsiella* spp. (MIC 0.015-0.062 μg/mL), *Enterococcus faecalis* (MIC 1 mg/mL; MIC 2.4 mg/mL), *E. coli* (MIC 1 mg/mL; MIC 2-2.3 mg/mL; MIC 5 μL/mL), *F. gramineareum* (300 μg/mL), *F. proliferatum* (MIC/MLC 0.05/0.1%), *F. oxysporum* (IC_{50} 18 μg/mL), *F. sporotrichioides* (MIC/MFC 0.5/1 μL/mL), *F. tricinctum* (MIC/MFC 0.25/1 μL/mL), *Lactobacillus* spp. (MIC/MBC 60/120 μL/L), *Lasiodiplodia theobromae* (MIC/MLC 0.045/0.06%), *L. monocytogenes* (MIC 1.4 mg/mL), *M. mucedo* (MIC/MFC 0.25 μL/mL), *Penicillium* spp. (MIC 1 μL/mL; MIC/MFC 0.5 μL/mL), *P. helianthi* (MIC/MFC 0.1/0.25 μL/mL), *P. magdonaldii* (MIC/MFC 0.25 μL/mL), *P. aeruginosa* (MIC 2.2 mg/mL; MIC 0.015 μg/mL; MIC 9 μL/mL), *S. typhimurium* (MIC 3.6 mg/mL), *S. typhi* (MIC 3.2 mg/mL; MIC 625 μg/mL), *S. enteritidis* (MIC 625 μg/mL), *S. aureus* (MIC 4-10 mg/mL; MIC 1.5 mg/mL; MIC 625 μg/mL; MIC 5 μL/mL), *S.*

warneri (MIC 2.7 mg/mL), *Streptococcus* spp. (MIC 0.015-0.062 μg/mL; MIC/MBC 30/60-80 μL/L), *Trichoderma viride* (MIC/MFC 2.5 μL/mL), *T. mentografites* (MIC/MFC 0.5 μL/mL), *Vibrio* spp. (MIC 0.015 μg/mL)] and antioxidants [DPPH· (509 ± 5 μmol/g; 12.5 μg/mL, % inh. > 80), $ABTS^{+\cdot}$ (IC_{50} 8.5 μg/mL; TAA 11900 ± 164 mmol Trolox®/kg EO), $O_2^{-\cdot}$ (IC_{50} 58 μg/mL)]; other remarkable biological effects were larvicidal [*A. aegypti* (LC_{50}/LC_{95} 125/180 μg/mL; LC_{50} 93 μg/mL) and *C. quinquefasciatus* (LC_{50} 124 μg/mL)], antidiabetic (IC_{50} 74 μg/mL) and cytotoxic [HMEC-1 (LC_{50} 0.018%), HNDF (LC_{50} 0.025%) and 153BR (LC_{50} 0.017%)].

On the other hand, the antimicrobial efficacy of sassafras EO was demonstrated on 17 strains [*A. alternate* (MIC/MFC 5-10/10 μL/mL), *A. flavus* (MIC/MFC 15 μL/mL), *A. niger* (MIC/MFC 15 μL/mL), *A. ochraceus* (MIC/MFC 15/25 μL/mL), *A. pullulans* (MIC/MFC 5-10/25 μL/mL), *A. terreus* (MIC/MFC 10-25/30 μL/mL), *A. versicolor* (MIC/MFC 10-25/25 μL/mL), *C. cladosporioides* (MIC/MFC 5-10/15 μL/mL), *C. fulvium* (MIC/MFC 5-10/10 μL/mL), *F. sporotrichoides* (MIC/MFC 10-25/25 μL/mL), *F. tricinctum* (MIC/MFC 10/25 μL/mL), *M. mucedo* (MIC/MFC 5-10/15 μL/mL), *Penicillium funiculosum* (MIC/MFC 10-25/25 μL/mL), *P. helianthi* (MIC/MFC 5/10 μL/mL), *P. magdonaldii* (MIC/MFC 5-10/10 μL/mL), *Penicillium ochrochloron* (MIC 15-25/25 μg/mL) and *T. viride* (MIC/MFC 10-25/30 μL/mL)].

In line with description made above for clove and EO/eugenol, in a similar way, lemongrass (*C. citratus*), its EO and the terpenoids citral A (geranial)/citral B (neral) (*quasi*-biomarkers for this species) are also broadly distributed and recognized. The relative amounts of geranial and neral found in these EO were 25-53% and 20-60%, respectively, with EO yields of 0.2-1.5%. The promising bioproperties attested were antimicrobial [*A. flavus* (20-60 μL, ϕ inh. 60-90 mm; MIC 118 mg/mL), *A. fumigatus* (20-60 μL, ϕ inh. 50-90 mm; MIC 59 mg/mL), *A. niger* (20-60 μL, ϕ inh. 25-90 mm; MIC 15 mg/mL), *A. ochraceus* (MIC 59 mg/mL), *A. parasiticus* (MIC 59 mg/mL), *A. terreus* (20-60 μL, ϕ inh. 65-90 mm), *C. albicans* (20-60 μL, ϕ inh. 33-90 mm), *C. parapsilosis* (20-60 μL, ϕ inh. 15-90 mm), *C. tropicalis* (20-60 μL, ϕ inh. 36-90 mm; MIC/MFC 1-4 μL/mL), *E. aerogenes* (MIC 13.3 ± 0.4 mg/mL), *E. coli* (MIC 10 mg/mL), *E. faecalis* (MIC 1 mg/mL),

L. monocytogenes (MIC 8.3 ± 0.2 mg/mL), *Mucro* sp. (20-60 μL, ϕ inh. 35-48 mm), *Penicillium* sp. (20-60 μL, ϕ inh. 90 mm), *P. expansum* (1000 μg/mL, NDR cfu/mL 0.36 ± 0.04 - 0.48 ± 0.03), *Phytophthora capsici* (30 μg/mL, GI > 60%), *P. drechsleri* (80 μg/mL, GI > 60%), *P. melonis* (44 μg/mL, GI > 60%), *Shigella sonnei* (IC_{50} 1.6%), *S. aureus* (MIC 2.5 mg/mL), *S. dysenteria* (MIC 8.3 ± 0.2 mg/mL), *S. enterica* (MIC 2.1 ± 0.1 mg/mL), *S. typhimurium* (MIC 2.5 mg/mL)], antiparasitic [*Trypanosoma brucei brucei* (IC_{50} 1.8 ± 0.1 μg/mL), *Plasmodium falciparum* chloroquine-sensitive (IC_{50} 48 ± 13 μg/mL); *P. berghei* (200-500 mg/kg, 62-87% suppression)], cytotoxic [CHO (IC_{50} 10.6 ± 0.7 μg/mL), WI38 (IC_{50} 40 ± 3 μg/mL), HaCat (39-66 μg/mL; IC_{50} 150 μL/mL), LDH (130-138 μg/mL); MCF-7 (IC_{50} 47 μg/mL), HCT-16 (IC_{50} 32 μg/mL)], analgesic (2-3 g/kg, tail-flick test (staying period): 6 ± 1 - 8 ± 2 s; reduction number of cramps 39 ± 3 - 30 ± 2), antiinflammatory [40-200 μL, 2.7 ± 0.1 - 2.88 ± 0.01 mm of left hind paw thickness (% inh. 67-97%); 2-3 g/kg, reduction edema volume (37.0 ± 0.3)], anticonvulsant [0.5-1 g/kg, not convulsive/anxiolytic on mice], antinociceptive [50-100 mg/kg, 50-80% increased reaction time; 10-50 mg/kg, produced 46-70% inh. (formalin test)], antiangiogenic (IC_{50} 52 μg/mL), antidiabetic [400-800 mg, 29-47% decrease glucose, 22-24% decrease insulin], and insecticidal [*Podisus nigrispinus* (1st-5th instar, LD_{50}/LD_{90} 1-139/2-192 μg/insect); *Frankliniella schultzei* (LC_{50} 1.5%), *Myzus persicae* (LC_{50} 0.3%); *A. aegypti* (LC_{50}/LC_{90} 94-123/163-243 μg/mL)]/repellent [*Brevicoryne brassicae* (0.01-0.1%, 5 ± 2 - 2 ± 2 aphids, 24-48 h); *Tribolium castaneum* (RD_{50} 0.016-0.021)]/larvicidal [*Musca domestica* (LC_{50}/LC_{90} 3-4/92-83%); *M. domestica* (LC_{50}/LC_{90} 0.4-5/1-10 $\mu L/cm^2$)].

Other species belonging to the genus *Cymbopogon* is *C. martinii*, whose chemical composition has been mainly characterized by geraniol (52-81%), and with EO yields that varied between 0.2-2.0%. The EO from species have demonstrated biological effects such as anthelmintic [*Haemonchus contortus*/*Trichostrogylus* spp. (LC_{50}/LC_{99} 30-150/170-610 μg/mL larval instar)], antimicrobial [*C. albicans* (MIC 2.4 μg/mL), *E. coli* (MIC 100-900 μg/mL; MIC 1.54 ± 0.07 μg/mL), *Pityrosporum ovale* (MIC 1.20 ± 0.07

μg/mL), *Propionibacterium acnes* (MIC 0.91 ± 0.07 μg/mL), *S. aureus* (MIC 1.04 ± 0.07 μg/mL), *Saccharomyces cerevisiae* (5 μL, 85% growth inh.)], antiinflammatory [5 μg/mL, stimulated production of TNF-α level; 5-lipoxygenase inh. (IC_{50} 1.50 ± 0.04 μg/mL)], and antioxidant [DPPH· (IC_{50} 51 ± 1 μg/mL), NO· (IC_{50} 56.9 ± 0.4 μg/mL), β-carotene/linoleic acid (IC_{50} 0.99 ± 0.03 μg/mL)].

The EO from *C. nardus* species contained mainly citronellal (13-42%) along with other terpene alcohols [geraniol (11-36%), nerol (22-24%), citronellol] and aldehydes (geranial/neral); the EO yields ranged among 0.1-3%. These EO also had biological effectiveness as antiparasitic [*T. brucei brucei* (IC_{50} 8 ± 1 μg/mL), *P. falciparum* chloroquine-sensitive (IC_{50} 53 ± 5 μg/mL)], analgesic [acetic acid-induced writhing test (2 mL/kg, 37-51% inh.)], antimicrobial [*Aeromonas* spp. (MIC 0.5-1 μg/mL), *A. candidus* (250 μg/mL, 100% inh.), *A. flavus* (250 μg/mL, 100% inh.), *A. niger* (MIC 400 μg/mL), *B. subtilis* (MIC 0.5 μg/mL), *A. versicolor* (250 μg/mL, 100% inh.), *C. albicans* (5x-10x MBC/MFC, 30-47% red.; MIC 25 μg/mL), *C. glabrata* (MIC 50 μg/mL), *C. tropicalis* (MIC 50 μg/mL), *C. freundii* (MIC 0.2 μg/mL), *Edwardsiella* spp. (MIC 0.2-1 μg/mL), *E. faecalis* (MIC 0.5 μg/mL), *E. coli* (MIC 0.2-0.5 μg/mL), *Eurotium amstelodami* (250 μg/mL, 100% inh.), *E. chevalieri* (250 μg/mL, 100% inh.), *Flavobacterium* spp. (MIC 1 μg/mL), *L. monocytones* (MIC 0.7 μg/mL), *Penicillium adametzii* (250 μg/mL, 100% inh.), *P. citrinum* (250 μg/mL, 100% inh.), *P. griseofulvum* (250 μg/mL, 100% inh.), *P. islandicum* (250 μg/mL, 100% inh.), *Pseudomonas* spp. (MIC 0.2 μg/mL), *P. aeruginosa* (MIC 0.2 μg/mL), *Salmonella* spp. (MIC 0.2-0.5 μg/mL), *S. typhinurium* (MIC 6 μg/mL), *S. agona* (MIC 8 μg/mL), *S. aureus* (5x-10x MBC/MFC, 23-40% red.; MIC 0.7 μg/mL), *S. epidermidis* (MIC 3 μg/mL), *Streptococcus* spp. (MIC 0.5 μg/mL), *S. agalactiae* (MIC 0.2 μg/mL), *Vibrio* spp. (MIC 0.2-0.5 μg/mL), *Yersinia enterocolitica* (MIC 0.5 μg/mL)], cytotoxic [HaCat (12.5%, 40% cell viability; IC_{50} 450 μL/mL)]/toxic [*Artemia salina* (LC_{50} (24/48 h) 12-20/5-12 μg/mL)], insecticidal [*Coptotermes curvignathus* (LC_{50} 4%)]/repellent [*C. curvignathus* (4%, 59% repellency)], and antioxidant [ORAC (13645 ± 1168 μmol TE/g dew, 190 ± 25 μmol TE/g dmw), and TBARS (CE_{50} 310-860 μg/mL)].

In reference to the EO from lemon balm (*M. officinalis*), its chemical compositions were also represented by terpene aldehydes, geranial (20-65%) and neral (14-39%), and some minor variability in the terpene chemistry (e.g., terpinen-4-ol, nerol, mentha-1,2,3-triol, β-caryophyllene, β-cubebene) and yields (0.09-1%). Their significant bioactivities were: antimicrobial [*B. subtilis* (MIC 2 μL/mL; 20-50%, ϕ inh. 28 ± 2 - 29.6 ± 0.9 mm), *B. cinerea* (2 μL/mL, 77 ± 2% growth inh.), *C. albicans* (MIC 3 μL/mL; MIC/MFC 30/60 μL), *Epidermophyton floccosum* (MIC/MFC 30/60 μL), *E. coli* (MIC 2 μL/mL; 20-50%, ϕ inh. 14.8 ± 0.8 - 40 ± 1 mm), *F. oxysporum albedinis* (MIC 2 μL/mL), *F. oxysporum lini* (MIC 1 μL/mL), *Haemophilus influenzae* (MIC/MBC 0.02/0.03%), *K. pneumoniae* (MIC 3 μL/mL), *L. monocytogenes* (MIC 2 μL/mL), MRSA (MIC/MBC 0.1%), *M. canis* (MIC/MFC 30 μL), *Micrococcus flavus* (20-50%, ϕ inh. 27.4 ± 0.9 - 30 ± 0 mm), *Moraxella catarrhalis* (MIC/MBC 0.02-0.03/0.02%), *Mucor ramannianus* (MIC 1 μL/mL), *P. expansum* (1 μL/mL, 100% growth inh.), *P. aeruginosa* (MIC 2 μL/mL; 20-50%, ϕ inh. 13.4 ± 0.9 - 15.6 ± 0.6 mm), *Rhizopus stolonifer* (2 μL/mL, 100% growth inh.), *S. cerevisiae* (MIC 2 μL/mL), *S. enterica* (MIC 5 μL/mL), *S. enteritidis* (20-50%, ϕ inh. 15.2 ± 0.4 - 16.2 ± 0.8 mm), *Sarcina lutea* (20-50%, ϕ inh. 25 ± 2 - 27 ± 1 mm), *S. aureus* (MIC 3 μL/mL; MIC/MBC 0.1%; 20-50%, ϕ inh. 19.4 ± 0.9 - 24 ± 1 mm), *S. epidermidis* (20-50%, ϕ inh. 18 ± 2 - 27 ± 2 mm), *Streptococcus pyogenes* (MIC/MBC 0.06%), *S. pneumoniae* (MIC/MBC 0.03/0.06%), *S. sonei* (20-50%, ϕ inh. 37 ± 2 - 38 ± 2 mm), *S. typhi* (20-50%, ϕ inh. 19.8 ± 0.4 - 24.4 ± 0.9 mm), *T. mentagrophytes* var. *mentagrophytes* (MIC/MFC 15/30 μL), *T. rubrum* (MIC/MFC 15/30 μL), *T. tonsurans* (MIC/MFC 15 μL)], antitumoral [A549 (0.05%, >90% inh), MCF-7 (0.05%, >90% inh), Caco-2 (0.05%, >80% inh), HL-60 (0.01%, 80% inh.), K562 (0.01%, 94% inh.), HaCat (CC_{50} 0.01-0.002%), HEp-2 (>100 μg/mL, toxic), B16F10 (0.01%, >60% inh), BEAS-2B (CC_{50} 0.04-0.001%)], antiviral [HSV-1/HSV-2 (IC_{50} 0.0004/0.00008%); HSV-2 (1-100TCD_{50} 78-23% decr. infectivity)], larvicidal (*C. pipiens*, LC_{50}/LC_{90} 61/87 μg/mL), antispasmodic (ileum contraction of rats, IC_{50} 19 ± 2 ng/mL), antihyperglycaemic (250 mg/kg o.a., decreasing blood glucose levels and increasing serum insulin levels), antiinflammatory (200-400 mg/kg p.o., 62-71/65-77% inh.

inflammation induced by carrageenan), toxicity [*A. salina* (LC_{50} 39 μg/mL), BALB/c mice (LD_{50} 2.6 g/kg)], and antioxidant [DPPH· (EC_{50} 2 μL; IC_{50} 7.6 μg/mL)].

Finally, the essential oils from *P. amboinicus* consisted predominantly of carvacrol (19-98%) and in some cases, by its structural isomer thymol (22-79%). These EO had relatively low yields (0.04-1.6%) and the noteworthy biological effects were allelopathic [*Lactuca sativa* (0.12%, 0% germination), *Sorghum bicolor* (0.12%, 23% germination)], cytotoxic [B16F-10 (5-50 μg, 27-65% cell death)], antimicrobial [*Aeromonas caviae* (10%, ϕ inh. 17.5 ± 0.7 mm), *A. flavus* (10 μL, 55% inh. mycelial growth), *A. niger* (10%, ϕ inh. 17.3 ± 0.6 mm; 10 μL, 64% inh. mycelial growth), *A. ochraceus* (10 μL, 60% inh. mycelial growth), *C. albicans* (MIC 80 μg/mL; MIC 12 mg/mL), *C. gattii* (MIC 30 μg/mL), *C. tropicalis* (MIC 6 mg/mL), *C. versatilis* (10 μL, 43% inh. mycelial growth), *C. neoformans* (MIC 10 μg/mL), *E. coli* (MIC 128 μg/mL; MIC 780 μg/mL; MIC 0.2%; MIC/MBC 1/2%; MIC 10 μg/mL; 10 μL, ϕ inh. 3.8 ± 0.2 - 22.7 ± 0.7 mm), *E. faecalis* (MIC/MBC 0.5/1%; MIC 30 μg/mL), *F. oxysporum* (10 μL, 55% inh. mycelial growth), *K. pneumoniae* (MIC/MCB 0.09 ± 0.01%; MIC 10 μg/mL), MRSA (MIC 6 mg/mL; MIC/MBC 2%), *Penicillium* sp. (10 μL, 60% inh. mycelial growth), *P. aeruginosa* (MIC/MBC 0.5/1%; 10 μL, ϕ inh. 15.4 ± 0.3 - 36 ± 1 mm), *P. vulgaris* (10%, ϕ inh. 24.5 ± 0.7 mm; MIC 6 mg/mL), *S. cerevisae* (MIC 20 μg/mL), *S. aureus* (MIC/MBC 0.25-0.5/1-2 mg/mL; 10%, ϕ inh. 25.5 ± 0.7 mm; MIC 12 mg/mL; MIC 0.1%; MIC/MBC 0.06%; MIC 20 μg/mL; 10 μL, ϕ inh. 21.6 ± 0.8 - 26.1 ± 0.3 mm), *S. cerevisiae* (10 μL, 45% inh. mycelial growth), *S. epidermidis* (MIC 31 μg/mL; MIC 25 mg/mL; MIC/MBC 0.03/0.1%), *Streptococcus pyogens* (10 μL, ϕ inh. 13.2 ± 0.4 - 28.3 ± 0.4 mm), *S. typhi* (MIC 10 μg/mL)], antioxidant [$ABTS^{+\cdot}$ (TAA 4800 ± 198 mmol Trolox®/kg), DPPH· (200 μg/mL, 88% inh.; 10-100 μg/mL, 41.1 ± 0.4 - 89.4 ± 0.8% inh.)], and larvicidal [*Anopheles stephensi* (LC_{50}/LC_{90} 28-34/59-70 μg/mL), *A. albopictus* (LC_{50}/LC_{90} 52-64/80-104 μg/mL), *A. aegypti* (LC_{50}/LC_{90} 43-45/62-64 μg/mL), *C. quinquefasciatus* (LC_{50}/LC_{90} 23/38-39 μg/mL)].

Renewable Starting Materials for Different Chemical Synthesis

Throughout the ages, humans have relied on natural products from plants. Nonetheless, chemists have studied plants to find new molecules, which could be useful for practical applications. During this long and hard process, numerous natural products were isolated and characterized for the first time, and subsequently applied to human needs, especially medicine [140]; thus, natural products and their related moieties have been an extraordinary source of therapeutic agents. However, research of natural products in the pharmaceutical industry has declined in the last 5-10 years, but despite this fact, natural products remain a predominant source of novel leading drugs [141].

Currently, other "urgent" guideline of modern chemistry that has caught the researchers' attention is the use of biomass (and in an ecological way), which is not only a source of food, medicines, fragrances and energy, but also of fine chemicals [142]. Interest in the value chain of biomass-to-chemicals increased as the chemical industry accelerated the development of sustainable manufacturing processes; this is mainly due to the requirement to decrease society's dependence on crude oil. In effect, some easily isolated biomass components are now used as chemical reagents in the synthesis of novel products with higher added value, replacing chemical substances based on petroleum source. For instance, ethanol, furans, glycerol, lactic acid, succinic acid, hydroxypropionic acid/aldehyde, levulinic acid, sorbitol and xylitol are all important platform molecules or building blocks for the synthesis of bio-based chemicals [143]. In contrast to the vast vegetable components such as carbohydrates, proteins, fats and some terpenoids, the EO, which are natural products of the secondary metabolism of "aromatic" plants, were poorly explored in this context [143, 144].

Even with the diverse bio-medical applications, EO could also be appropriate materials to be utilized as suitable/particular chemical agents. Being terpenic and/or phenolic in nature with additional functional groups, the constituents of essential oils appear as attractive renewable precursors in the construction of new and varied molecules with novel structural/skeletal diversity and greater added value (pharmacological, biological, physical properties) [145, 146].

FINE SYNTHESIS OF HETEROCYCLES

Some of the essential oils mentioned above (e.g., star anise and clove essential oils) are considered suitable sources of raw-material for heterocyclic synthesis [147, 148]. The olefinic nature of the main components of these EO allows its use in the construction of diverse heterocyclic ring systems, which are common scaffolds of numerous natural products, e.g., alkaloid or phenol metabolites/groups.

The significance of heterocycles is very complex to explain; they are of immense biological and industrial importance, and overriding for the functioning of any developed human society. Most biologically active pharmaceutical and agrochemical products are heterocyclic, as are countless additives and modifiers used in industries as varied as cosmetics, reprography, information storage, and plastics [149].

Tetrahydroquinolines

Quinolines and tetrahydroquinolines are important ubiquitous structural motifs in biologically active natural products and pharmacologically relevant therapeutic agents due to their broad spectrum of activities, which include antiparasitic, antibiotic, antifungal, antiviral, antioxidant, anti-tuberculous, anticancer, inter alia [150-152].

Taking into consideration this information, the Kouznetsov´s group has demonstrated for the first time the synthetic applicability of star anise and clove bud EO for these heterocycles. First, a three-component condensation ([4+2] cycloaddition reaction) starting from anise EO (Route a) or star anise fruit under $scCO_2$ conditions (Route b), i.e., (*E*)-anethole (1), anilines (13), and benzaldehydes (14) in the presence of a Lewis acid catalyst ($BF_3·OEt_2$) produced polyfuncionalized *cis*-2,4-diaryl-3-methyl-tetrahydroquinolines (15) in a very simple and efficient manner [153] (Figure 3).

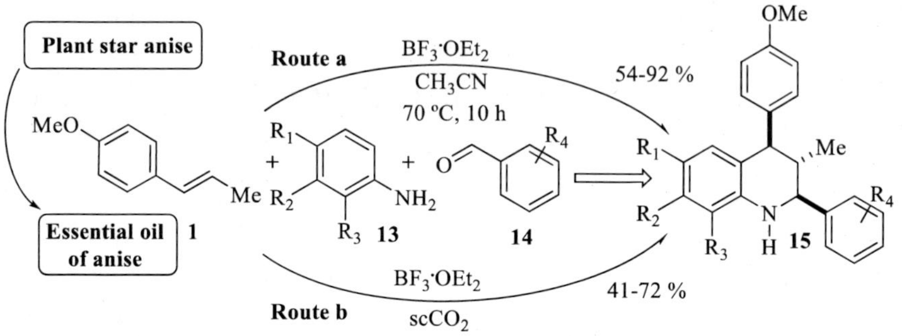

Figure 3. Chemical transformations of star anise EO towards new 2,4-diaryl-3-methyl-tetrahydroquinolines, interesting rigid molecules in pharmacological studies.

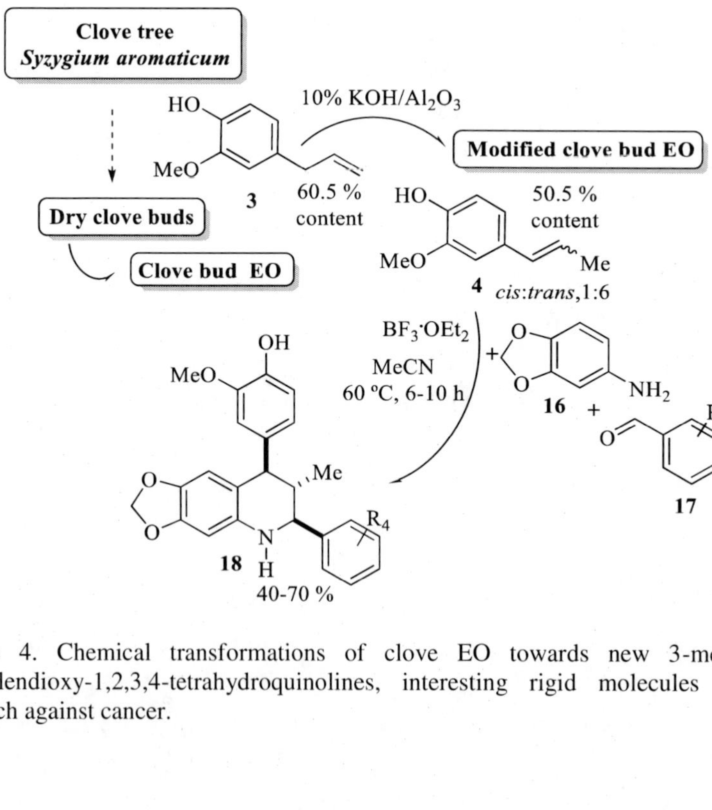

Figure 4. Chemical transformations of clove EO towards new 3-methyl-6,7-methylendioxy-1,2,3,4-tetrahydroquinolines, interesting rigid molecules in drug research against cancer.

Therefore, star anise EO was used as a renewable material in which the main component [(*E*)-anethole] acted as a chemical reagent (dienophile) in this type of cycloaddition reaction. Remarkable features of these procedures were mild and green reaction conditions, good yields and reaction rates, and cleaner reaction profiles.

Clove EO, which contains eugenol as its main component could also be an appropriate reagent for the synthesis of (tetrahydro)quinolines. Although eugenol (3) has an olefinic nature like (*E*)-anethole, it could not be used in the transformations described in Figure 3. To be useful as a dienophile, eugenol should become (*E*)-isoeugenol (4) (e.g., transformed clove bud EO).

The latter phenolic compound smoothly reacted with anilines (16), and benzaldehydes (17) to provide tetrahydroquinoline molecules with phenolic and dioxymethylene moieties (18). This three-component condensation was catalized by $BF_3{\cdot}OEt_2$, a low-cost catalyst [154] (Figure 4).

It is noteworthy that the transformations of allylbenzenes such as (3) in the corresponding 1-propenyl derivatives, e.g., (4), is a clear example of the synthetic utility of this textbook reaction, since the latter are common starting materials in the flavor and fragrance industries, as well as advanced intermediates for the preparation of a wide variety of biologically active compounds.

Following this idea, the isomerization reaction of clove bud EO (eugenol) was performed with potassium hydroxide (10% KOH) supported on alumina, which allowed to obtain a modified clove EO with 50.5% (*Z*)/(*E*)-isoeugenol (4) in a 1:6 (*Z*)/(*E*)-ratio. This last product was used in the aforementioned transformation without prior purification [154].

As depicted in Figure 4, a modified clove OE was used as a dienophile component (4) in the [4+2] cycloaddition reaction with an aldimine derived from 3,4-(methylenedioxy)aniline (16) and benzaldehydes (17) to produce new heterolignan-like 3-methyl-1,2,3,4-tetrahydroquinolines (18), which could be prospective and safe agents for adjuvant cancer therapy [51, 155, 156]. Some of these 3-methyl-6,7-methylendioxy-1,2,3,4-tetrahydroquinoline derivatives resulted in active compounds having a greater selectivity index compared to colchicine and doxorubicin, reference compounds that confirm their potential in the treatment of cancer [157].

Isoindoloquinolinones

Isoindoloquinolinones, in particular, dihydroisoindolo[2,1-*a*]quinolin-11(5*H*)-ones are complex heterocyclic molecules based on the isoindoline substructure fused with the tetrahydroquinoline skeleton. These heterocycles are found in many natural products and bioactive synthetic compounds, for example, alkaloid nuevamine, a molecule of medicinal importance isolated from *Berberis darwinii* (shrub). Berberine alkaloid analogues act as inhibitors of N_2-induced hypoxia and human topoisomerase-II.

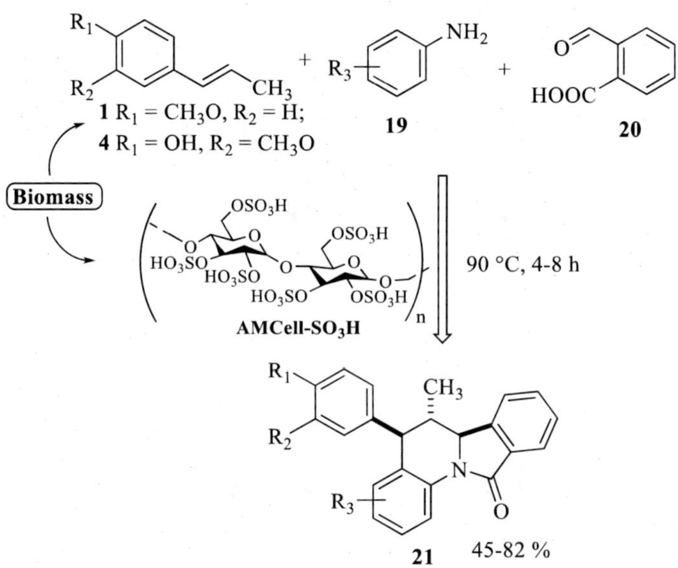

Figure 5. Highly green construction of the isoindolo[2,1-*a*]quinolinone skeleton using EO containing arylpropanoids (1) and (4).

Due to the biological significance of these heterocycles, their synthetic methods are constantly being developed. One of them is based on the acid-catalyzed three-component condensation and included the utilization of renewable and nontoxic phenylpropanoids (1) and (4), main components of star anise and clove EO, respectively. The simple and effective construction of isoindolo[2,1-*a*]quinolin-11(5*H*)-one derivatives (21), new pharmacologically important rigid molecules, was easily achieved by means of cycloaddition/intramolecular amide cyclization cascade reactions of these phenylpropanoids, anilines (19) and 2-formylbenzoic acid (20) without solvent and with AMCell-SO_3H (catalytic amorphous milled cellulose sulfonic acid) [158] (Figure 5).

The last example is worth mentioning, biomass was not used only as starting fine chemical reagents (eg, activated alkenes (1) and (4) from star anise and clove EO), but also as substrates for recoverable heterogeneous acid-catalysts (eg, modified cellulose-based acids such as AMCell-SO_3H). As the most abundant renewable feedstock derived from plants, cellulose derivatives and EO are attractive for the heterocyclic synthesis of new chemical entities using green processes.

Dihydrobenzofuranols

In the nature collection of biologically active heterocyclic metabolites, benzofuran derivatives constitute an interesting group, as they are very important phenolic compounds. The broad spectrum of pharmacological activities in individual benzofurans indicates that this series of compounds is of undoubted interest [159, 160].

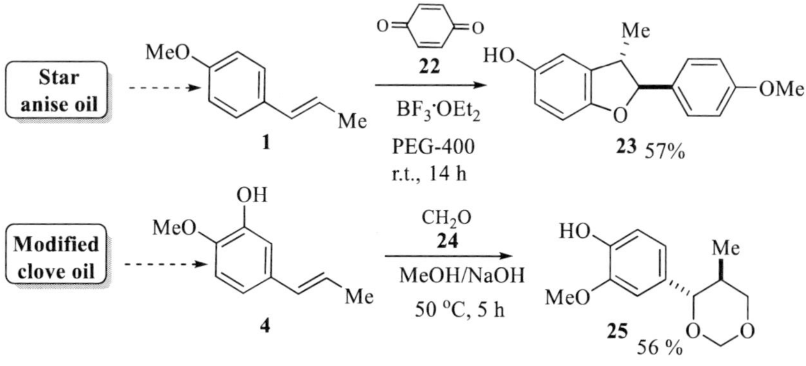

Figure 6. Chemical transformations of phenylpropanoid-based EO towards new oxygenated heterocycles of phenolic nature.

One of the most efficient preparation of such oxygenated heterocycles is a $BF_3 \cdot OEt_2$-promoted [3+2] cycloaddition reaction between (*E*)-anethole (1) or star anise oil and 1,4-benzoquinone (22) on PEG-400 to result in the corresponding *trans*-2,3-dihydrobenzo[*b*]furan-5-ol (23) with good yields [161] (Figure 6).

A simple processing of the isoeugenol molecule, obtained from the modified clove EO (see Figure 4), with formaldehyde (24) in methanol under basic conditions provided a new 2-methoxy-4-(5-methyl-1,3-dioxan-4-yl)phenol (25), which exhibited a strong antioxidant activity that was ca. 3-fold more effective than vitamin E [51]. An easy preparation and remarkable antioxidant property of this 1,3-dioxane phenolic derivative make it attractive as a molecular model in pharmacological research. Therefore, both star anise and clove bud EO resulted in suitable starting materials for the preparation of more complex phenolic compounds with potential biological activities.

Iridoids

Iridoids represent an interesting class of cyclopentano[*c*]pyran monoterpenoid compounds that display hepatoprotective, choleretic, vasoconstriction, anti-viral, anti-microbial, anti-inflammatory and analgesic activities. They also act as chemical agents for defense against herbivores and pathogens. Some synthetic methods for its preparations include the use of citronella EO, extracted mainly from *Cymbopogon nardus*. The annual production of this valuable renewable feedstock is around 2300 metric tons. Its main constituent (40-50%), citronellal, is typically isolated as a non-racemic mixture of its *R*- and *S*- enantiomers by steam distillation or solvent extraction.

This acyclic monoterpene is recognized as a raw material for commodities such as isopulegol, menthol, α-tocopherol, and irones [162]. Nonetheless, its use in heterocyclic synthesis is still underdeveloped. Among the first reported heterocyclic synthesis based on citronellal, the highly efficient synthesis of isoiridomyrmecin (26), defensive iridoid of

Iridomyrmex ants [163] and nepetalactone (27), sex attractant of aphids [164] should be mentioned. Synthesis of the iridoid molecule (26) involved three consequent cyclocondensation reactions starting with (*R*)-citronellal (8) (Figure 7, Route a); while production of iridoid lactone (27) using (*S*)-citronellal (9) is based on intramolecular [4+2] cycloaddition reactions (Figure 7, Route b) [165, 166].

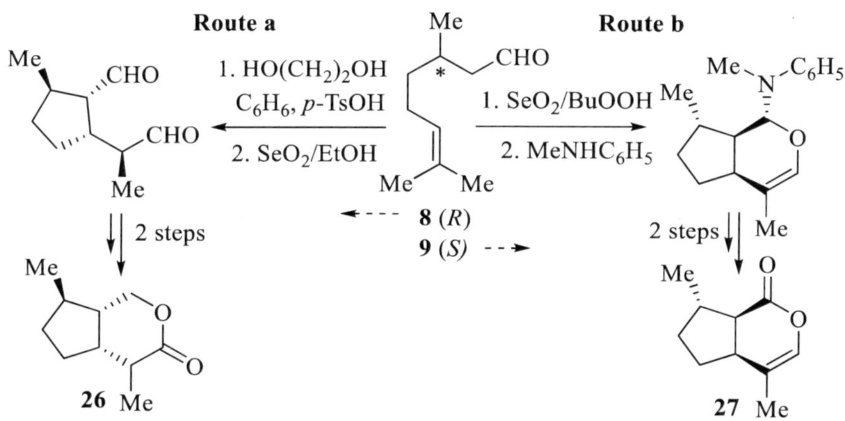

Figure 7. Use of citronellal-based EO in the synthesis of biologically important iridoid molecules.

It should be noted that citronellal and citronella oil are not only valuable materials for oxygenated heterocycles, but also for nitrogen-containing cyclic molecules.

Octahydroacridines

Among the nitrogen-containing heterocycles, octahydroacridines (OHA) stand out as a pharmacologically interesting class of linear tricyclic molecules [167]. In addition, acridine derivatives have been used to synthesize labeled conjugates with peptides, proteins and nucleic acids that exhibit antitumor and DNA-binding properties. OHA molecules could be prepared using citronellal and citronella EO.

For example, the preparation of OHA (29) consisted of a simple interaction between citronellal (8) [or (9)] and aniline derivatives (28) through the intramolecular imino Diels-Alder reaction in the presence of acid catalysts (Figure 8).

This approach is the most atom-economic and provides OHA with high yields (78-85%). The use of citronella EO, obtained from Brazilian *Cymbopogon nardus* (L.) Rendle, as a chemical reagent in this reaction makes it "greener." In fact, this eco-friendly protocol was successfully applied to the synthesis of 20 OHA by using anilines and crude citronella oil, avoiding the need for separation of citronellal [168] (Figure 8).

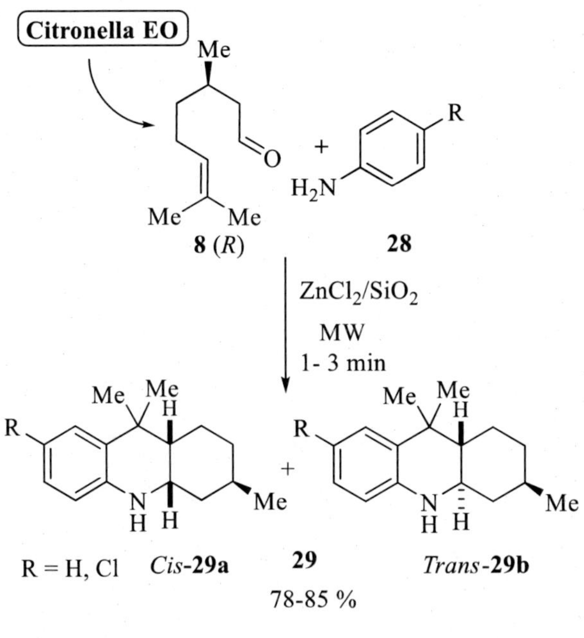

Figure 8. Intramolecular imino Diels-Alder reaction with citronella EO as a raw material.

It should be noted that the used EO contained 40-51% of (*R*)-citronellal (8). However, the formation of *cis/trans* OHA (29a/29b) (1:1 *cis/trans* ratio) occurred under reaction conditions. The diastereoselectivity of the *cis/trans* OHA product using this reaction appears as a central problem for synthetic organic and medicinal chemists.

Fortunately, the bulky *N*-substituent group (allyl, propargyl and/or benzyl substituents) in anilines played a key role in the formation of the *cis/trans* ratio of OHA. The authors [169] found that the use of *N*-benzylanilines (30) and citronella EO (containing 46% of citronellal) allowed to complete a highly diastereoselective process, which offered the easily separable *trans*-fused *N*-benzyl substituted OHA (31), with good yields (Figure 9).

Although chiral chromatographic analysis is not yet available for Colombian *Cymbopogon nardus* EO (the enantiomeric content of citronellal is unknown in the mixture), this essential oil proved to be a cost-effective renewable source of citronellal to successfully create diverse functionalized OHA products as potential bioassays substrates [170].

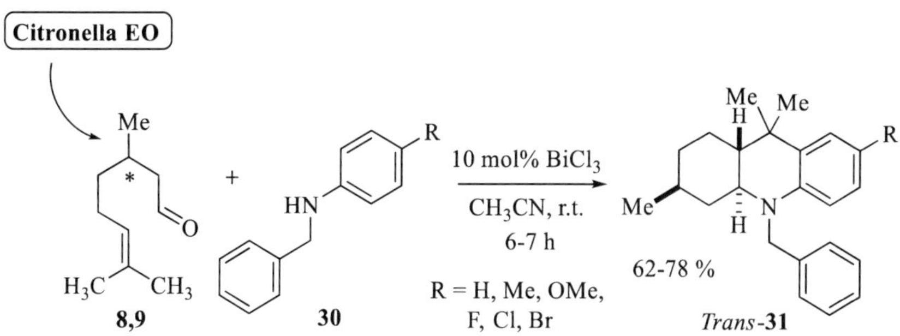

Figure 9. Preparation of trans N-benzyl OHA from citronella EO.

Trioxanes/Oxiranes

Like citronellal, geraniol is a biologically and synthetically important acyclic monoterpene, which occurs as a main component of palm rose EO (*Cymbopogon martinii*). This terpenoid is of pharmacological and commercial importance due to the numerous and different biological properties (Table 1). In addition, their esters of carboxylic acids, such as geranyl acetate, are important constituents of many natural fragrances used in the food, cosmetic and pharmaceutical industries.

Thus, the laboratory preparation of these monoterpenoids and their chemical transformations into new geraniol-based heterocyclic molecules are an important and prospective task. Being a naturally-occurring allylic alcohol of abundant availability, geraniol has been used as a starting material to prepare diverse potentially bioactive heterocycles, e.g., geraniol-based 1,2,4-trioxanes with potent *in vivo* antimalarial activity [171] or (2*R*,3*R*)-3-methyl-3-hydroxypipecolic acid, a key intermediate in the synthesis of dual MMP-13/aggrecanase inhibitors [172].

In addition, the best-known oxidized derivatives of geraniol are iridoids with important medicinal properties [173]. However, there is only one report that describes the use of palmarosa EO as raw material for the synthesis of new heterocyclic molecules [174].

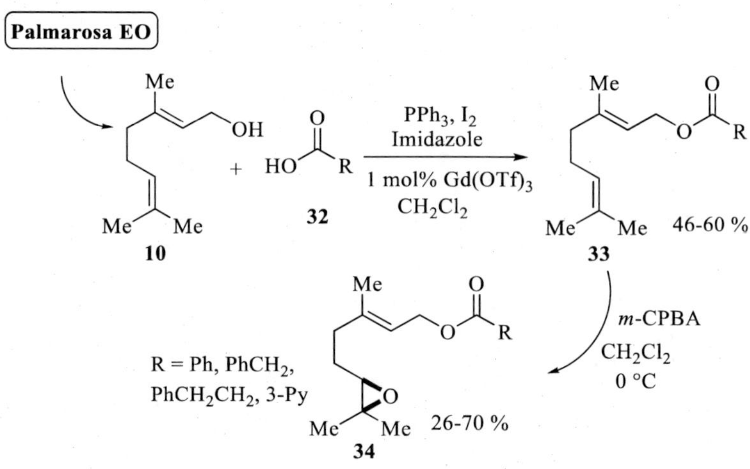

Figure 10. Preparation of geranyl esters using palmarosa EO and its oxidation reaction to geraniol esters-based oxiranes.

In this work, the authors developed a new sustainable and eco-friendly protocol for the novel geraniol esters-based oxiranes (34) using EO of palmarosa (*C. martinii*), enriched (84%) with geraniol (10). This protocol involved the $Gd(OTf)_3$-catalyzed esterification reaction of palmarosa EO (e.g., 10) and different carboxylic acids (RCOOH, 32) in the presence of PPh_3-I_2-imidazole [as an activating system, to produce geraniol esters (33)], along with the Prilezhaev reaction (*m*-chloroperoxybenzoic acid, *m*-CPBA at 0 °C in dichloromethane) (Figure 10).

The final products, 6,7-epoxy geranyl esters (34) are interesting models for pharmacological studies, as well as for the synthesis of novel compounds with a complex molecular architecture.

Benzochromene Derivatives

Benzochromenes are important pharmacophores associated with a broad range of pharmacological activities, such as antimicrobial, anticancer, hypolipidemic, antioxidant, analgesic, antileishmanial, estrogenic, anticoagulant and antispasmolytic, as well as vascular-disrupting and platelet-antiaggregating effects [175]. Thus, the synthesis of benzochromene compounds has been well developed by way of mainly multicomponent reaction strategies, which involved some phenolic molecules [176].

It is interesting to note that carvacrol and carvacrol-rich EO (e.g., *Plectranthus amboinicus* from Colombia) have not been used in the preparation of 6*H*-benzo[*c*]chromene prior to Kouznetsov' work reported in 2017 [177]. In this work, the authors described a preparative method for the new oxygenated heterocycle, 1-isopropyl-4-methyl-6*H*-benzo[*c*]chromene (37), using a two-step linear synthesis including carvacrol (12) and carvacrol-rich EO as green starting materials (Figure 11).

This synthetic tactic involved the O-benzyl alkylation of this EO with 2-((2-bromobenzyl)oxy)-4-isopropyl-1-methylbenzene (35) to provide a modified EO containing O-benzyl substituted carvacrol (2-((2-bromobenzyl)oxy)-4-isopropyl-1-methylbenzene, (36) and its cyclocondensation conversion to an oxygenated heterocycle (37) [177]. Interestingly, thymol also reacted easily in this scheme to produce an analogous benzo[*c*]chromene derivative. Moreover, similar sequence reactions of clove bud EO with its main component eugenol offer polyfunctionalized benzo[c]chromenes, interesting molecules for biological research.

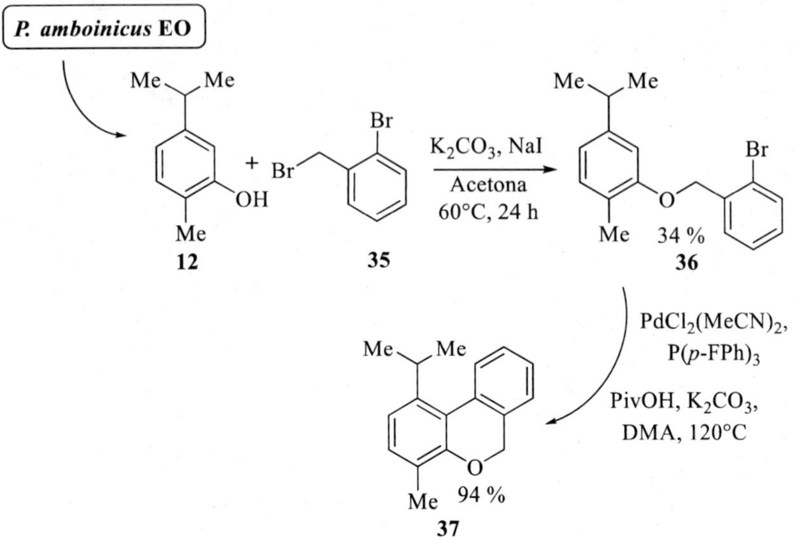

Figure 11. Use of *P. amboinicus* EO to construct 6*H*-benzo[*c*]chromene ring.

CONCLUSION

The imperative need to develop green and sustainable processes for the conversion of renewable biomass into commodity chemicals is now commonly recognized. In fact, some easily isolated biomass components are used as fine reagents in the preparation of higher value-added chemicals, replacing existing petroleum-based chemicals. In this context, the implementation and sustainable exploitation of essential oils as a valuable chemical resource for the design of chemical/structural platforms has been underdeveloped. The key problems identified for its synthetic uses are generally related to low yield of isolation (<0.5%, in some cases) and multi-component chemical nature (>20 constituents, in certain cases). However, as it was demonstrated here, certain EO (rich in eugenol, anethole or citronellal) could be successfully used in the preparation of potentially bioactive heterocycles.

Finally, in the search for more adaptable and sustainable protocols for obtaining new heterocyclic molecules, these EO are incorporated as reagents/raw materials of alternative and efficient methodologies as a possible replacement for fossil resource-based production of commodity chemicals. Without any doubts, the most sustainable technologies based on renewable biomass, including EO, will continue to grow in the future, on the road to a more sustainable bio-based economy.

ACKNOWLEDGMENTS

V. V. K. is grateful to the Colombian Institute for Science and Research (COLCIENCIAS) for financial support (project No. RC-007-2017, Cod. 110274558597). In addition, authors would like to thank to Universidad Santo Tomás by the use of the Bibliometric Unit.

REFERENCES

[1] De Solla Price, D. J. "*Little science, big science*." New York, NY: Columbia University Press, (1963).

[2] Ilijeva, R. and Buchbauer, G. "Biological properties of some volatile phenylpropanoids." *Natural Product Communications* (2016): 1619-1629. URL: http://journals.sagepub.com/doi/10.1177/1934578X1601101041.

[3] Figueiredo, A. C. "Biological properties of essential oils and volatiles: sources of variability." *Natural Volatiles & Essential Oils* (2017): 1-13. URL: http://nveo.org/wp-content/uploads/2019/03/ NVEO-2017-Volume-4-Issue-4-Pages-1-13.pdf.

[4] Bakkali, F., Averbeck, S., Averbeck, D. and Idaomar, M. "Biological effects of essential oils - a review." *Food and Chemical Toxicology* (2008): 446-475. URL:http://www.sciencedirect.com/ science/ article/pii/S0278691507004541.

[5] Adorjan, B. and Buchbauer, G. "Biological properties of essential oils: an updated review." *Flavour and Fragrance Journal* (2010):

407-426. URL: https://onlinelibrary.wiley.com/doi/epdf/10.1002/ffj.2024.

[6] Lima, R., Cardoso, M. G., Moraes, J., Vieira, S., Melo, B. and Filgueiras, C. "Composition of the essential oils from the Japanese star anise *Illicium verum* L. and lemon grass *Cymbopogon citratus* (DC.) Stapf: evaluation of their repellent effects on *Brevicoryne brassicae* (L.) (Hemiptera: Aphididae)." *BioAssay* (2008): 1-6. URL: https://www.bioassay.org.br/bioassay/article/view/56.

[7] Freire, J. M. Cardoso, M. G., Batista, L. R. and Andrade, M. A. "Essential oil of *Origanum majorana* L., *Illicium verum* Hook. f. and *Cinnamomum zeylanicum* Blume: chemical and antimicrobial characterization." *Brazilian Journal of Medicinal Plants* (2011): 209-214. URL: http://www.scielo.br/scielo.php?script=sci_arttext&pid=S1516-05722011000200013.

[8] Voris, D. G. R., Dias, L. S., Lima, J. A., Lima, K. S. C., Lima, J. B. P. and Lima, A. L. S. "Evaluation of larvicidal, adulticidal, and anticholinesterase activities of essential oils of *Illicium verum* Hook. f., *Pimenta dioica* (L.) Merr., and *Myristica fragrans* Houtt. against Zika virus vectors." *Environmental Sciences and Pollution Research* (2018): 22541-22551. URL: https://link.springer.com/article/10.1007/s11356-018-2362-y.

[9] Liu, Z., Huang, C., Tian, Y. and Xu, Z. "Studies on the chemical components and antimicrobial activities of volatile oil from *Illicium verum* Hook.f.." *China Condiment* (2009): 52-55. URL: https://caod.oriprobe.com/articles/16816587/Studies_on_the_chemical_components_and_antimicrobi.htm.

[10] Huang, Y., Zhao, J., Zhou, L., Wang, J., Gong, Y., Chen, X., Guo, Z., Wang, Q. and Jiang, W. "Antifungal activity of the essential oil of *Illicium verum* fruit and its main component *trans*-anethole." *Molecules* (2010): 7558-7569. URL: https://www.ncbi.nlm.nih.gov/pmc/articles/PMC6259245/pdf/molecules-15-07558.pdf.

[11] Muñoz-Acevedo, A., Kouznetsov, V. and Stashenko, E. "Composition and *in-vitro* antioxidant capacity of essential oils rich in thymol, carvacrol, *trans*-anethole or estragole." *Journal of the*

Industrial University of Santander. Health (2009) 287-294. URL: http://www.scielo.org.co/scielo.php?script=sci_arttext&pid=S0121-08072009000300012.

[12] Aly, S. E., Sabry, B. A., Shaheen, M. S. and Hathout, A. S. "Assessment of antimycotoxigenic and antioxidant activity of star anise (*Illicium verum*) *in vitro*." *Journal of the Saudi Society of Agricultural Sciences* (2016): 20-27. URL: https://www.sciencedirect.com/science/article/pii/S1658077X14000368.

[13] Kimbaris, A. C., Koliopoulos, G., Michaelakis, A. and Konstantopoulou, M. A. "Bioactivity of *Dianthus caryophyllus*, *Lepidium sativum*, *Pimpinella anisum*, and *Illicium verum* essential oils and their major components against the West Nile vector *Culex pipiens*." *Parasitology Research* (2012): 2403-2410. URL: https://link.springer.com/article/10.1007%2Fs00436-012-3097-1.

[14] Padmashree, A., Roopa, N., Semwal, A. D., Sharma, G. K., Agathian, G. and Bawa, A. S. "Star-anise (*Illicium verum*) and black caraway (*Carum nigrum*) as natural antioxidants." *Food Chemistry* (2007): 59-66. URL: http://www.sciencedirect.com/science/article/ pii/ S0308814606008594.

[15] Asif, M., Yehya, A. H. S., Al-Mansoub, M. A., Revadigar, V., Ezzat, M. O., Ahamed, M. B. K., Oon, C. E., Murugaiyah, V., Majid, A. S. A. and Majid, A. M. S. A. "Anticancer attributes of *Illicium verum* essential oils against colon cancer" *South African Journal of Botany* (2016): 156-161. URL: http://www. sciencedirect.com/science/article/pii/S0254629915004111.

[16] Dzamic, A., Sokovic, M., Ristic, M. S., Grijic-Jovanovic, S., Vukojevic, J. and Marin, P. D. "Chemical composition and antifungal activity of *Illicium verum* and *Eugenia caryophyllata* essential oils." *Chemistry of Natural Compounds* (2009): 259-261. URL: https://link.springer.com/article/10.1007/s10600-009-9283-4.

[17] Park, C. G., Shin, E. and Kim, J. "Insecticidal activities of essential oils, *Gaultheria fragrantissima* and *Illicium verum*, their components and analogs against *Callosobruchus chinensis* adults." *Journal of Asia-Pacific Entomology* (2016): 269-273. URL:

http://www.sciencedirect.com/science/article/pii/S122686151530242.

[18] Pavela, R. "Insecticidal properties of *Pimpinella anisum* essential oils against the *Culex quinquefasciatus* and the non-target organism *Daphnia magna*." *Journal of Asia-Pacific Entomology* (2014): 287-293. URL: http://www.sciencedirect.com/science/article/pii/S122686151400017X.

[19] Fitsiou, E., Mitropoulou, G., Spyridopoulou, K., Tiptiri-Kourpeti, A., Vamvakias, M., Bardouki, H., Panayiotidis, M. I., Galanis, A., Kourkoutas, Y., Chlichlia, K. and Pappa, A. "Phytochemical profile and evaluation of the biological activities of essential oils derived from the Greek aromatic plant species *Ocimum basilicum*, *Mentha spicata*, *Pimpinella anisum* and *Fortunella margarita*." *Molecules* (2016): E1069. URL: https://www.ncbi.nlm.nih.gov/pmc/articles/PMC6274325/pdf/molecules-21-01069.pdf.

[20] Singh, G., Kapoor, I. P. S., Singh, P., de Heluani, C. S. and Catalan, C. A. N. "Chemical composition and antioxidant potential of essential oil and oleoresins from anise seeds (*Pimpinella anisum* L.)." *International Journal of Essential Oil Therapeutics* (2008): 122-130. URL: https://pdfs.nutramedix.ec/Pimpinella%20anisum%20-%20Antioxidant%20(comp).pdf.

[21] Obaid, A. J., Al-Janabi, J. K. A. and Taj-Aldin, W. R. "Chemical composition and bioactivity characteristics of *Pimpinella anisum* essential oil against *Trichophyton rubrum*." *Journal of Global Pharma Technology* (2017): 44-56. URL: https://pdfs.semanticscholar.org/fa48/143a388c0e0cd490445259068fdd0ecce70d.pdf?_ga=2.52014636.487138250.1580750037-1540240380.1536612776.

[22] Park, I. K., Choi, K. S., Kim, D. H., Choi, I. H., Kim, L. S., Bak, W. C., Choi, J. W. and Shin, S. C. "Fumigant activity of plant essential oils and components from horseradish (*Armoracia rusticana*), anise (*Pimpinella anisum*) and garlic (*Allium sativum*) oils against *Lycoriella ingenua* (Diptera: Sciaridae)." *Pest Management Science*

(2006): 723-728. URL: https://onlinelibrary.wiley.com/doi/full/10.1002/ps.1228.

[23] Fatemi, H., Aminifard, M. H. and Mohammadi, S. "Efficacy of plant essential oils on post-harvest control of rot caused by *Botrytis cinerea* on kiwi fruits." *Archives of Phytopathology and Plant Protection* (2013): 536-547 URL: https://www.tandfonline.com/ doi/full/10.1080/03235408.2012.749687.

[24] Özcan, M. M. and Chalchat, J. C. "Chemical composition and antifungal effect of anise (*Pimpinella anisum* L.) fruit oil at ripening stage." *Annals of Microbiology* (2006): 353-358. URL: https://link.springer.com/article/10.1007/BF03175031.

[25] Tepe, B., Akpulat, H. A., Sokmen, M., Daferera, D., Yumrutas, O., Aydin, E., Polissiou, M. and Sokmen, A. "Screening of the antioxidative and antimicrobial properties of the essential oils of *Pimpinella anisetum* and *Pimpinella flabellifolia* from Turkey." *Food Chemistry* (2006): 719-724. URL: http://www.sciencedirect.com/science/article/pii/S0308814605004450.

[26] Lopes-Lutz, D., Alviano, D. S., Alviano, C. S. and Kolodziejczyk, P. P. "Screening of chemical composition, antimicrobial and antioxidant activities of *Artemisia* essential oils." *Phytochemistry* (2008): 1732-1738. URL: https://www.sciencedirect.com/science/ article/pii/S0031942208001076.

[27] Liu, T., Lin, P., Bao, T., Ding, Y., Lha, Q., Nan, P., Huang, Y., Gu, Z. and Zhong, Y., "Essential oil composition and antimicrobial activity of *Artemisia dracunculus* L. var. *qinghaiensis* YR. Ling (Asteraceae) from Qinghai-Tibet Plateau." *Industrial Crops and Products* (2018): 1-4. URL: https://www.sciencedirect.com/science/article/pii/S0926669018307842.

[28] Bandeira Reidel, R. V., Nardoni, S., Mancianti, F., Anedda, C., El Gendy, A. E. G., Omer, E. A. and Pistelli, L. "Chemical composition and antifungal activity of essential oils from four Asteraceae plants grown in Egypt." *Zeitschrift für Naturforschung C, Journal of Biosciences* (2018): 313-318. URL: https://www.

degruyter.com/ view/j/znc.2018.73.issue-7-8/znc-2017-0219/znc-2017-0219.xml?format=INT.

[29] Dohi, S. Terasaki, M. and Makino, M. "Acetylcholinesterase inhibitory activity and chemical composition of commercial essential oils" *Journal of Agricultural and Food Chemistry* (2009): 4313-4318. URL: https://pubs.acs.org/doi/10.1021/jf804013j.

[30] Bahmani, L., Aboonajmi, M., Arabhosseini, A. and Mirsaeedghazi, H. "Effects of ultrasound pre-treatment on quantity and quality of essential oil of tarragon (*Artemisia dracunculus* L.) leaves." *Journal of Applied Research on Medicinal and Aromatic Plants* (2018): 47-52. URL: https://www.sciencedirect.com/science/article/pii/S2214786117305077.

[31] Ayoughi, F., Barzegar, M., Sahari, M. A. and Naghdibadi, H. "Chemical compositions of essential oils of *Artemisia dracunculus* L. and endemic *Matricaria chamomilla* L. and an evaluation of their antioxidative effects." *Journal of Agricultural Science and Technology* (2011): 79-88. URL: https://pdfs.semanticscholar.org/35cd/20d6c1e4a0864a84d12687596854d5e310bb.pdf?_ga=2.221557277.487138250.1580750037-1540240380.1536612776.

[32] Sharafati Chaleshtori, R., Rokni, N., Razavilar, V. and Rafieian Kopaei, M. "The evaluation of the antibacterial and antioxidant activity of tarragon (*Artemisia dracunculus* L.) essential oil and its chemical composition." *Jundishapur Journal of Microbiology* (2013): e7877. URL: http://jjmicrobiol.com/en/articles/18591.html.

[33] Sayyah, M., Nadjafnia, L. and Kamalinejad, M. "Anticonvulsant activity and chemical composition of *Artemisia dracunculus* L. essential oil." *Journal of Ethnopharmacology* (2004): 283-287. URL: https://www.sciencedirect.com/science/article/pii/S0378874104002880.

[34] Osanloo, M., Amani, A., Sereshti, H., Abai, M. R., Esmaeili, F. and Sedaghat, M. M. "Preparation and optimization nanoemulsion of Tarragon (*Artemisia dracunculus*) essential oil as effective herbal larvicide against *Anopheles stephensi*." *Industrial Crops and*

Products (2017): 214-219. URL: https://www.sciencedirect.com/science/article/pii/S0926669017305484.

[35] Sharafati Chaleshtori, R., Taghizadeh, M., Mazroii Arani, N. and Sharafati Chaleshtori, F. "A comparative study on the antibacterial activity of *Artemisia dracunculus* and *Ocimum basilicum* essential oils on multidrug resistant bacteria isolated from ready to eat foods." *Journal of Essential Oil Bearing Plants* (2018): 701-712. URL: https://www.tandfonline.com/doi/abs/10.1080/0972060X.2018.1491328.

[36] Obolskiy, D., Pischel, I., Feistel, B., Glotov, N. and Heinrich, M. "*Artemisia dracunculus* L. (tarragon): a critical review of its traditional use, chemical composition, pharmacology, and safety," *Journal of Agricultural and Food Chemistry* (2011): 11367-11384. URL: https://pubs.acs.org/doi/10.1021/jf202277w.

[37] Szczepanik, M., Walczak, M., Zawitowska, B., Michalska-Sionkowska, M., Szumny, A., Wawrzeńczyk, C. and Brzezinska, M. S. "Chemical composition, antimicrobial activity and insecticidal activity against the lesser mealworm *Alphitobius diaperinus* (Panzer) (Coleoptera: Tenebrionidae) of *Origanum vulgare* L. ssp. *hirtum* (Link) and *Artemisia dracunculus* L. essential oils." *Journal of the Science of Food and Agriculture* (2018): 767-774. URL: https://onlinelibrary.wiley.com/doi/full/10.1002/jsfa.8524.

[38] Fildan, A. P., Ioan, P., Stoin, D., Bujanca, G., Lukinich-Gruia, A. T., Jianu, C., Jianu, A. M., Radulescu, M. and Tofolean, D. E. "*Artemisia dracunculus* essential oil chemical composition and antioxidant properties." *Revista de Chimie* (2019): 59-62. URL: https://revistadechimie.ro/pdf/13%20FILDAN%201%2019.pdf.

[39] Kordali, S., Kotan, R., Mavi, A., Cakir, A., Ala, A and Yildirim, A. "Determination of the chemical composition and antioxidant activity of the essential oil of *Artemisia dracunculus* and of the antifungal and antibacterial activities of Turkish *Artemisia absinthium*, *A. dracunculu*s, *Artemisia santonicum*, and *Artemisia spicigera* essential oils." *Journal of Agricultural and Food Chemistry* (2005): 9452-9458. URL: https://pubs.acs.org/doi/10.1021/jf0516538.

[40] Vera, S. S., Zambrano, D. F., Méndez-Sanchez, S. C., Rodríguez-Sanabria, F., Stashenko, E. E. and Duque Luna, J. E. "Essential oils with insecticidal activity against larvae of *Aedes aegypti* (Diptera: Culicidae)." *Parasitology Research* (2014): 2647-2654. URL: https://link.springer.com/article/10.1007%2Fs00436-014-3917-6.

[41] Sepúlveda-Arias, J. C., Veloza, L. A., Escobar, L. M., Orozco, L. M. and Lopera, I. A. "Anti-inflammatory effects of the main constituents and epoxides derived from the essential oils obtained from *Tagetes lucida*, *Cymbopogon citratus*, *Lippia alba* and *Eucalyptus citriodora*." *Journal of Essential Oil Research* (2013): 186-193. URL: https://www.tandfonline.com/doi/full/10.1080/10412905.2012.751556.

[42] Olivero-Verbel, J., González-Cervera, T., Güette-Fernandez, J., Jaramillo-Colorado, B. and Stashenko, E. "Chemical composition and antioxidant activity of essential oils isolated from Colombian plants." *Brazilian Journal of Pharmacognosy* (2010): 568-574. URL: http://www.scielo.br/pdf/rbfar/v20n4/v20n4a16.pdf.

[43] Regalado, E. L., Fernández, M. D., Pino, J. A., Mendiola, J. and Echemendia, O. A. "Chemical composition and biological properties of the leaf essential oil of *Tagetes lucida* Cav. from Cuba." *Journal of Essential Oil Research* (2011): 63-67. URL: https://www.tandfonline.com/doi/pdf/10.1080/10412905.2011.9700485.

[44] Mendoza-García E. E., Ortega-Arenas, L. D., Serrato-Cruz, M. A., Villanueva-Jiménez, J. A., López-Arroyo, J. I. and Pérez-Pacheco, R. "Chemical composition, toxicity, and repellence of plant essential oils against *Diaphorina citri* (Hemiptera: Liviidae)." *Chilean Journal of Agricultural Research* (2019): 636-647. URL: https://scielo.conicyt.cl/pdf/chiljar/v79n4/0718-5839-chiljar-79-04-00636.pdf.

[45] López López, E., Peña Ortega, M. G., Colinas León, M. T. B., Díaz Cedillo, F. and Serrato Cruz, M. A. "Fungistasis of essential oil extrated from a *Tagetes lucida* population of Hidalgo, México." *Mexican Journal of Agricultural Sciences* (2018): 329-341. URL:

http://www.scielo.org.mx/pdf/remexca/v9n2/2007-0934-remexca-9-02-329-en.pdf.

[46] Scopel, R., Falcão, M. A., Lucas, A. M., Almeida, R. N., Gandolfi, P. H. K., Cassel, E. and Vargas, R. M. F. "Supercritical fluid extraction from *Syzygium aromaticum* buds: Phase equilibrium, mathematical modeling and antimicrobial activity." The *Journal of Supercritical Fluids* (2014): 223-230. URL: https://www. sciencedirect.com/ science/article/pii/S0896844614001594.

[47] Eboumbou Massodi, M. L., Mime, L. C., Dongmo Fogang, H. P., Djikeng, F. T., Karuna, M. S. L. and Womeni, H. M. "Chemical composition and antioxidant activity of *Syzygium aromaticum* and *Monodora myristica* essential oils from Cameroon." *Journal of Food Stability* (2018): 1-13. URL: https://www.semanticscholar. org/ paper/Chemical-Composition-and-Antioxidant-Activity-of-Lucrece-Cecilia/49434f9bfd65a65494509b71c5921e76f05f3b88.

[48] Ismail, M., Kemegne, G. A., Njayou, F. N., Penlap, V., Mbacham, W. F. and Kamdem, S. L. S. "Chemical composition, antibiotic promotion and *in vivo* toxicity of *Piper nigrum* and *Syzygium aromaticum* essential oil" *African Journal of Biochemsitry Research* (2017): 58-71. URL: https://www.semanticscholar.org/paper/ Chemical-composition%2C-antibiotic-promotion-and-in-Ismail-Kemegne/9b998508b8f73b015ae53d8e42fd6e0d92ad6ae5.

[49] Huang, X. W., Feng, Y. C., Huang, Y. and Li, H. L. "Chemical composition, antioxidant and the possible use as skin-care ingredient of clove oil (*Syzygium aromaticum* (L.) Merr. & Perry) and citronella oil (*Cymbopogon goeringii*) from China." *Journal of Essential Oil Research* (2013): 315-323. URL: https://www. tandfonline.com/ doi/full/10.1080/10412905.2013.775082.

[50] Sutthanont, N., Choochote, W., Tuetun, B., Junkum, A., Jitpakdi, A., Chaithong, U., Riyong, D. and Pitasawat, B. "Chemical composition and larvicidal activity of edible plant-derived essential oils against the pyrethroid-susceptible and -resistant strains of *Aedes aegypti* (Diptera: Culicidae)." *Journal of Vector Ecology* (2010): 106-115.

URL: https://onlinelibrary.wiley.com/doi/epdf/10.1111/j.1948-7134.2010.00066.x.

[51] Merchán Arenas, D. R., Muñoz Acevedo, A., Vargas Méndez, L. Y. and Kouznetsov, V. V. "Scavenger activity evaluation of the clove bud essential oil (*Eugenia caryophyllus*) and eugenol derivatives employing $ABTS^{+\bullet}$ decolorization." *Scientia Pharmaceutica* (2011): 779-791. URL: https://www.ncbi.nlm.nih.gov/pmc/articles/PMC3221489/pdf/scipharm-2011-79-779.pdf.

[52] Politeo, O., Jukić, M. and Miloš, M. "Chemical composition and antioxidant activity of essential oils of twelve spice plants." *Croatica Chemica Acta* (2006): 545-552. URL: https://bib.irb.hr/datoteka/296564.39.pdf.

[53] Nassar, M. I., Gaara, A. H., El-Ghorab, A. H., Farrag, A. R. H., Shen, H., Huq, E. and Mabry, T. J. "Chemical constituents of clove (*Syzygium aromaticum*, Fam. Myrtaceae) and their antioxidant activity." *Latin American Journal of Chemistry* (2007): 47-57. URL: https://pdfs.semanticscholar.org/8980/8a009ebed204d1d98c0b206f0655de4ca2fd.pdf?_ga=2.140572402.1399158524.1580707167-1009408842.1550543375.

[54] Barakat, H. "Composition, antioxidant, antibacterial activities and mode of action of clove (*Syzygium aromaticum* L.) buds essential oil." *Bristish Journal of Applied Science and Technology* (2014): 1934-1951. URL: https://pdfs.semanticscholar.org/3185/3fc417007e2cddee02698c258e5d16ecfad0.pdf?_ga=2.109238853.1399158524.1580707167-1009408842.1550543375.

[55] Sharma, A., Rajendran, S., Srivastava, A., Sharma, S. and Kundu, B. "Antifungal activities of selected essential oils against *Fusarium oxysporum* f. sp. lycopersici 1322, with emphasis on *Syzygium aromaticum* essential oil." *Journal of Bioscience and Bioengineering* (2017): 308-313. URL: https://www.sciencedirect. com/science/article/pii/S1389172316303097.

[56] Park, M. J., Gwak, K. S., Yang, I., Choi, W. S., Jo, H. J., Chang, J.W., Jeung, E. B. and Choi, I. G. "Antifungal activities of the essential oils in *Syzygium aromaticum* (L.) Merr. Et Perry and *Leptospermum*

petersonii Bailey and their constituents against various dermatophytes." *Korean Journal of Microbiology* (2007): 460-465. URL: http://www.msk.or.kr/jsp/view_old_journalD.asp?THEIDX=2589.

[57] Lee, S., Najiah, M., Wendy, W. and Nadirah, M. "Chemical composition and antimicrobial activity of the essential oil of *Syzygium aromaticum* flower bud (Clove) against fish systemic bacteria isolated from aquaculture sites." *Frontiers of Agriculture in China* (2009): 332-336. URL: https://link.springer.com/article/10. 1007/s11703-009-0052-8.

[58] Aguilar-González, A. E., Palou, E. and López-Malo, A., "Antifungal activity of essential oils of clove (*Syzygium aromaticum*) and/or mustard (*Brassica nigra*) in vapor phase against gray mold (*Botrytis cinerea*) in strawberries." *Innovation Food Science and Emerging Technologies* (2015): 181-185. URL: http://www.sciencedirect.com/science/article/pii/S1466856415001654.

[59] Fayemiwo, K. A., Adeleke, M. A., Okoro, O. P., Awojide, S. H. and Awoniyi, I. O. "Larvicidal efficacies and chemical composition of essential oils of *Pinus sylvestris* and *Syzygium aromaticum* against mosquitoes." *Asian Pacific Journal of Tropical Biomedicine* (2014): 30-34. URL: http://www.sciencedirect.com/science/article/pii/S2221169114602045.

[60] Jimoh, S. O., Arowolo, L. A. and Alabi, K. A. "Phytochemical screening and antimicrobial evaluation of *Syzygium aromaticum* extract and essential oil." *International Journal of Current Microbiology and Applied Sciences* (2017): 4557-4567. URL: https://www.ijcmas.com/6-7-2017/Simiat%20Olanike%20Jimoh,%20et%20al.pdf.

[61] Tahir, H. U., Sarfraz, R. A., Ashraf, A. and Adil, S. "Chemical composition and antidiabetic activity of essential oils obtained from two spices (*Syzygium aromaticum* and *Cuminum cyminum*)." *International Journal of Food Properties* (2016): 2156-2164. URL: http://www.tandfonline.com/doi/full/10.1080/10942912.2015.1110166.

[62] Alshaikh, N. and Perveen, K. "Anti-candidal activity and chemical composition of essential oil of clove (*Syzygium aromaticum*)." *Journal of Essential Oil Bearing Plants* (2017): 951-958. URL: https://www.tandfonline.com/doi/full/10.1080/0972060X.2017.1375867.

[63] Santamarina, M. P., Roselló, J., Giménez, S. and Blázquez, M.A. "Commercial *Laurus nobilis* L. and *Syzygium aromaticum* L. Merr. & Perry essential oils against post-harvest phytopathogenic fungi on rice." *LWT - Food Science and Technology* (2016): 325-332. URL: http://www.sciencedirect.com/science/article/pii/S0023643815301341.

[64] Ranasinghe, L., Jayawardena, B. and Abeywickrama, K. "Fungicidal activity of essential oils of *Cinnamomum zeylanicum* (L.) and *Syzygium aromaticum* (L.) Merr et L. M. Perry against crown rot and anthracnose pathogens isolated from banana." *Letters in Applied Microbiology* (2002): 208-211. URL: https://sfamjournals.onlinelibrary.wiley.com/doi/epdf/10.1046/j.1472-765X.2002.01165.x.

[65] Koba, K., Nenonene, A. Y., Raynaud, C., Chaumont, J. P. and Sanda, K. "Antibacterial activities of the buds essential oil of *Syzygium aromaticum* (L.) Merr. & Perry from Togo." *Journal of Biologically Active Products from Nature* (2011): 42-51. URL: http://www.tandfonline.com/doi/full/10.1080/22311866.2011.10719072.

[66] Chaieb, K., Hajlaoui, H., Zmantar, T., Kahla-Nakbi, A. B., Rouabhia, M., Mahdouani, K. and Bakhrouf, A. "The chemical composition and biological activity of clove essential oil, *Eugenia caryophyllata* (*Syzigium aromaticum* L. Myrtaceae): a short review." *Phytotherapy Research* (2007): 501-506. URL: https://onlinelibrary.wiley.com/doi/abs/10.1002/ptr.2124.

[67] Prashar, A., Locke, I. C. and Evans, C. S. "Cytotoxicity of clove (*Syzygium aromaticum*) oil and its major components to human skin cells." *Cell Proliferation* (2006): 241-248. URL: https://

onlinelibrary.wiley.com/doi/epdf/10.1111/j.1365-2184.2006.00384.x.

[68] Simić, A., Soković, M. D., Ristić, M., Grujić-Jovanović, S., Vukojević, J. and Marin, P. D. "The chemical composition of some Lauraceae essential oils and their antifungal activities." *Phytotherapy Research* (2004): 713-717. URL: https://onlinelibrary.wiley.com/doi/epdf/10.1002/ptr.1516.

[69] Boukhatem, M. N., Ferhat, M. A., Kameli, A., Saidi, F. and Kebir, H. T. "Lemon grass (*Cymbopogon citratus*) essential oil as a potent anti-inflammatory and antifungal drugs." *Libyan Journal of Medicine* (2014): 25431. URL: https://www.ncbi.nlm.nih.gov/pmc/articles/PMC4170112/pdf/LJM-9-25431.pdf.

[70] Kpoviessi, S., Bero, J., Agbani, P., Gbaguidi, F., Kpadonou-Kpoviessi, B., Sinsin, B., Accrombessi, G., Frédérich, M., Moudachirou, M. and Quetin-Leclercq, J. "Chemical composition, cytotoxicity and *in vitro* antitrypanosomal and antiplasmodial activity of the essential oils of four *Cymbopogon* species from Benin." *Journal of Ethnopharmacology* (2014): 652-659. URL: https://www.sciencedirect.com/science/article/pii/S0378874113008210.

[71] Gbenou, J. D., Ahounou, J. F., Akakpo, H. B., Laleye, A., Yayi, E., Gbaguidi, F., Baba-Moussa, L., Darboux, R., Dansou, P., Moudachirou, M. and Kotchoni, S. O. "Phytochemical composition of *Cymbopogon citratus* and *Eucalyptus citriodora* essential oils and their anti-inflammatory and analgesic properties on Wistar rats." *Molecular Biology Reports* (2013): 1127-1134. URL: https://link.springer.com/article/10.1007%2Fs11033-012-2155-1.

[72] Almeida, K. B., Ramos, A. S., Nunes, J. B. B., Silva, B. O., Ferraz, E. R. A., Fernandes, A. S., Felzenszwalb, I., Amaral, A. C. F., Roullin, V. G. and Falcão, D. Q. "PLGA nanoparticles optimized by Box-Behnken for efficient encapsulation of therapeutic *Cymbopogon citratus* essential oil." *Colloids and Surfaces B: Biointerfaces* (2019): 935-942. URL: https://www.sciencedirect. com/science/article/pii/S0927776519304084.

[73] Brügger, B. P., Martínez, L. C., Plata-Rueda, A., e Castro, B. M. C., Soares, M. A., Wilcken, C. F., Carvalho, A. G., Serrão, J. E. and Zanuncio, J. C. "Bioactivity of the *Cymbopogon citratus* (Poaceae) essential oil and its terpenoid constituents on the predatory bug, *Podisus nigrispinus* (Heteroptera: Pentatomidae)." *Scientific Reports* (2019): 8358. URL: https://www.nature.com/articles/s41598-019-44709-y.

[74] Blanco, M. M., Costa, C. A. R. A., Freire, A. O., Santos, J. G. and Costa, M. "Neurobehavioral effect of essential oil of *Cymbopogon citratus* in mice." *Phytomedicine* (2009): 265-270. URL: https://www.sciencedirect.com/science/article/pii/S0944711307000712.

[75] Costa, A. V., Pinheiro, P. F., Rondelli, V. M., de Queiroz, V. T., Tuler, A. C., Britto, K. B., Stiguel, P. and Pratissolli, D. "*Cymbopogon citratus* (Poaceae) essential oil on *Frankliniella schultzei* (Thysanoptera: Thripidae) and *Myzus persicae* (Hemiptera: Aphididae)." *Bioscience Journal* (2013): 1840-1847. URL: http://www.seer.ufu.br/index.php/biosciencejournal/article/view/22052/13422.

[76] Viana, G. S. B., Vale, T. G., Pinho, R. S. N. and Matos, F. J. A. "Antinociceptive effect of the essential oil from *Cymbopogon citratus* in mice." *Journal of Ethnopharmacology* (2000): 323-327. URL: https://www.sciencedirect.com/science/article/pii/S0378874199001683.

[77] Moreira, F. V., Bastos, J. F. A., Blank, A. F., Alves, P. B. and Santos, M. R. V. "Chemical composition and cardiovascular effects induced by the essential oil of *Cymbopogon citratus* DC. Stapf, Poaceae, in rats." *Brazilian Journal of Pharmacognosy* (2010): 904-909. URL: http://www.scielo.br/pdf/rbfar/v20n6/aop1210.pdf.

[78] Pinto, Z. T., Sánchez, F. F., dos Santos, A. R., Amaral, A. C. F., Ferreira, J. L. P., Escalona-Arranz, J. C. and Queiroz, M. M. C. "Chemical composition and insecticidal activity of *Cymbopogon citratus* essential oil from Cuba and Brazil against housefly."

Brazilian Journal of Veterinary Parasitology (2015): 36-44. URL: http://www.scielo.br/pdf/rbpv/v24n1/1984-2961-rbpv-24-1-36.pdf.

[79] Bassolé, I. H. N., Lamien-Meda, A., Bayala, B., Obame, L. C., Ilboudo, A. J., Franz, C., Novak, J., Nebié, R. C. and Dicko, M. H. "Chemical composition and antimicrobial activity of *Cymbopogon citratus* and *Cymbopogon giganteus* essential oils alone and in combination." *Phytomedicine* (2011): 1070-1074. URL: http://www.sciencedirect.com/science/article/pii/S0944711311001565.

[80] Menut, C., Bessiére, J. M., Samaté, D., Djibo, A. K., Buchbauer, G and Schopper, B. "Aromatic plants of tropical West Africa. XI. Chemical composition, antioxidant and antiradical properties of the essential oils of three *Cymbopogon* species from Burkina Faso." *Journal of Essential Oil Research* (2000): 207-212. URL: https://www.tandfonline.com/doi/full/10.1080/10412905.2000.9699499.

[81] Nguefack, J., Tamgue, O., Lekagne Dongmo, J. B., Dakole, C. D., Leth, V., Vismer, H. F., Amvam Zollo, P. H. and Nkengfack, A. E. "Synergistic action between fractions of essential oils from *Cymbopogon citratus*, *Ocimum gratissimum* and *Thymus vulgaris* against *Penicillium expansum*." *Food Control* (2012): 377-383. URL: https://www.sciencedirect.com/science/article/pii/S0956713511003100.

[82] Olivero-Verbel, J., Nerio, L. S. and Stashenko, E. E. "Bioactivity against *Tribolium castaneum* Herbst (Coleoptera: Tenebrionidae) of *Cymbopogon citratus* and *Eucalyptus citriodora* essential oils grown in Colombia." *Pest Management Science* (2010): 664-668. URL: https://onlinelibrary.wiley.com/doi/epdf/10.1002/ps.1927.

[83] Lulekal, E., Tesfaye, S., Gebrechristos, S., Dires, K., Zenebe, T., Zegeye, N., Feleke, G., Kassahun, A., Shiferaw, Y. and Mekonnen, A., "Phytochemical analysis and evaluation of skin irritation, acute and sub-acute toxicity of *Cymbopogon citratus* essential oil in mice and rabbits." *Toxicology Reports* (2019): 1289-1294. URL: https://www.sciencedirect.com/science/article/pii/S2214750019302525.

[84] Tchoumbougnang, F., Zollo, P. H. A., Dagne, E. and Mekonnen, Y. "*In vivo* antimalarial activity of essential oils from *Cymbopogon citratus* and *Ocimum gratissimum* on mice infected with *Plasmodium berghei*." *Planta Medica* (2005): 20-23. URL: https://www.thieme-connect.com/products/ejournals/abstract/10. 1055/s-2005-837745.

[85] Bharti, S. K., Kumar, A., Prakash, O., Krishnan, S. and Gupta, A. K. "Essential oil of *Cymbopogon Citratus* against diabetes: validation by *in vivo* experiments and computational studies." *Journal of Bioanalysis and Biomedicine* (2013): 194-203. URL: https://www. hilarispublisher.com/open-access/essential-oil-of-cymbopogon-citratus-against-diabetes-validation-by-in-vivo-experiments-and-computational-studies-1948-593X.1000098.pdf.

[86] Kumar, P., Mishra, S., Malik, A. and Satya, S. "Housefly (Musca domestica L.) control potential of *Cymbopogon citratus* Stapf. (Poales: Poaceae) essential oil and monoterpenes (citral and 1,8-cineole)." *Parasitology Research* (2013): 69-76. URL: https://link.springer.com/article/10.1007%2Fs00436-012-3105-5.

[87] Farhang, V., Amini, J., Javadi, T., Nazemi, J. and Ebadollahi, A. "Chemical composition and antifungal activity of essential oil of *Cymbopogon citratus* (DC.) stapf. against three *phytophthora* species." *Greener Journal of Biological Sciences* (2013): 292-298. URL: https://pdfs.semanticscholar.org/5b06/4c2f97d23f77e986 92490971fc42851771cb.pdf.

[88] Matasyoh, J. C., Wagara, I. N., Nakavuma, J. L. and Kiburai, A. M. "Chemical composition of *Cymbopogon citratus* essential oil and its effect on mycotoxigenic *Aspergillus* species." *African Journal of Food Science* (2011): 138-142. URL: https://academicjournals. org/article/article1379515549_Matasyoh%20et%20al.pdf.

[89] Piaru, S. P., Perumal, S., Cai, L. W., Mahmud, R., Majid, A. M. S. A., Ismail, S. and Man, C. N. "Chemical composition, anti-angiogenic and cytotoxicity activities of the essential oils of *Cymbopogan citratus* (lemon grass) against colorectal and breast carcinoma cell lines." *Journal of Essential Oil Research* (2012): 453-459.

URL: https://www.tandfonline.com/doi/full/10.1080/10412905.2012.703496.

[90] Sahal, G., Woerdenbag, H. J., Hinrichs, W. L. J., Visser, A., Tepper, P. G., Quax, W. J., van der Mei, H. C. and Bilkay, I. S. "Antifungal and biofilm inhibitory effect of *Cymbopogon citratus* (lemongrass) essential oil on biofilm forming by *Candida tropicalis* isolates; an *in vitro* study." *Journal of Ethnopharmacology* (2020): 112188. URL: https://www.sciencedirect.com/science/article/pii/S0378874119320641.

[91] Adesegun, A. S., Samuel, F. O., Olawale, R. G. and Funmilola, S. A. "Antioxidant activity of the volatile oil of *Cymbopogon citratus* and its inhibition of the partially purified and characterized extracellular protease of *Shigella sonnei*." *American Journal of Research Communication* (2013): 31-45. URL: http://www.usa-journals.com/wp-content/uploads/2012/12/Adesegun_Vol11.pdf.

[92] Koba, K., Sanda, K., Guyon, C., Delgado Raynaud, C., Chaumont, J. P. and Nicod, L. "*In vitro* cytotoxic activity of *Cymbopogon citratus* L. and *Cymbopogon nardus* L. essential oils from Togo." *Bangladesh Journal of Pharmacology* (2009): 29-34. URL: https://www.banglajol.info/index.php/BJP/article/view/1040/1107.

[93] Katiki, L. M., Chagas, A. C. S., Bizzo, H. R., Ferreira, J. F. S. and Amarante, A. F. T. "Anthelmintic activity of *Cymbopogon martinii*, *Cymbopogon schoenanthus* and *Mentha piperita* essential oils evaluated in four different *in vitro* tests." *Veterinary Parasitology* (2011): 103-108. URL: http://www.sciencedirect.com/science/article/pii/S0304401711004705.

[94] Duarte, M. C. T., Leme, E. E. Delarmelina, C., Soares, A. A., Figueira, G. M. and Sartoratto, A. "Activity of essential oils from Brazilian medicinal plants on *Escherichia coli*." *Journal of Ethnopharmacology* (2007): 197-201. URL: http://www.sciencedirect.com/science/article/pii/S0378874106005939.

[95] Andrade, B. F. M. T., Conti, B. J., Santiago, K. B., Fernandes Júnior, A. and Sforcin, J. M. "*Cymbopogon martinii* essential oil and geraniol at noncytotoxic concentrations exerted immunomodulatory/anti-

inflammatory effects in human monocytes." *Journal of Pharmacy and Pharmacology* (2014): 1491-1496. URL: https://onlinelibrary.wiley.com/doi/epdf/10.1111/ jphp.12278.

[96] Prasad, C. S., Shukla, R., Kumar, A. and Dubey, N. K. "*In vitro* and *in vivo* antifungal activity of essential oils of *Cymbopogon martini* and *Chenopodium ambrosioides* and their synergism against dermatophytes." *Mycoses* (2010): 123-129. URL: https:// onlinelibrary.wiley.com/doi/epdf/10.1111/j.1439-0507.2008. 01676.x.

[97] Tsai, M. L., Lin, C. C., Lin, W. C. and Yang, C. H. "Antimicrobial, antioxidant, and anti-inflammatory activities of essential oils from five selected herbs." *Bioscience, Biotechnology and Biochemistry* (2011): 1977-1983. URL: https://www.tandfonline.com/doi/pdf/ 10.1271/bbb.110377?needAccess=true.

[98] Prashar, A., Hili, P., Veness, R. G. and Evans, C. S. "Antimicrobial action of palmarosa oil (*Cymbopogon martinii*) on *Saccharomyces cerevisiae*." *Phytochemistry* (2013): 569-575. URL: http://www. sciencedirect.com/science/article/pii/S0031942203002267.

[99] Abena, A. A., Gbenou, J. D., Yayi, E., Moudachirou, M., Ongoka, R. P., Ouamba, J. M. and Silou, T. "Comparative chemical and analgesic properties of essential oils of *Cymbopogon nardus* (L) rendle of Benin and Congo." *African Journal of Traditional, Complementaty and Alternatives Medicines* (2007): 267-272. URL: https://www.ncbi.nlm.nih.gov/pmc/articles/PMC2816489/pdf/AJT0 403-0267.pdf.

[100] Cunha, B. G., Duque, C., Caiaffa, K. S., Massunari, L., Catanoze, I. A., Dos Santos, D. M., de Oliveira, S. H. P. and Guiotti, A. M. "Cytotoxicity and antimicrobial effects of citronella oil (*Cymbopogon nardus*) and commercial mouthwashes on *S. aureus* and *C. albicans* biofilms in prosthetic materials." *Archives of Oral Biology* (2020): 104577. URL: http://www.sciencedirect.com/ science/article/pii/S0003996919304340.

[101] Clain, E, Baranauskienė, R., Kraujalis, P., Šipailienė, A., Maždžierienė, R., Kazernavičiūtė, R., El Kalamouni, C. and

Venskutonis, P. R. "Biorefining of *Cymbopogon nardus* from Reunion Island into essential oil and antioxidant fractions by conventional and high-pressure extraction methods." *Industrial Crops and Products* (2018): 158-167. URL: http://www.sciencedirect.com/science/article/pii/S0926669018308781.

[102] De Billerbeck, V. G., Roques, C. G., Bessière, J. M., Fonvieille, J. L. and Dargent, R. "Effects of *Cymbopogon nardus* (L.) W. Watson essential oil on the growth and morphogenesis of *Aspergillus niger*." *Canadian Journal of Microbiology* (2001): 9-17. URL: http://www.nrcresearchpress.com/doi/10.1139/w00-117.

[103] Kandimalla, R., Kalita, S., Choudhury, B., Dash, S., Kalita, K and Kotoky, J. "Chemical composition and anti-candidiasis mediated wound healing property of *Cymbopogon nardus* essential oil on chronic diabetic wounds." *Frontiers in Pharmacology* (2016): 198. URL: https://www.ncbi.nlm.nih.gov/pmc/articles/PMC4928018/pdf/fphar-07-00198.pdf.

[104] Wei, L. S. and Wee, W. "Chemical composition and antimicrobial activity of *Cymbopogon nardus* citronella essential oil against systemic bacteria of aquatic animals." *Iranian Journal of Microbiology* (2013): 147-152. URL: https://www.ncbi.nlm.nih.gov/pmc/articles/PMC3696851/pdf/IJM-5-147.pdf.

[105] Roszaini, K., Nor Azah, M. A., Mailina, J., Zaini, S. and Faridz, Z. M. "Toxicity and antitermite activity of the essential oils from *Cinnamomum camphora*, *Cymbopogon nardus*, *Melaleuca cajuputi* and *Dipterocarpus* sp. against *Coptotermes curvignathus*." *Wood Science and Technology* (2013): 1273-1284. URL: https://link.springer.com/article/10.1007/s00226-013-0576-1.

[106] Nakahara, K., Alzoreky, N. S., Yoshihashi, T., Nguyen, H. T. T. and Trakoontivakorn, G. "Chemical composition and antifungal activity of essential oil from *Cymbopogon nardus* (Citronella Grass)." *Japan. Agricultural Research Quarterly* (2003): 249-252. URL: https://www.jstage.jst.go.jp/article/jarq/37/4/37_249/_article.

[107] Abdellatif, F., Boudjella, H., Zitouni, A. and Hassani, A. "Chemical composition and antimicrobial activity of the essential oil from leaves

of Algerian *Melissa officinalis* L.." *EXCLI Journal* (2014): 772-781. URL: https://www.ncbi.nlm.nih.gov/pmc/articles/PMC4464394/pdf/EXCLI-13-772.pdf.

[108] De Sousa, A. C., Gattass, C. R., Alviano, D. S., Alviano, C. S., Blank, A. F. and Alves, P. B. "*Melissa officinalis* L. essential oil: antitumoral and antioxidant activities." *Journal of Pharmacy and Pharmacology* (2004): 677-681. URL: https://onlinelibrary.wiley.com/doi/epdf/10.1211/0022357023321.

[109] Schnitzler, P., Schuhmacher, A., Astani, A. and Reichling, J. "*Melissa officinalis* oil affects infectivity of enveloped herpesviruses." *Phytomedicine* (2008): 734-740. URL: https://www.sciencedirect.com/science/article/pii/S0944711308001128.

[110] Suschke, U., Sporer, F., Schneele, J., Geiss, H. K. and Reichling, J. "Antibacterial and cytotoxic activity of *Nepeta Cataria* L., *N. Cataria* Var. *Citriodora* (Beck.) Balb. and *Melissa officinalis* L. essential oils." *Natural Product Communications* (2007): 1277-1286. URL: https://journals.sagepub.com/doi/pdf/10.1177/1934578X0700201218.

[111] Koliopoulos, G., Pitarokili, D., Kioulos, E., Michaelakis, A. and Tzakou, O. "Chemical composition and larvicidal evaluation of Mentha, Salvia, and Melissa essential oils against the West Nile virus mosquito *Culex pipiens*." *Parasitology Research* (2010): 327-335. URL: https://link.springer.com/article/10.1007%2Fs00436-010-1865-3.

[112] Sadraei, H., Ghannadi, A. and Malekshahi, K. "Relaxant effect of essential oil of *Melissa officinalis* and citral on rat ileum contractions." *Fitoterapia* (2003): 445-452. URL: https://www.sciencedirect.com/science/article/pii/S0367326X03001096.

[113] Chung, M. J., Cho, S. Y., Bhuiyan, M. J. H., Kim, K. H. and Lee, S. J. "Anti-diabetic effects of lemon balm (*Melissa officinalis*) essential oil on glucose- and lipid-regulating enzymes in type 2 diabetic mice." *British Journal of Nutrition* (2010): 180-188. URL: https://www.cambridge.org/core/journals/british-journal-of-nutrition/article/antidiabetic-effects-of-lemon-balm-melissa-

officinalis-essential-oil-on-glucose-and-lipidregulating-enzymes-in-type-2-diabetic-mice/C840A043880C7883DFF8DE0F249AA0AC.

[114] Bounihi, A., Hajjaj, G., Alnamer, R., Cherrah, Y. and Zellou, A. "*In vivo* potential anti-inflammatory activity of *Melissa officinalis* L. essential oil." *Advances in Pharmacologica Science* (2013): 101759. URL: https://www.ncbi.nlm.nih.gov/pmc/articles/PMC3870089/pdf/APS2013-101759.pdf.

[115] El Ouadi, Y., Manssouri, M., Bouyanzer, A., Majidi, L., Bendaif, H., Elmsellem, H., Shariati, M. A., Melhaoui, A. and Hammouti, B. "Essential oil composition and antifungal activity of *Melissa officinalis* originating from north-Est Morocco, against postharvest phytopathogenic fungi in apples." *Microbial Pathogenesis* (2017): 321-326. URL: https://www.sciencedirect.com/science/article/pii/S0882401017302759.

[116] Stojanović, N. M., Randjelović, P. J., Mladenović, M. Z., Ilić, I. R., Petrović, V., Stojiljković, N., Ilić, S. and Radulović, N. S. "Toxic essential oils, part VI: Acute oral toxicity of lemon balm (*Melissa officinalis* L.) essential oil in BALB/c mice." *Food and Chemical Toxicology* (2019): 110794. URL: https://www.sciencedirect.com/science/article/pii/S0278691519305848.

[117] Mimica-Dukic, N., Bozin, B., Sokovic, M. and Simin, N. "Antimicrobial and antioxidant activities of *Melissa officinalis* L. (Lamiaceae) essential oil." *Journal of Agricultural and Food Chemistry* (2004): 2485-2489. URL: https://pubs.acs.org/doi/10.1021/jf030698a.

[118] Allahverdiyev, A., Duran, N., Ozguven, M. and Koltas, S. "Antiviral activity of the volatile oils of *Melissa officinalis* L. against *Herpes simplex* virus type-2." *Phytomedicine* (2004): 657-661. URL: https://www.sciencedirect.com/science/article/pii/S094471130400100X.

[119] Pinheiro, P. F., Costa, A. V., Alves, T. A., Galter, I. N., Pinheiro, C. A., Pereira, A. F., Oliveira, C. M. R. and Fontes, M. M. P. "Phytotoxicity and cytotoxicity of essential oil from leaves of *Plectranthus amboinicus*, carvacrol, and thymol in plant bioassays."

Journal of Agricultural and Food Chemistry (2015): 8981-8990 URL: https://pubs.acs.org/doi/10.1021/acs.jafc.5b03049.

[120] Gonçalves, T. B., Braga, M. A., de Oliveira, F. F. M., Santiago, G. M. P., Carvalho, C. B. M., e Cabral, P. B., Santiago, T. M., Sousa, J. S., Barros, E. B., do Nascimento, R. F. and Nagao-Dias, A. T. "Effect of subinihibitory and inhibitory concentrations of *Plectranthus amboinicus* (Lour.) Spreng essential oil on *Klebsiella pneumoniae*." *Phytomedicine* (2012): 962-968. URL: http://www.sciencedirect.com/science/article/pii/S0944711312001912.

[121] Aguiar, J. J. S., Sousa, C. P. B., Araruna, M. K. A., Silva, M. K. N., Portelo, A., Lopes, J. C., Carvalho, V. R. A., Figueredo, F. G., Bitu, V. C. N., Coutinho, H. D. M., Miranda, T. A. S. and Matias, E. F. F. "Antibacterial and modifying-antibiotic activities of the essential oils of *Ocimum gratissimum* L. and *Plectranthus amboinicus* L.." *European Journal of Integrative Medicine* (2015): 151-156. URL: http://www.sciencedirect.com/science/article/pii/S1876382014003084.

[122] Vasconcelos, S. E. C. B., Melo, H. M., Cavalcante, T. T. A., Catunda Júnior, F. E. A., de Carvalho, M. G., Menezes, F. G. R., de Sousa, O. V. and Costa, R. A. "*Plectranthus amboinicus* essential oil and carvacrol bioactive against planktonic and biofilm of oxacillin- and vancomycin-resistant *Staphylococcus aureus*." *BMC Complementary and Alternative Medicine* (2017): 462. URL: https://bmccomplementmedtherapies.biomedcentral.com/track/pdf/10.1186/s12906-017-1968-9.

[123] Da Costa, J. G. M., Pereira, C. K. B., Rodrigues, F. F. G. and de Lima, S. G. "Chemical composition, antibacterial and fungicidal activities of leaf oil of *Plectranthus amboinicus* (Lour.) Spreng.." *Journal of Essential Oil Research* (2010): 183-185. URL: http://www.tandfonline.com/doi/pdfs/10.1080/10412905.2010.9700298.

[124] Dos Santos, N. O., Mariane, B., Lago, J. H. G., Sartorelli, P., Rosa, W., Soares, M. G., da Silva, A. M., Lorenzi, H., Vallim, M. A. and Pascon, R. C. "Assessing the chemical composition and antimicrobial

activity of essential oils from Brazilian plants-*Eremanthus erythropappus* (Asteraceae), *Plectrantuns barbatus*, and *P. amboinicus* (Lamiaceae)." *Molecules* (2015): 8440-8452. URL: https://www.ncbi.nlm.nih.gov/pmc/articles/PMC6272540/pdf/molecules-20-08440.pdf.

[125] Senthilkumar, A. and Venkatesalu, V. "Chemical composition and larvicidal activity of the essential oil of *Plectranthus amboinicus* (Lour.) Spreng against *Anopheles stephensi*: a malarial vector mosquito." *Parasitology Resesarch* (2010): 1275-1278. URL: https://link.springer.com/article/10.1007%2Fs00436-010-1996-6.

[126] Murthy, P. S., Ramalakshmi, K. and Srinivas, P. "Fungitoxic activity of Indian borage (*Plectranthus amboinicus*) volatiles." *Food Chemistry* (2009): 1014-1018. URL: http://www.sciencedirect.com/science/article/pii/S030881460801282X.

[127] Manjamalai, A. and Berlin Grace, V. M. "The chemotherapeutic effect of essential oil of *Plectranthus amboinicus* (Lour) on lung metastasis developed by B16F-10 cell line in C57BL/6 mice." *Cancer Investigation* (2013): 74-82. URL: https://www.tandfonline.com/doi/full/10.3109/07357907.2012.749268.

[128] Erny Sabrina, M. N., Razali, M., Mirfat, A. H. S. and Mohd Shukri, M. A. "Antimicrobial activity and bioactive evaluation of *Plectranthus amboinicus* essential oil." *American Journal of Research Communication* (2014): 121-127. URL: http://www.usa-journals.com/wp-content/uploads/2014/11/Erny_Vol212.pdf.

[129] Hassani Said, M., Zainati, I., Zrira, S., Mahdi, S. and Oukessou, M. "Chemical composition and antimicrobial activity of *Plectranthus amboinicus* (Lour) Spring. essential oil from Archipelago of Comoros." *Journal of Essential Oil Bearing Plants* (2012): 637-644. URL: http://www.tandfonline.com/doi/pdf/10.1080/0972060X.2012.10644098.

[130] Bugayong, A. M., Cruz, P. and Padilla, P. I. "Antibacterial activity and chemical composition of essential oils from leaves of some aromatic plants of Philippines." *Journal of Essential Oil Bearing*

Plants (2019): 932-946. URL: https://www.tandfonline.com/doi/pdf/10.1080/0972060X.2019.1682683.

[131] Huang, H. T., Lin, C. C., Kuo, T. C., Chen, S. J. and Huang, R. N. "Phytochemical composition and larvicidal activity of essential oils from herbal plants." *Planta* (2019): 59-68. URL: https://link.springer.com/article/10.1007%2Fs00425-019-03147-w.

[132] Velasco, J., Rojas, L. B., Díaz, T. and Usubillaga, A. "Chemical composition and antibacterial activity of the essential oil of *Coleus amboinicus* Lour., against enteric pathogens." *Journal of Essential Oil Bearing Plants* (2009): 453-461. URL: http://www.tandfonline.com/doi/pdf/10.1080/0972060X.2009.10643744.

[133] Hussein, K., Ahmed, A. H. and Algabali, S. "Antibacterial/radical scavenging activities, content, chemotaxonomy and chemical components of volatile oils of two *Plectranthus amboinicus* (Lour.) Spreng. (Lamiaceae), grown in Yemen." *American Journal of Essential Oils and Natural Products* (2017): 12-18. URL: http://www.essencejournal.com/pdf/2017/vol5issue2/PartA/5-1-4-650.pdf.

[134] Liu, H. X., He, D. M., Huang, C. S., Sun, Z. J. and Lin, S. "Chemical component analysis of volatile oil from *Illicium verum* Hook.f. seed by gas chromatography-mass spectrometry." *Food Science* (2009). URL: http://en.cnki.com.cn/Article_en/ CJFDTOTAL-SPKX200922074.htm.

[135] Zhai, Y., Sun, S., Wang, Z., Cheng, J., Sun, Y., Wang, L., Zhang, Y., Zhang, H. and Yu, A. "Microwave extraction of essential oils from dried fruits of *Illicium verum* Hook. f. and *Cuminum cyminum* L. using ionic liquid as the microwave absorption medium." *Journal of Separation Science* (2009): 3544-3549. URL: https://onlinelibrary.wiley.com/doi/epdf/10.1002/jssc.200910204.

[136] De, M., De, A. K., Sen, P., Banerjee, A. B. "Antimicrobial properties of star anise (*Illicium verum* Hook f)." *Phytotherapy Research* (2002): 94-95. URL: https://onlinelibrary.wiley.com/doi/epdf/10.1002/ptr.989.

[137] Chauhan, R.S., Kitchlu, S., Ram, G., Kaul, M. K. and Tava, A. "Chemical composition of capillene chemotype of *Artemisia dracunculus* L. from North-West Himalaya, India." *Industrial Crops and Products* (2010): 546-549. URL: https://www.sciencedirect.com/science/article/pii/S0926669010000336.

[138] Olszewska-Kaczynska, I. and Suchorska, K. "Evaluation of three cultivated forms of tarragon (*Artemisia dracunculus* L.)." *Folia Horticulturae* (1996): 29-37.

[139] Pappas, R. S. and Sturtz, G. "Unusual alkynes found in the essential oil of *Artemisia dracunculus* L. var. *dracunculus* from the Pacific Northwest." *Journal of Essential Oil Research* (2001): 187-188. URL: https://www.tandfonline.com/doi/pdf/10.1080/10412905.2001.9699657.

[140] Dias, D.A., Urban, S. and Roessner. U. "A historical overview of natural products in drug discovery." *Metabolites* (2012): 303-336. URL: https://www.mdpi.com/2218-1989/2/2/303.

[141] David, B., Wolfender, J. L. and Dias, D. A. "The pharmaceutical industry and natural products: historical status and new trends." *Phytochemistry Reviews* (2015): 299-315. URL: https://link.springer.com/article/10.1007/s11101-014-9367-z.

[142] Bozell, J. J. and Petersen, G. R. "Technology development for the production of biobased products from biorefinery carbohydrates-the US Department of Energy's "Top 10" revisited." *Green Chemistry* (2010): 539-554. URL: https://pubs.rsc.org/en/content/articlelanding/2010/GC/b922014c.

[143] Sheldon, R. A. "Green and sustainable manufacture of chemicals from biomass: state of the art." *Green Chemistry* (2014): 950-963. URL: https://pubs.rsc.org/en/content/articlelanding/2014/gc/c3gc41935e.

[144] Li, Y., Fabiano-Tixier, A. S. and Chemat, F. "*Essential oils as reagents in green chemistry.*" Springer, Berlin, (2014):1-71.

[145] Kouznetsov, V. V. "Biology and chemistry connection via organic synthesis aimed at molecular diversity." *Journal of the Colombian*

Academy of Exact, Physical and Natural Sciences (2014): 129-141. URL: https://www.raccefyn.co/index.php/raccefyn/article/ view/159.

[146] Kouznetsov, V. V. "Essential oils as chemical reagents in heterocyclic synthesis." *Natural Product Communications* (2019): 91-96. URL: https://journals.sagepub.com/doi/pdf/10.1177/ 1934578X1901400124.

[147] Taylor, A. P., Robinson, R. P., Fobian, Y. M., Blakemore, D. C., Jones, L. H. and Fadeyi, O. "Modern advances in heterocyclic chemistry in drug discovery." *Organic and Biomolecular Chemistry* (2016): 6611-6637. URL: https://pubs.rsc.org/en/content/ articlelanding/2016/ob/c6ob00936k.

[148] Cabrele, C. and Reiser. O. "The modern face of synthetic heterocyclic chemistry." *Journal of Organic Chemistry* (2016): 10109-10125. URL: https://pubs.acs.org/doi/pdf/10.1021/acs.joc. 6b02034.

[149] Katritzky, A. R. "Introduction: heterocycles." *Chemical Reviews* (2004): 2125-2126. URL: https://pubs.acs.org/doi/full/10.1021/ cr0406413.

[150] Kumar, S., Bawa, S. and Gupta, H. "Biological activities of quinoline derivatives." *Mini Reviews Medicinal Chemistry* (2009): 1648-1654. URL: http://www.eurekaselect.com/86038/article.

[151] Solomon, V. R. and Lee, H. "Quinoline as a privileged scaffold in cancer drug discovery." *Current Medicinal Chemistry* (2011): 1488-1508. URL: http://www.eurekaselect.com/73766/article.

[152] Keri, R. S. and Patil, S. A. "Quinoline: a promising antitubercular target." *Biomedicine and Pharmacotherapy* (2014): 1161-1175. URL: https://www.sciencedirect.com/science/article/pii/S075333 221400136X.

[153] Kouznetsov, V. V., Bohorquez-Romero, A. R. and Stashenko, EE. "Three-component imino Diels-Alder reaction with essential oil and seeds of anise: generation of new tetrahydroquinolines." *Tetrahedron Letters* (2007): 8855-8860. URL: https://www. sciencedirect.com/science/article/pii/S0040403907020588.

[154] Merchan-Arenas, D. R., Rojas-Ruíz, F. A. and Kouznetsov, V. V. "Highly diastereoselective synthesis of new heterolignan-like 6,7-

methylendioxy-tetrahydroquinolines using the clove bud essential oil as raw material." *Tetrahedron Letters* (2011): 1388-1391. URL: https://www.sciencedirect.com/science/article/pii/S0040403911001110.

[155] Kouznetsov, V. V., Merchan-Arenas, D. R., Arvelo, F., Bello-Forero, J. S., Sojo, F. and Muñoz, A. "4-Hydroxy-3-methoxyphenyl substituted 3-methyl-tetrahydroquinoline derivatives obtained through imino Diels-Alder reactions as potential antitumoral agents." *Letter in Drug Design and Discovery* (2010): 632-639. URL: https://www.ingentaconnect.com/content/ben/lddd/2010/00000007/00000009/003aj.

[156] Muñoz, A., Sojo, F., Merchan-Arenas, D. R., Kouznetsov, V. V. and Arvelo, F. "Cytotoxic effects of new *trans*-2,4-diaryl-r-3-methyl-1,2,3,4-tetrahydroquinolines and their interaction with antitumoral drugs gemcitabine and paclitaxel on cellular lines of human breast cancer." *Chemico-Biological Interactions* (2011): 215-221. URL: https://www.sciencedirect.com/science/article/pii/S000927971000637X.

[157] Kouznetsov, V. V., Merchan-Arenas, D. R., Tangarife-Castaño, V., Correa-Royero, J. and Betancur-Galvis, L. "Synthesis and cytotoxic evaluation of novel 2-aryl-4-(4-hydroxy-3-methoxyphenyl)-3-methyl-6,7-methylendioxy-1,2,3,4-tetrahydroquinolines, podophyllotoxin-like molecules." *Medicinal Chemistry Research* (2016): 429-437. URL: https://link.springer.com/article/10.1007/s00044-015-1486-6.

[158] Merchan-Arenas, D. R. and Kouznetsov, V. V. "Diastereoselective synthesis of dihydroisoindolo[2,1-*a*]quinolin-11-ones by solvent-free AMCell-SO_3H-catalyzed imino Diels-Alder/intramolecular amide cyclization cascade reactions." *Journal of Organic Chemistry* (2014): 5327-5333. URL: https://pubs.acs.org/doi/pdf/10.1021/ jo500516c.

[159] Dawood, K. M. "Benzofuran derivatives: a patent review." *Expert Opinion on Therapeutic Patents* (2013): 1133-1156. URL: https://www.tandfonline.com/doi/full/10.1517/13543776.2013.801455.

[160] Khanam, H. and Shamsuzzaman. "Bioactive benzofuran derivatives: A review." *European Journal of Medicinal Chemistry* (2015): 483-504. URL: https://www.sciencedirect.com/science/article/pii/S022352341401071X.

[161] Kouznetsov, V. V., Merchan-Arenas, D. R. and Bohorquez-Romero, A. R. "PEG-400 as green reaction medium for Lewis acid-promoted cycloaddition reactions with isoeugenol and anethole." *Tetrahedron Letters* (2008): 3097-3100. URL: https://www.sciencedirect.com/science/article/pii/S0040403908004899.

[162] Lenardao, E. J., Botteselle, G. V., de Azambuja, F., Perin, G. and Jacob, R. G. "Citronellal as key compound in organic synthesis." *Tetrahedron* (2007): 6671-6712. URL: https://www.sciencedirect.com/science/article/abs/pii/S0040402007006138.

[163] Tundis, R., Loizzo, M. R., Menichini, F., Statti, G. A. and Menichini, F. "Biological and pharmacological activities of iridoids: recent developments." *Mini Reviews in Medicinal Chemistry* (2008): 399-420. URL: http://www.eurekaselect.com/82422/article.

[164] Dawson, G. W., Pickett, J. A. and Smiley, D. W. M. "The aphid sex pheromone cyclopentanoids: synthesis in the elucidation of structure and biosynthetic pathways." *Bioorganic and Medicinal Chemistry* (1996): 351-361. URL: https://www.sciencedirect.com/science/article/pii/0968089696000120.

[165] Schreiber, S. L., Meyers, H. V. and Wiberg, K. B. "Stereochemistry of the intramolecular enamine/enal (enone) cycloaddition reaction and subsequent transformations." *Journal of the American Chemical Society* (1986): 8274-8277. URL: https://pubs.acs.org/doi/pdf/10.1021/ja00286a034.

[166] Nangia, A., Prasuna, G. and Rao, P. B. "Synthesis of cyclopenta[*c*]pyran skeleton of iridoid lactones." *Tetrahedron* (1997): 14507-14545. URL: https://www.sciencedirect.com/science/article/pii/S0040402097007485.

[167] Del Giudice, M. R., Borioni, A., Mustazza, C. and Gatta, F. "Synthesis of 9-amino-, 9-aminomethyl-1,2,3,4-tetrahydro- and 1,2,3,4,5,6,7,8-octahydroacridine derivatives." *Journal of*

Heterocyclic Chemistry (1997): 1661-1667. URL: https://onlinelibrary.wiley.com/doi/epdf/10.1002/jhet.5570340604.

[168] Jacob, R. G., Perin, G., Botteselle, G. V. and Lenardão, E.J. "Clean and atom-economic synthesis of octahydroacridines: application to essential oil of citronella." *Tetrahedron Letters* (2003): 6809-6812. URL: https://www.sciencedirect.com/science/article/pii/S0040403903017490.

[169] Acelas, M., Romero Bohórquez, A. R. and Kouznetsov, V. V. "Highly diastereoselective synthesis of new *trans*-fused octahydroacridines via intramolecular cationic imino Diels-Alder reaction of *N*-protected anilines and citronellal or citronella essential oil." *Synthesis* (2017): 2153-2162. URL: https://www.thieme-connect.com/products/ejournals/abstract/10.1055/s-0036-1588713.

[170] Acelas, M., Kouznetsov, V. V. and Romero Bohórquez, A. R. "Facile and highly diastereo and regioselective synthesis of novel octahydroacridine-isoxazole and octahydroacridine-1,2,3-triazole molecular hybrids from citronella essential oil." *Molecular Diversity* (2019): 183-193. URL: https://link.springer.com/article/10.1007/s11030-018-9863-y.

[171] Singh, C., Gupta, N. and Puri, S. K. "Geraniol-derived 1,2,4-trioxanes with potent *in-vivo* antimalarial activity." *Bioorganic and Medicinal Chemistry Letters* (2003): 3447-3450. URL: https://www.sciencedirect.com/science/article/pii/S0960894X03007820.

[172] Noe, M. C., Hawkins, J. M., Snow, S. L. and Wolf-Gouveia, L. "A short enantioselective synthesis of N-Boc-(2R,3R)-3-methyl-3-hydroxypipecolic acid from geraniol." *Journal of Organic Chemistry* (2008): 3295-3298. URL: https://pubs.acs.org/doi/pdf/10.1021/jo800080t.

[173] Ilc, T., Parage, C., Boachon, B., Navrot, N. and Werck-Reichhart, D. "Monoterpenol oxidative metabolism: role in plant adaptation and potential applications." *Frontier in Plant Science* (2016): 509. URL: https://www.frontiersin.org/articles/10.3389/fpls.2016.00509/full.

[174] García Santos, W. H., Galvis-Puerto, C. E. and Kouznetsov, V. V. "Gd(OTf)$_3$-catalyzed synthesis of geranyl esters for the intramolecular radical cyclization of their epoxides mediated by titanocene (III)." *Organic and Biomolecular Chemistry* (2015): 1358-1366. URL: https://pubs.rsc.org/en/content/articlelanding/2015/ob/c4ob02312a.

[175] Okasha, R. M., Alblewi, F. F., Afifi, T. H., Naqvi, A., Fouda, A. M., Al-Dies, A. A. M. and El-Agrody, A. M. "Design of new benzo[*h*]chromene derivatives: Antitumor activities and structure-activity relationships of the 2,3-positions and fused rings at the 2,3-positions." *Molecules* (2017): 479. URL: https://www.mdpi.com/1420-3049/22/3/479.

[176] Elinson, M. N., Ilovaisky, A. I., Merkulova, V. M., Belyakov, P. A., Chizhov, A. O. and Nikishin, G. I. "Solvent-free cascade reaction: Direct multicomponent assembling of 2-amino-4*H*-chromene scaffold from salicylaldehyde, malononitrile or cyanoacetate and nitroalkanes." *Tetrahedron* (2010): 4043-4048. URL: https://www.sciencedirect.com/science/article//pii/S0040402010005673.

[177] Ortiz-Villamizar, M. C., Zubkov, F. I., Puerto-Galvis, C. E., Vargas-Méndez, L. Y. and Kouznetsov, V. V. "The study of metal-free and palladium-catalysed synthesis of benzochromenes via direct C-H arylation using unactivated aryl benzyl ethers derived from essential oils as raw materials." *Organic Chemistry Frontiers* (2017): 1736-1744. URL: https://pubs.rsc.org/en/content/articlelanding/2017/qo/c7qo00232g.

INDEX

A

B

C

E